2007
YEAR BOOK OF
NEONATAL AND
PERINATAL MEDICINE®

The 2007 Year Book Series

Year Book of Anesthesiology and Pain Management™: Drs Chestnut, Abram, Black, Gravlee, Lee, Mathru, and Roizen

Year Book of Cardiology®: Drs Gersh, Cheitlin, Elliott, Graham, Sundt, and Waldo

Year Book of Critical Care Medicine®: Drs Dellinger, Parrillo, Balk, Bekes, Dorman, and Dries

Year Book of Dentistry®: Drs McIntyre, Belvedere, Buhite, Davis, Henderson, Johnson, Ohrbach, Olin, Scott, Spencer, and Zakariasen

Year Book of Dermatology and Dermatologic Surgery™: Drs Thiers and Lang

Year Book of Diagnostic Radiology®: Drs Osborn, Abbara, Birdwell, Dalinka, Elster, Gardiner, Levy, Oestreich, and Rosado de Christenson

Year Book of Emergency Medicine®: Drs Hamilton, Bruno, Handly, Quintana, and Werner

Year Book of Endocrinology®: Drs Mazzaferri, Bessesen, Clarke, Howard, Kennedy, Leahy, Meikle, Molitch, Rogol, and Schteingart

Year Book of Family Practice®: Drs Bowman, Apgar, Bouchard, Dexter, Neill, Scherger, and Zink

Year Book of Gastroenterology™: Drs Lichtenstein, Chang, Dempsey, Drebin, Jaffe, Katzka, Kochman, Makar, Morris, Osterman, Rombeau, Shah, and Stein

Year Book of Hand and Upper Limb Surgery®: Drs Chang and Steinmann

Year Book of Medicine®: Drs Barkin, Berney, Frishman, Garrick, Loehrer, Mazzaferri, Phillips, and Snydman

Year Book of Neonatal and Perinatal Medicine®: Drs Fanaroff, Ehrenkranz, and Stevenson

Year Book of Neurology and Neurosurgery®: Drs Kim and Verma

Year Book of Nuclear Medicine®: Drs Coleman, Blaufox, Royal, Strauss, and Zubal

Year Book of Obstetrics, Gynecology, and Women's Health®: Dr Shulman

Year Book of Oncology®: Drs Loehrer, Arceci, Glatstein, Gordon, Hanna, Morrow, and Thigpen

Year Book of Ophthalmology®: Drs Rapuano, Cohen, Eagle, Flanders, Hammersmith, Myers, Nelson, Penne, Sergott, Shields, Tipperman, and Vander

Year Book of Orthopedics®: Drs Morrey, Beauchamp, Huddleston, Peterson, Swiontkowski, and Trigg

Year Book of Otolaryngology-Head and Neck Surgery®: Drs Paparella, Gapany, and Keefe

Year Book of Pathology and Laboratory Medicine®: Drs Raab, Parwani, Bejarano, and Bissell

2007

The Year Book of NEONATAL AND PERINATAL MEDICINE®

Editors
Avroy A. Fanaroff, MD, FRCPE, FRCPCH
Gertrude Lee Chandler Tucker Professor and Chair, Department of Pediatrics and Reproductive Biology, Case Western Reserve University School of Medicine; Eliza Henry Barnes Chair of Neonatology, Physician in Chief, Rainbow Babies and Children's Hospital, Cleveland, Ohio
Richard A. Ehrenkranz, MD
Professor of Pediatrics, Obstetrics and Gynecology, and Reproductive Sciences, Department of Pediatrics, Yale University School of Medicine, New Haven, Connecticut
David K. Stevenson, MD
Harold K. Faber Professor of Pediatrics, Vice Dean and Senior Associate Dean for Academic Affairs; Chief, Division of Neonatal and Developmental Medicine, Department of Pediatrics; Director, Charles B. and Ann L. Johnson Center for Pregnancy and Newborn Services, Stanford University School of Medicine, Stanford, California

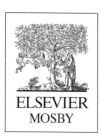

ELSEVIER
MOSBY

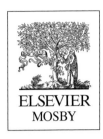

ELSEVIER
MOSBY

Vice President, Continuity: John A. Schrefer
Editor: Carla Holloway
Production Supervisor, Electronic Year Books: Donna M. Adamson
Electronic Article Manager: Jennifer C. Pitts
Illustrations and Permissions Coordinator: Dawn Vohsen

2007 EDITION

Printed in the United States of America
Composition by Thomas Technology Solutions, Inc.
Printing/binding by Sheridan Books, Inc.

Editorial Office:
Elsevier
Suite 1800
1600 John F. Kennedy Blvd.
Philadelphia, PA 19106-3399

International Standard Serial Number: 8756-5005
International Standard Book Number: 978-0-323-04658-9

Contributing Editors

Namasivayam Ambalavanan, MD
Associate Professor of Pediatrics and Cell Biology, University of Alabama at Birmingham, Birmingham, Alabama

James E. Arnold, MD
Professor, Pediatrics; Chair, Department of Otolaryngology Case Western Reserve University School of Medicine, Rainbow Babies and Children's Hospital, Cleveland, Ohio

David J. Aughton, MD
Professor, Pediatrics; Chief, Division of Genetics, Department of Pediatrics, William Beaumont Hospital, Royal Oak, Michigan

Mert Ozan Bahtiyar, MD
Assistant Professor of Obstetrics and Gynecology and Reproductive Sciences, Yale University School of Medicine, New Haven, Connecticut

Cynthia F. Bearer, MD, PhD
Associate Professor, Pediatrics, Neurosciences and Environmental Health Sciences; Associate Director, Medical Scientist Training Program, Case Western Reserve University School of Medicine; Director of Medical Education, Mary Ann Swetland Center for Environmental Health; Director, Neonatology Fellowship Training Program, Rainbow Babies and Children's Hospital, Cleveland, Ohio

William E. Benitz, MD
Philip Sunshine, MD, Professor in Neonatology, Division of Neonatal and Developmental Medicine, Department of Pediatrics; Director of Nurseries, Stanford University School of Medicine, Stanford, California

Melvin Berger, MD, PhD
Professor, Pediatrics and Pathology, Case Western Reserve University School of Medicine; Director, Jeffrey Modell Center for Primary Immune Deficiencies, Division of Allergy-Immunology, Rainbow Babies and Children's Hospital, Cleveland, Ohio

William Berquist, MD
Professor of Pediatrics, Stanford University School of Medicine, Stanford, California

Vineet Bhandari, MD, DM
Assistant Professor of Pediatrics, Yale University School of Medicine, New Haven, Connecticut

Matthew J. Bizzarro, MD
Assistant Professor of Pediatrics, Yale University School of Medicine, New Haven, Connecticut

Martin L. Blakely, MD
University of Tennessee Health Science Center, Department of Surgery, Division of Pediatric Surgery, Memphis, Tennessee

Richard D. Bland, MD
Professor (Research) of Pediatrics, Division of Neonatal and Developmental Medicine, Department of Pediatrics, Stanford University School of Medicine, Stanford, California

Michael B. Bracken, PhD, MPH
Susan Dwight Bliss Professor of Epidemiology, Yale University School of Medicine, New Haven, Connecticut

Rachel L. Chapman, MD
Assistant Professor of Pediatrics, Yale University School of Medicine, New Haven, Connecticut

Valerie Chock, MD
Department of Pediatrics, Stanford University School of Medicine, Stanford, California

Eve R. Colson, MD
Associate Professor of Pediatrics, Yale University School of Medicine, New Haven, Connecticut

Joshua A. Copel, MD
Professor of Obstetrics and Gynecology, Yale University School of Medicine, New Haven, Connecticut

David N. Cornfield, MD
Professor of Pediatrics, Stanford University School of Medicine, Stanford, California

Olaf Dammann, Dr med, SM
Director of Clinical Research, Division of Newborn Medicine, Tufts-New England Medical Center, Boston, Massachusetts

Carl T. D'Angio, MD
Assistant Professor of Pediatrics, University of Rochester School of Medicine and Dentistry, Rochester, New York

Katherine M. Dell, MD
Assistant Professor, Pediatrics, Case Western Reserve University School of Medicine; Division of Pediatric Nephrology, Rainbow Babies and Children's Hospital, Cleveland, Ohio

Gregory M. Enns, MB, ChB
Associate Professor of Pediatrics, Stanford University School of Medicine, Stanford, California

Heidi M. Feldman, MD, PhD
Ballinger-Swindells Endowed Professor in Behavioral and Developmental Pediatrics, Stanford University School of Medicine, Stanford, California

Edmund F. Funai, MD
Associate Chair, Clinical Affairs; Associate Professor, Department of Obstetrics and Gynecology, Yale University School of Medicine, New Haven, Connecticut

Lydia M. Furman, MD

Assistant Professor, Pediatrics, Rainbow Babies and Children's Hospital, Cleveland, Ohio

Patrick G. Gallagher, MD

Associate Professor of Pediatrics, Yale University School of Medicine, New Haven, Connecticut

Jeffrey B. Gould, MD, MPH

Robert L. Hess Professor in Pediatrics, Division of Neonatal and Developmental Medicine, Department of Pediatrics; Director of Perinatal Epidemiology and Outcomes Research Unit of the Johnson Center, Stanford University School of Medicine, Stanford, California

Frank R. Greer, MD

Professor of Pediatrics, University of Wisconsin-Madison, Madison, Wisconsin

Ian Gross, MD

Professor of Pediatrics and Obstetrics and Gynecology, Yale University School of Medicine, New Haven, Connecticut

Jeffrey R. Gruen, MD

Associate Professor, Pediatrics, Genetics, and Investigative Medicine, Yale University School of Medicine, New Haven, Connecticut

Maureen Hack, MD

Professor, Pediatrics, Case Western Reserve University School of Medicine; Director, High Risk Follow-up Program, Rainbow Babies and Children's Hospital, Cleveland, Ohio

Jonathan Hellmann, MBBCh, FCP(SA), FRCPC

Professor of Paediatrics, University of Toronto; Clinical Director, NICU, The Hospital for Sick Children, Toronto, Ontario, Canada

Susan R. Hintz, MD, MS

Assistant Professor of Pediatrics, Division of Neonatal and Developmental Medicine, Department of Pediatrics, Stanford University School of Medicine, Stanford, California

Claudia Hoyen, MD

Assistant Professor, Pediatrics, Case Western Reserve University School of Medicine; Division of Infectious Diseases, Rainbow Babies and Children's Hospital, Cleveland, Ohio

Terrie E. Inder, MD

Associate Professor, Pediatrics, Washington University School of Medicine; St. Louis Children's Hospital, St. Louis, Missouri

Harris C. Jacobs, MD

Clinical Professor of Pediatrics, Yale University School of Medicine, New Haven, Connecticut; Associate Director, NICU, Bridgeport Hospital, Bridgeport, Connecticut

Carolyn M. Kercsmar, MD

Professor, Pediatrics, Case Western Reserve University School of Medicine; Rainbow Babies and Children's Hospital, Cleveland, Ohio

Lisa Kobrynski, MD, MPH
Assistant Professor, Pediatrics, Division of Allergy and Immunology, Emory University, Atlanta, Georgia

Abbot Laptook, MD
Professor of Pediatrics, Brown Medical School, Providence, Rhode Island

Henry C. Lee, MD
Clinical Instructor, Stanford University School of Medicine, Stanford, California

Deirdre J. Lyell, MD
Assistant Professor of Obstetrics and Gynecology, Stanford University School of Medicine, Stanford, California

Ashima Madan, MD
Associate Professor of Pediatrics, Division of Neonatal and Developmental Medicine, Department of Pediatrics, Stanford University School of Medicine, Stanford, California

M. Jeffrey Maisels, MB, BCh
Professor and Chairman, Department of Pediatrics, William Beaumont Hospital, Royal Oak, Michigan

Richard J. Martin, MD
Professor, Pediatrics, Reproductive Biology, and Physiology and Biophysics, Druminsky-Fanaroff Professor in Neonatology, Case Western Reserve University School of Medicine; Director, Division of Neonatology, Rainbow Babies and Children's Hospital, Cleveland, Ohio

Paula P. Meier, RN, DNSc
Director for Clinical Research and Lactation, Rush University Medical Center, Chicago, Illinois

Mark R. Mercurio, MD, MA
Associate Professor of Pediatrics, Yale University School of Medicine, New Haven, Connecticut

Jane Morton, MD
Clinical Professor of Pediatrics, Stanford University School of Medicine, Stanford, California

Errol R. Norwitz, MD, PhD
Associate Professor of Obstetrics, Gynecology and Reproductive Sciences; Co-Director, Division of Maternal-Fetal Medicine, Yale University School of Medicine, New Haven, Connecticut

Anna Penn, MD, PhD
Assistant Professor of Pediatrics, Division of Neonatal and Developmental Medicine, Department of Pediatrics, Stanford University School of Medicine, Stanford, California

Steven M. Peterec, MD
Assistant Clinical Professor, Pediatrics, Yale University School of Medicine, New Haven, Connecticut; Director, Neonatology, Lawrence and Memorial Hospitals, New London, Connecticut

Emese Pinter, MD
Associate Research Scientist, Division of Perinatal Medicine, Yale University School of Medicine, New Haven, Connecticut

Charles G. Prober, MD
Professor of Pediatrics, Microbiology and Immunology, Stanford University School of Medicine, Stanford, California

Michael D. Reed, PharmD, FCCP, FCP
Professor, Pediatrics, Case Western Reserve University School of Medicine; Director, Pediatric Clinical Pharmacology and Toxicology, Rainbow Babies and Children's Hospital, Cleveland, Ohio

William D. Rhine, MD
Professor of Pediatrics, Division of Neonatal and Developmental Medicine, Department of Pediatrics; Director, Neonatal Intensive Care Unit, Stanford University School of Medicine, Stanford, California

Seetha Shankaran, MD
Professor, Pediatrics, Wayne State University School of Medicine; Director, Neonatal-Perinatal Medicine, Children's Hospital of Michigan and Hutzel Women's Hospital, Detroit, Michigan

Ann Stark, MD
Professor, Pediatrics, Baylor College of Medicine; Texas Children's Hospital, Houston, Texas

Eileen K. Stork, MD
Professor, Pediatrics, Case Western Reserve University School of Medicine; Director, Neonatal Program, Rainbow Babies and Children's Hospital, Cleveland, Ohio

Trenna L. Sutcliffe, MD, MSc, FRCPC
Instructor, Pediatrics, Division of Neonatal and Developmental Medicine, Department of Pediatrics, Stanford University School of Medicine, Stanford, California

Karl G. Sylvester, MD
Lucile Packard Children's Hospital, Stanford University School of Medicine, Stanford, California

Philip H. Toltzis, MD
Associate Professor, Pediatrics, Case Western Reserve University School of Medicine; Division of Infectious Diseases, Rainbow Babies and Children's Hospital, Cleveland, Ohio

Marietta Vázquez, MD
Assistant Professor, Pediatrics, Yale University School of Medicine, New Haven, Connecticut

Betty R. Vohr, MD
Professor, Pediatrics, Brown Medical School, Providence, Rhode Island

Hendrik J. Vreman, PhD
Senior Research Scientist, Department of Pediatrics, Stanford University School of Medicine, Stanford, California

Richard J. Wong

Senior Research Scientist, Department of Pediatrics, Stanford University School of Medicine, Stanford, California

Linda Wright, MD

Deputy Director, Center for Research for Mothers and Children, National Institute of Child Health and Human Development, National Institutes of Health, Rockville, Maryland

Table of Contents

Journals Represented

Journals represented in this YEAR BOOK are listed below.

Acta Obstetricia et Gynecologica Scandinavica
Acta Orthopaedica Scandinavica
Acta Paediatrica
American Journal of Epidemiology
American Journal of Obstetrics and Gynecology
American Journal of Perinatology
American Journal of Physiology-Lung Cellular and Molecular Physiology
American Journal of Respiratory and Critical Care Medicine
Anesthesiology
Annals of Thorasic Surgery
Archives of Disease in Childhood
Archives of Disease in Childhood. Fetal and Neonatal Edition
Archives of General Psychiatry
Archives of Ophthalmology
Archives of Pediatrics and Adolescent Medicine
Brain
Brain Research
British Medical Journal
Canadian Medical Association Journal
Circulation
Clinical Journal of Pain
Diabetes Care
European Journal of Obstetrics, Gynecology and Reproductive Biology
European Journal of Radiology
Intensive Care Medicine
International Journal of Gynecology & Obstetrics
Journal of Clinical Endocrinology and Metabolism
Journal of Immunology
Journal of Neurology, Neurosurgery and Psychiatry
Journal of Neurosurgery
Journal of Pediatric Gastroenterology and Nutrition
Journal of Pediatric Orthopaedics
Journal of Pediatric Surgery
Journal of Pediatrics
Journal of Urology
Journal of the American Medical Association
Journal of the American Society of Nephrology
Journal of the National Cancer Institute
Lancet
Medical Care
Neurology
Neurosurgery
New England Journal of Medicine
Obstetrics and Gynecology
Pediatric Infectious Disease Journal
Pediatric Radiology
Pediatric Research
Pediatrics
Revista panamericana de salud/Pan American Journal of Public Health

Social Science and Medicine
The Laryngoscope Journal
Thorax
Ultrasound in Obstetrics and Gynecology

STANDARD ABBREVIATIONS

The following terms are abbreviated in this edition: acquired immunodeficiency syndrome (AIDS), cardiopulmonary resuscitation (CPR), central nervous system (CNS), cerebrospinal fluid (CSF), computed tomography (CT), deoxyribonucleic acid (DNA), electrocardiography (ECG), health maintenance organization (HMO), human immunodeficiency virus (HIV), intensive care unit (ICU), intramuscular (IM), intravenous (IV), magnetic resonance (MR) imaging (MRI), ribonucleic acid (RNA), and ultrasound (US).

NOTE

The YEAR BOOK OF NEONATAL AND PERINATAL MEDICINE® is a literature survey service providing abstracts of articles published in the professional literature. Every effort is made to assure the accuracy of the information presented in these pages. Neither the editors nor the publisher of the YEAR BOOK OF NEONATAL AND PERINATAL MEDICINE® can be responsible for errors in the original materials. The editors' comments are their own opinions. Mention of specific products within this publication does not constitute endorsement.

To facilitate the use of the YEAR BOOK OF NEONATAL AND PERINATAL MEDICINE® as a reference tool, all illustrations and tables included in this publication are now identified as they appear in the original article. This change is meant to help the reader recognize that any illustration or table appearing in the YEAR BOOK OF NEONATAL AND PERINATAL MEDICINE® may be only one of many in the original article. For this reason, figure and table numbers will often appear to be out of sequence within the YEAR BOOK OF NEONATAL AND PERINATAL MEDICINE®.

Introduction

Perhaps this will be the final occasion in which we will have assembled the YEAR BOOK OF NEONATAL AND PERINATAL MEDICINE in the same manner as the past 20 years. The editorial change of Richard A. Ehrenkranz from Yale University replacing Jeffrey Maisels has been accomplished seamlessly and effortlessly. Elsevier, the publisher of the YEAR BOOK, is determined to bring the reader all the information in a timelier manner. In the very near future, the information will be available online prior to the publication of the book. Furthermore, all the articles will be graded. For the editors, this will present new challenges as we change our behavior patterns, but we anticipate that the process will be more efficient and the commentaries will be available soon after the publication of the original manuscripts. To accomplish this, we will need more section editors, and we are very receptive to volunteers.

This edition of the YEAR BOOK highlights advances in neonatal perinatal medicine. It publishes at a critical time for health care in the USA. The NIH funding is restricted, and a record number of Americans are without health insurance. The problems of the uninsured are particularly acute among children. Between 2005 and 2006, the number of children without health insurance increased from 8 million to 8.7 million representing 11.7% of the nation's children. Together, with the President's threat to veto the State Children's Health Insurance Program, we are facing a crisis. It is important for all readers to keep your legislators informed and urge them to support health care programs and insurance for women and children. We must also plead for increased NIH funding so that we can continue to push the envelope and further improve perinatal outcomes. Not only must the research focus on translation from bench to bedside, but better efforts must be made to ensure that knowledge is disseminated to all health care providers in a timely manner.

This issue of the YEAR BOOK contains the usual admixture of randomized trials and database explorations. There is a balance between the basic sciences and therapeutic innovations together with many reports on the long-term outcome of preterm infants. We remain indebted to the many contributors who willingly give of their time and expertise. We thank Jonathan Hellman for his continued leadership of the ethical section. We also thank the Elsevier YEAR BOOK team, headed by Tim Maxwell and Carla Holloway for their patience, assistance, and support, resulting in the high quality of the final product.

Avroy A. Fanaroff, MD, FRCPE, FRCPCH

Richard A. Ehrenkranz, MD

David K. Stevenson, MD

Chromosomal Microarray Analysis Is Replacing the Karyotype in the Evaluation of Neonates

ARTHUR L. BEAUDET, MD

Chromosome analysis has played an important role in prenatal and neonatal diagnosis for decades now. Over the years, the high-resolution banded karyotype, region-specific fluorescence in situ hybridization (FISH) testing, and telomere FISH have increased the ability to detect significant abnormalities. Now a new method termed either array comparative genomic hybridization (array CGH) or genomic copy number analysis is bringing the most dramatic revolutionary advance to date. The term chromosomal microarray analysis (CMA) is used here to include both array CGH and similar non-CGH array methods. The most widely used form of the CMA at present is array CGH, in which a patient's DNA is labeled with one fluorescent dye (eg, red) and a control DNA is labeled with another dye (eg, green). The 2 DNAs are then mixed and hybridized to long DNA molecules (bacterial artificial chromosome clones [BACs]) or short DNA molecules (oligonucleotides) fixed in spots on a solid phase, usually a glass slide. In the case of array CGH, if the patient has a deletion for a chromosomal region, the intensity of the dye for the control will be greater than that for the patient—green greater than red, according to the colors noted above. In contrast, if the patient has a duplication, the intensity for the dyes will be greater for the patient relative to the control, or red greater than green. Exactly which clones or oligonucleotides show the changes define the specific regions of deletion or duplication. This methodology allows the performance of the equivalent of hundreds or even thousands of FISH tests on a single slide. Agilent Technologies (Santa Clara, Calif) and NimbleGen Systems (Madison, Wis) offer arrays and reagents suitable for use in clinical CGH analyses.

The arrays in clinical use typically have a few thousand probes for large genomic clones such as BACs, and those with oligonucleotides typically have from 15,000 to more than 1 million probes. Clinical arrays may be low density, with probes clustered in disease regions and at telomeres, in which case they are described as targeted arrays, or they may have much higher density of probes throughout the genome, in which case they may be referred to as tiling arrays. With one commercial platform, the solid phase can be 3-μm silica beads in wells on a slide rather than the glass surface of the slide itself. In some variations, genomic copy number is quantified directly without comparison with a control so that the method is technically not CGH, although the resulting data are comparable. Such non-CGH methods are offered by Illumina (San Diego, Calif) with bead arrays and by Affymetrix (Santa Clara, Calif) with copy number analysis.

The major advantage of CMA is that it can diagnose a multitude of abnormalities that are not detectable by a routine Giemsa-banded karyotype. In contrast, there are very few clinically relevant abnormalities that are detected by karyotype but not by CMA. Karyotype still has a role in selected cases, such as in distinguishing translocation from free trisomy causing

Down syndrome; a karyotype, not CMA, should be requested as the first test in infants with a very high suspicion of Down syndrome. In virtually all other clinical settings, including suspected trisomy 13 or 18, CMA will increasingly be requested as the first-line test, particularly if important decisions about management are a consideration. Some experts recommend requesting both CMA and a karyotype concurrently. It is debatable whether a karyotype should be requested if CMA is normal because balanced translocations and inversions will be undetected by the CMA, and the chromosomal breakpoints occasionally will disrupt a gene or disturb gene function by a position effect on an adjacent gene. However, this yield will be low, and performing a higher resolution CMA may be more fruitful. At present, the primary advantages of karyotype analysis is that it is often locally available, and payers are familiar with karyotype costs. Payers are just beginning to become familiar with the advantages of CMA. At present, CMA currently costs two to three times that of a karyotype, but this is expected to change because CMA is intrinsically less expensive in terms of technician time required and the professional time required for interpretation, especially for normal results. The CMA method is amenable to automation, and the yield of informative data relative to the cost of the test should be increasingly favorable in the future.

Some of the most common diagnoses that will be made by CMA are deletions or duplications of the DiGeorge/velocardial facial region, the Williams syndrome region, and the Prader-Willi/Angelman region. Other common abnormalities will include telomeric deletions or duplications for many chromosomes. Although the largest of these can be detected by karyotype and more than 90% can be detected by telomere FISH, CMA is superior to all other methods for detection of telomeric abnormalities because clinical arrays have tens (for BACs) or hundreds (for oligonucleotide) of probes for each telomeric region. Another relatively common abnormality detected by the array methods is multigenic duplications, including the *MECP2* (Rett) gene in males. These infants have relatively severe neurological symptoms, and mothers are most often healthy carriers of the X-linked duplication, making genetic counseling very important.

The introduction of array-based methods for genomic analysis has revealed a surprising extent of copy number variants (CNVs) in the normal population. In one of the most detailed analyses to date,[1] almost 1500 CNVs were found among 270 normal individuals, with each individual having 24 to 70 such variations compared with a consensus genome. The CNV regions involved cover 12% of the genome and lead to hundreds of genes being present at one or three copies in an individual compared with the usual two copies for most autosomal genes. Most of these CNVs do not have obvious phenotypic effects, although some may contribute to the predispositions for common diseases. The clinical relevance of CNVs is that CMA, particularly when performed at high density of probes, detects gains and losses of copy number in the genome of normal individuals. The pathological changes will generally be larger in size, will most often be de novo (eg, not present in either parent), and will often occur in known disease regions (eg, the DiGeorge/velocardiofacial region). Occasionally it can be difficult to be certain whether a gain or loss of copy number in a region is a benign CNV or is the cause of the abnormal phenotype in the child. By using targeted arrays, the detection of benign CNVs can be minimized. Many CNVs will be detected in all individuals if high-density tiling arrays are used. Proper interpretation may then require routine parental analyses to distinguish benign CNVs inherited from a healthy parent from de novo events, which are far more likely to be the cause of phenotypic abnormalities.

The most recent trends in CMA are: (1) a rapidly increasing number of laboratories are offering the test for the first time; (2) BAC arrays were initially used almost exclusively, but oligonucleotide arrays now predominate; (3) higher and higher density coverage focused on disease-prone regions but with increasingly good "backbone" coverage of the entire genome is the rule. Current oligonucleotide arrays for routine clinical care typically have 30,000 to 70,000 oligos, but research arrays with hundreds of thousands or even 1 million oligonucleotides are in widespread research use. These higher density arrays will move into the clinic, although the detection of benign CNVs may slow this trend. CMA will almost certainly supplant karyotype analysis for prenatal diagnosis as well as postnatal diagnosis, and more infants will be delivered with known cytogenetic diagnoses established by CMA while the infant was in utero.

In summary, new array-based methods are rapidly replacing banded karyotype analysis as the method of choice for detecting chromosomal abnormalities in patients of all ages. Detection of chromosomal abnormalities is very common in the neonatal ICU,[2,3] and the availability of CMA will lead to expanded detection compared with the experience with karyotype analysis. The frequency of detecting chromosomal abnormalities generally is higher for samples submitted in the newborn period than later in infancy and childhood because the proportion of infants with multiple malformations tested in the newborn period is higher in the neonatal setting compared with milder developmental phenotypes being tested at later ages. This makes CMA particularly relevant to neonatal care. Soon neonatologists will routinely request CMA for indications for which they might have previously requested karyotype or various FISH tests. More detailed reviews are available, although not focused specifically on neonatal applications.[4-6]

Arthur L. Beaudet, MD

Professor and Chair, Department of Molecular and Human Genetics, and Professor of Pediatrics, Baylor College of Medicine and Texas Children's Hospital, Houston, Texas

References

1. Redon R, Ishikawa S, Fitch KR, et al. Global variation in copy number in the human genome. *Nature*. 2006;444:444-454.
2. Hudome SM, Kirby RS, Senner JW, et al. Contribution of genetic disorders to neonatal mortality in a regional intensive care setting. *Am J Perinatol*. 1994;11:100-103.
3. Stevenson DA, Carey JC. Contribution of malformations and genetic disorders to mortality in a children's hospital. *Am J Med Genet A*. 2004;126:393-397.
4. Shaffer LG, Kashork CD, Saleki R, et al. Targeted genomic microarray analysis for identification of chromosome abnormalities in 1500 consecutive clinical cases. *J Pediatr*. 2006;149:98-102.
5. Lu X, Shaw CA, Patel A, et al. Clinical implementation of chromosomal microarray analysis: Summary of 2513 postnatal cases. *PLoS ONE*. 2007;2:e327.
6. Stankiewicz P, Beaudet AL. Use of array CGH in the evaluation of dysmorphology, malformations, developmental delay, and idiopathic mental retardation. *Curr Opin Genet Dev*. 2007;17:182-192.

1 The Fetus

Ultrasound screening for fetal anomalies in Southern Sweden: a population-based study
Nikkilä A, Rydhstroem H, Källén B, et al (Lund Univ, Sweden; Helsingborg Gen Central Hosp, Sweden; Univ of Lund, Sweden; et al)
Acta Obstet Gynecol Scand 85:688-693, 2006   1–1

Background.—The accuracy of ultrasound in the diagnosis of congenital malformations has been the subject of many studies. Most of these are hospital-based studies over a limited period of years presenting high detection rates and also relatively high incidence of major malformations. We present here a large population-based study over a long period of years.

Methods.—The prenatal diagnoses are compared with the diagnoses of the newborns and aborted fetuses, including autopsy results. The detection rate of some common structural malformations is studied.

Results.—The overall detection rate of malformations in our study was 28.4%. We noticed an improved detection rate of heart defects and cleft lip during the study period. The prevalence of malformations in the population was 2.6%. The false positive diagnoses were few, 54 cases, and mainly of a mild nature.

Conclusions.—Ultrasound screening of fetal malformations in our population has a low false positive rate and even though the overall sensitivity is low, 28.4%, the detection rate for many common structural malformations is relatively good.

▶ There has been remarkable progress in the field of ultrasonography. In the 1960s investigators were barely able to detect the number of fetuses and detection of fetal anomalies was too great a stretch. The routine use of ultrasound for antenatal examination is, today, a virtually universal procedure. Additionally, it is not restricted to a single scan as most women receive an early scan to establish gestational age, followed by an anatomical survey to look for anomalies and then ultrasonographic evaluation of fetal well being. Ultrasonography is also used to detect multiple gestations, estimate fetal weight, detect placental location in addition to guiding amniocentesis, cordocentesis and chorionic villus sampling.

In 1994 Crane et al,[1] in a randomized clinical trial, tested the hypothesis that antenatal detection of fetal congenital malformations by means of ultrasonographic screening would significantly alter perinatal outcome. Although ultrasound helped detect more anomalies (35% of anomalies detected in the screened group versus 11% in the controls), they were unable to validate their hypothesis and concluded that ultrasonography had no major impact on the frequency of abortion for fetal anomalies. Survival rates for anomalous fetuses were also unaffected by screening. Nonetheless, antenatal ultrasound has become established as an integral component of antenatal care. It has become almost absurd that shopping malls offer "photographs" of the fetus and a vigorous new industry has emerged.

Most studies are local or regional, so it is refreshing to come across a study covering large populations because, whereas the data from tertiary centers has generally been reliable, multicenter studies have reported lower detection rates.[1,2] Nikkilä et al[3] note that screening for fetal malformations had a low sensitivity, but there was a low false-positive rate (not diagnosing conditions that did not exist nor causing undue anxiety for the parents) and the prevalence of malformations (2.6%) exceeds the "standardized prevalence" of 2% as proposed by Levi.[4]

Nikkilä et al[3] also reported on a population-based study of the prenatal diagnosis of spina bifida in Sweden over a period of 31 years. They compared the number of newborns with spina bifida and the elective terminations because of the prenatal diagnosis of spina bifida for different periods and, to no one's great surprise, observed that the rate of spina bifida among newborns diminished gradually from 0.55 per 1000 to 0.29 per 1000 during the study period.

When the definitive diagnosis of an anomaly is uncertain on ultrasound, MRI has been added to the diagnostic armamentarium (see Griffiths[5]).

A. A. Fanaroff, MD

References

1. Crane JP, LeFevre ML, Winborn RC, et al. A randomized trial of prenatal ultrasonographic screening: impact on the detection, management, and outcome of anomalous fetuses. The RADIUS Study Group. *Am J Obstet Gynecol.* 1994;171:392-399.
2. Ewigman BG, Crane JP, Frigoletto FD, LeFevre ML, Bain RP, McNellis D. Effect of prenatal ultrasound screening on perinatal outcome. RADIUS Study Group. *N Engl J Med.* 1993;32:821-827.
3. Nikkilä A, Rydhström H, Källén B. The incidence of spina bifida in Sweden 1973-2003: the effect of prenatal diagnosis. *Eur J Public Health.* 2006;16:660-662.
4. Levi S. Ultrasound in prenatal diagnosis: polemics around routine ultrasound screening for second trimester fetal malformations. *Prenat Diagn.* 2002;22:285-295.
5. Griffiths PD, Widjaja E, Paley MN, Whitby EH. Imaging the fetal spine using in utero MR: diagnostic accuracy and impact on management. *Pediatr Radiol.* 2006;36:927-933.

Accuracy of fetal echocardiography: a cardiac segment-specific analysis
Gottliebson WM, Border WL, Franklin CM, et al (Cincinnati Children's Hosp, Ohio)
Ultrasound Obstet Gynecol 28:15-21, 2006   1–2

Objective.—In patients with congenital heart disease, comprehensive, segment-specific analysis of cardiac anatomy has become 'the standard of care', largely as a result of improvements in cardiac imaging technology. Our aim was to apply segment-specific standards to assess the accuracy of fetal echocardiography.

Methods.—This was a retrospective review of all fetal echocardiograms (*n* = 915) performed at our center between August 1998 and June 2003. Of these, 100 studies had congenital heart disease findings and corresponding postnatal studies on the same patients for comparison. An expert independent pediatric echocardiologist, using the standards of accuracy expected of postnatal echocardiography, assessed the studies for the following cardiac segments: abdominal situs, systemic venous return (VR), pulmonary VR, atria, atrioventricular valves, ventricular septum, ventricular hypoplasia, ventricular morphology, semilunar valves, great arterial relation and aortic arch. Sensitivity, specificity, and positive and negative predictive values were calculated for each segment.

Results.—Specificity and negative predictive value were high for all cardiac segments (range, 82–100%). Sensitivity and positive predictive value were similarly high (range, 83–100%) for most cardiac segments, but were only 50–88% for systemic VR, pulmonary VR and aortic arch segments (Table 5).

Conclusions.—Fetal echocardiography has excellent diagnostic accuracy in describing intracardiac anatomy. However, despite both technological ad-

TABLE 5.—Sensitivity, Specificity and Positive (PPV) and Negative (NPV) Predictive Values of Fetal Echocardiography and Prevalence of Abnormalities, According to Anatomical Segment: Old Cohort (1998–2000; *n* = 48)

Segment	Sensitivity (%)	Specificity (%)	PPV (%)	NPV (%)	Prevalence (%)
Abdominal situs	100	100	100	100	12.5
Systemic venous return	56	88	83	64	53
Pulmonary venous return	67	100	100	92	21
Atria	90	100	100	97	25
Atrioventricular valves	97	91	97	91	73
Ventricular septum	81	94	94	81	54
Ventricular hypoplasia	96	100	100	94	62
Ventricular morphology	91	97	91	97	28
Semilunar valves	96	83	93	91	69
Great arterial relation	86	96	92	93	34
Aortic arch	71	94	92	75	52
Ductal arch	95	93	95	93	61

vances and improved physician awareness, assessment of systemic VR, pulmonary VR, and aortic arch anatomy remain challenging.

▶ Whereas there have been tremendous advances in the imaging modalities permitting accurate diagnosis of fetal malformation and function, it is important to know some of the limitations of the current state of the art. Gottliebson et al, in a methodical analysis of the evaluation of 100 patients with congenital heart disease, point out the weaknesses. The identification of structural anomalies is excellent with the exception of the aortic arch anomalies, and there are significant limitations in the assessment of both systemic and pulmonary venous return. No doubt these issues are being addressed and solutions can be anticipated in the near future. It is worth noting that in a regional study the overall detection rate of malformations was 28.4%.[1] Garne et al[2] wished to evaluate the prenatal diagnosis of congenital heart diseases by ultrasound investigation in well-defined European populations. They reviewed data from 20 registries of congenital malformations in 12 European countries. The prenatal ultrasound screening programs in the countries ranged from no routine screening to three ultrasound investigations per patient routinely performed. There were 2454 cases with congenital heart disease with an overall prenatal detection rate of 25%. Termination of pregnancy was performed in 293 cases (12%). Stoll et al,[3] utilizing the same database, noted that the proportion of prenatal diagnosis of associated congenital heart diseases varied in relation to the ultrasound screening policies from 18% in countries without routine screening (The Netherlands and Denmark) to 46% in countries with only one routine fetal scan, and 56% in countries with two or three routine fetal scans. They also noted that cardiac defects were more likely to be found if there were associated malformations and if the size of the ventricles was altered. Thus, despite all the technologic advances and increased screening, most congenital heart disease is not diagnosed in the fetus, but after birth. Our vigilance in this regard must remain high.

A. A. Fanaroff, MD

References

1. Nikkilä A, Rydhströem H, Källén B, Jörgensen C. Ultrasound screening for fetal anomalies in Southern Sweden: a population based study. *Acta Obstet Gynecol Scand.* 2006;85:688-693.
2. Garne E, Stoll C, Clementi M, for the EUROSCAN Group. Evaluation of prenatal diagnosis of congenital heart diseases by ultrasound: experience from 20 European registries. *Ultrasound Obstet Gynecol.* 2001;17:386-391.
3. Stoll C, Garne E, Clementi M, for the EUROSCAN Group. Evaluation of prenatal diagnosis of associated congenital heart diseases by fetal ultrasonographic examination in Europe. *Prenat Diagn.* 2001;21:243-252.

False-positive rate in prenatal diagnosis of surgical anomalies

Borsellino A, Zaccara A, Nahom A, et al (Bambino Gesù Pediatric Hosp, Roma, Italy; Artemisia Med Centre, Roma, Italy)
J Pediatr Surg 41:826-829, 2006   1–3

Background/Purpose.—Technical refinements and increasingly sophisticated equipment have led to higher sensitivity in prenatal diagnosis of congenital malformations; however, such progress may be accompanied by decreased specificity. The aim of this study is to evaluate evolution of prenatal diagnosis from the first sonographic suspicion of fetal anomaly until after delivery (diagnosis confirmed, resolution before birth, healthy baby, or affected with different disorder) to document rate of false-positive (FP) results.

Methods.—Retrospective review of prenatal ultrasound examinations performed at our institution between 2000 and 2002 was conducted. The series includes pregnancies referred to our department after detection of thoracic and abdominal anomalies at routine obstetrical sonography and with a follow-up comprising at least the first 6 months of life. Urologic malformations were excluded. Those fetuses who proved healthy at birth were considered FP results.

Results.—One hundred fifty-seven fetuses/neonates underwent complete follow-up. Prenatal diagnosis of esophageal atresia resulted in 3 (27%) of 11 FPs. Finding of dilated bowel, isolated or associated with hyperechogenicity or ascites, was not predictive of small bowel obstruction in 7 (41%) of 17 fetuses. No FPs were found with regard to abdominal wall defects (8 gastroschisis and 26 omphaloceles, all confirmed at birth). Concerning thoracic malformations, no FPs were seen among the 28 cases of congenital diaphragmatic hernia, whereas diagnosis of lung malformation presented a specificity of 97% (1/28 FP). Ovarian cysts accounted for an FP rate of 17% (4/23 FPs).

Overall, a percentage of FP of 12% (6/50) was seen in 2000, of 11% (5/44) in 2001, and 9% (6/63) in 2002, with no statistically significant difference.

Conclusions.—Because of the high FP rate regarding some particular anomalies, unnecessary psychological burden to prospective parents may ensue. This issue should be dealt with in future prospective studies.

▶ It is somewhat disconcerting to learn that the false-positive rate in the prenatal diagnosis of surgical conditions hovers around 10%. This number would, no doubt, have been much higher had urologic malformations been included. On the other hand, it is somewhat reassuring that abdominal wall defects and congenital diaphragmatic herniae were never incorrectly overdiagnosed. Hyperechogenic bowel is an unreliable indicator of a surgical condition and may be observed with infection, swallowed blood, cystic fibrosis, and obstructive bowel disease. Nikkilä et al[1] reported that the prevalence of malformation in a defined population (Southern Sweden) was 2.6%, and the overall detection rate of malformations prenatally was 28.4%. They noted few false-positive diagnoses (n = 54), which they described as mainly of a mild nature.

The birth incidence of neural tube defect (NTD) cases in North America is reported to be declining. This decline is being attributed to folic acid (FA) supplementation and food fortification, but second-trimester prenatal screening of pregnancies for NTDs and other congenital anomalies has increased during this timeframe, as well. Van Allen et al[2] reported that prenatal screening identified 86.1% (124/144) of NTD-affected pregnancies, with 72.6% (90/124) resulting in pregnancy termination, and 27.4% (34/124) continuing to term. Use of FA supplementation in the periconceptional period was recorded in only 36.4% of pregnancies (39/107). As a result, the NTD incidence at birth declined 60% from 1.16/1000 to 0.47/1000 live births due predominantly to pregnancy terminations following prenatal diagnosis, which reduces the NTD incidence by 60%, from 1.16/1000 to 0.47/10002. Nikkilä et al[3] have reported a similar experience.

If decisions to terminate pregnancies are made on the basis of prenatal ultrasound, it is imperative to eliminate false-positive diagnoses.

A. A. Fanaroff, MD

References

1. Nikkilä A, Rydhströem H, Källén B, Jörgensen C. Ultrasound screening for fetal anomalies in Southern Sweden: a population-based study. *Acta Obstet Gynecol Scand.* 2006;85:688-693.
2. Van Allen MI, Boyle E, Thiessen P, et al. The impact of prenatal diagnosis on neural tube defect (NTD) pregnancy versus birth incidence in British Columbia. *J Appl Genet.* 2006;47:151-158.
3. Nikkilä A, Rydhström H, Källén B. The incidence of spina bifida in Sweden 1973-2003: the effect of prenatal diagnosis. *Eur J Public Health.* 2006;16:660-662.

Nasal bone in first-trimester screening for trisomy 21
Cicero S, Avgidou K, Rembouskos G, et al (King's College, London)
Am J Obstet Gynecol 195:109-114, 2006   1–4

Objective.—This study was undertaken to investigate the impact of incorporating assessment of the nasal bone into first-trimester combined screening by fetal nuchal translucency (NT) thickness and maternal serum biochemistry.

Study Design.—In this prospective combined screening study for trisomy 21, the fetal nasal bone was also examined and classified as present or absent. A multivariate approach was used to calculate patient-specific risks for trisomy 21 and the detection rate (DR) and false-positive rate (FPR) were estimated. We examined 2 screening strategies; first, integrated first-trimester screening in all patients and second, first-stage screening of all patients using fetal NT and maternal serum free β-hCG and PAPP-A, followed by second-stage assessment of nasal bone only in those with an intermediate risk of 1 in 101 to 1 in 1000 after the first-stage.

Results.—The nasal bone was absent in 113 (0.6%) of the 20,165 chromosomally or phenotypically normal fetuses and in 87 (62.1%) of the 140 fetuses with trisomy 21. With combined first-trimester NT and serum

TABLE 1.—Prevalence of Absent Nasal Bone in
Chromosomally Normal and Abnormal Fetuses
at 11 to 13^{+6} Weeks

Fetal Karyotype	N	Absent Nasal Bone
Normal	20,165	113 (0.6%)
Trisomy 21	140	87 (62.1%)
Trisomy 18	40	22 (55.0%)
Trisomy 13	19	6 (31.6%)
Turner syndrome	13	5 (38.5%)
Triploidy	11	1 (9.1%)
Other*	30	4 (13.3%)
Total	20,418	238 (1.2%)

* Trisomies or sex chromosome aneuploidies other than above, unbalanced translocations, deletions, mosaics.

(Courtesy of Cicero S, Avgidou K, Rembouskos G, et al. Nasal bone in first-trimester screening for trisomy 21. *Am J Obstet Gynecol*. 195:109-114. Copyright 2006 by Elsevier.)

screening, the DR of 90% was achieved at a FPR of 5%. Inclusion of the nasal bone, either in all cases or in about 10% of the total in the 2-stage approach, halved the FPR to 2.5%.

Conclusion.—Inclusion of the nasal bone in first-trimester combined screening for trisomy 21 achieves a DR of 90% for a FPR of 2.5% (Table 1).

▶ In the general population, there is a 2% to 3% risk of birth defects, regardless of prior history, family history, maternal age, or lifestyle. Chromosomal abnormalities account for approximately 10% of birth defects but are important because of their high mortality and morbidity rates. A detailed fetal anatomical survey performed at 18 to 22 weeks remains the primary means for detecting the majority of serious "structural" birth defects; however, first-trimester screening at 11 to 14 weeks has developed into the initial screening test for many patients. A small nose is a common feature in trisomy 21 and radiologic, histomorphologic, and sonographic studies reveal that nasal bone abnormalities are significantly more common in fetuses with trisomy 21 than in euploid fetuses. In 2001, Sonek and Nicolaides[1] described the technique for prenatal sonographic assessment of the fetal nasal bones and reported that in 2 of 3 fetuses with trisomy 21 the nasal bone was absent and in 1, it was hypoplastic. The article by Cicero is a well-illustrated and tabulated review of the topic and makes a strong argument for inclusion of the nasal bone evaluation in the first-trimester combined screening for trisomy 21. At no risk to the fetus or mother, the detection rate is enhanced and the false-positive rate decreased—an ideal outcome. The article includes results from many ethnic groups with varied nasal shapes and sizes, so it is "generalizable."

A. A. Fanaroff, MD

Reference

1. Sonek J, Nicolaides K. Prenatal ultrasonographic diagnosis of nasal bones abnormalities in three fetuses with Down syndrome. *Am J Obstet Gynecol.* 2002;186: 139-141.

Is measurement of nuchal translucency thickness a useful screening tool for heart defects? A study of 16 383 fetuses
Westin M, Saltvedt S, Bergman G, et al (Lund Univ, Malmö, Sweden; South Stockholm Gen Hosp; Hosp of Astrid Lundgren, Sweden; et al)
Ultrasound Obstet Gynecol 27:632-639, 2006   1–5

Objective.—To determine the performance of nuchal translucency thickness (NT) measurement as a screening method for congenital heart defects (CHD) among fetuses with normal karyotype.

Methods.—An NT measurement was made in 16 383 consecutive euploid fetuses derived from an unselected pregnant population. The cut-offs for increased risk of heart defects, chosen a priori and tested prospectively, were: NT ≥95th centile for crown–rump length, NT ≥ 3 mm, and NT ≥3.5 mm. The sensitivity and false-positive rate (FPR; 1 minus specificity) of the risk cut-offs and their positive and negative likelihood ratios (+LR and −LR) with regard to CHD were calculated.

Results.—Among the 16 383 fetuses with an NT measurement there were 127 cases with a diagnosis of heart defect confirmed by cardiac investigations after birth or at autopsy. Of these, 55 defects were defined as major, of which 52 were isolated (no other defects or chromosomal aberrations), corresponding to a prevalence of major heart defects in chromosomally normal fetuses/newborns of 3.3/1000. The sensitivity, FPR, +LR and −LR for NT ≥95th centile with regard to an isolated major heart defect were: 13.5%, 2.6%, 5.2 and 0.9, respectively. For NT ≥3.0 mm these values were: 9.6%, 0.8%, 12.0 and 0.9, and for NT ≥3.5 mm they were: 5.8%, 0.3%, 19.3 and 0.9.

Conclusions.—NT measurement is a poor screening method for isolated major CHD. A method with a much higher detection rate and with a reasonably low FPR is needed. However, increased NT indicates increased risk of fetal heart defect, and women carrying fetuses with increased NT should be offered fetal echocardiography in the second trimester.

▶ This article addresses a similar theme to the Comstock article (Abstract 1–6). There have been several observations of an association between the degree of NT thickening and the risk of fetal cardiac anomalies in euploid fetuses. The levels of risk have clearly related to the severity of the NT enlargement, and a consequent question has been whether we could improve our ability to screen for fetal cardiac anomalies with NT. At present the literature suggests about 30% detection of cardiac anomalies with second-trimester USs incorporating a "4-chamber view" of the heart.[1] This is lower than early reports of detection rates as high as 55%[2]; however, a literature review incorporated into

Hyett's article suggests a composite detection rate of 37%. Data from the United States reported by Bahado-Singh et al[3] and by Simpson et al[4] have shown lower detection rates than Hyett.

The Westin article reports on a Swedish cohort of 16,383 low-risk fetuses who had NT measurements. There were 127 cases of congenital heart disease, 55 major and of these 52 were isolated heart defects. With the use of the 95th percentile (ie, 5% of the normal population would require fetal echocardiograms), only 13.5% of heart defects would be detected, higher cutoffs resulted in lower detection rates.

All of the articles noted here have had similar conclusions: although NT is not a good way to SCREEN for heart defects, elevated values are clearly associated with an increased RISK of heart defects. So, although there are excellent arguments to offer NT to the general population as an aneuploidy risk assessment tool, screening for heart disease is not part of the indication. At the same time, if the NT is elevated in fetuses with normal chromosomes, a fetal echocardiogram is clearly indicated. The International Society of Ultrasound in Obstetrics and Gynecology has suggested using a threshold of 3.5 mm for this purpose.[5]

J. A. Copel, MD

References

1. Todros T, Faggiano F, Chiappa E, Gaglioti P, Mitola B, Sciarrone A. Accuracy of routine ultrasonography in screening heart disease prenatally. Gruppo Piemontese for Prenatal Screening of Congenital Heart Disease. *Prenat Diagn.* 1997;17: 901-906.
2. Hyett J. Does nuchal translucency have a role in fetal cardiac screening? *Prenat Diagn.* 2004;24:1130-1135.
3. Bahado-Singh RO, Wapner R, Thom E, et al. Elevated first-trimester nuchal translucency increases the risk of congenital heart defects. *Am J Obstet Gynecol.* 2005;192:1357-1361.
4. Simpson LL, Malone FD, Bianchi DW, et al. Nuchal translucency and the risk of congenital heart disease. *Obstet Gynecol.* 2007;109:376-383.
5. International Society of Ultrasound in Obstetrics and Gynecology. Cardiac screening examination of the fetus: guidelines for performing the 'basic' and 'extended basic' cardiac scan. *Ultrasound Obstet Gynecol.* 2006;27:107-113.

Is there a nuchal translucency millimeter measurement above which there is no added benefit from first trimester serum screening?
Comstock CH, for the FASTER Research Consortium (William Beaumont Hosp, Royal Oak, Mich; et al)
Am J Obstet Gynecol 195:843-847, 2006   1–6

Objective.—The purpose of this study was to evaluate whether there is a nuchal translucency (NT) measurement, independent of gestational age, above which immediate diagnostic testing should be offered without waiting for first trimester serum markers.

Study Design.—Thirty-six thousand one hundred twenty patients had successful measurement of simple NT at 10 3/7 to 13 6/7 weeks and had first trimester serum screening. No risks were reported until second trimester serum screening was completed.

Results.—Thirty-two patients (0.09%) had NT ≥4.0 mm; the lowest combined first trimester trisomy 21 risk assessment in euploid cases was 1 in 8 and among aneuploidy cases was 7 in 8. One hundred twenty-eight patients (0.3%) had simple NT ≥3.0 mm: the lowest combined first trimester trisomy 21 risk assessment of any patient in this group was 1 in 1479 and the lowest risk assessment among aneuploid cases was 1 in 2. Ten patients (8%) had first trimester trisomy 21 risk assessments lowered to less that 1:200 and none of these 10 cases had an abnormal outcome.

Conclusion.—During first trimester Down syndrome screening, whenever an NT measurement of 3.0 mm or greater is obtained there is minimal benefit in waiting for serum screening results, and no benefit for NT of 4.0 mm or greater. Differentiation between cystic hygroma and enlarged simple NT (≥3.0 mm) is now a moot point as both are sufficiently high risk situations to warrant immediate CVS.

▶ The introduction of NT measurements in combination with serum analytes (usually pregnancy associated plasma protein A [PAPP-A] and either total human chorionic gonadotropin [HCG] or its free-β subunit) to practice in the United States has opened up the option of aneuploidy risk assessment in the first trimester. Results of the testing use the maternal age-related risk sequentially adjusted with likelihood ratios derived from the US and the serum analytes to provide a personal risk to the woman. It is critical to the success of the program that there be ongoing monitoring of the US results, optimally by epidemiologic surveillance of individual sonographers and sonologists.

In most parts of the country it is not yet possible to get serum results at the same time as the US is performed, although some areas have systems in place to draw maternal blood ahead of time and integrate the results with the US "on the fly." Coming months will see greater introduction of 1-stop approaches, either with advanced maternal blood draws, or on-site laboratory systems to process blood while the patient is being scanned.

One of the common questions that has been raised is what an elevated NT means by itself. This article asked whether there might be an NT measurement above which it was no longer necessary to draw blood at all, because the risks of aneuploidy would be high enough to lead women to ask for definitive testing in virtually all situations, and regardless of maternal age. The investigators in the First and Second Trimester Evaluation of Risk (FASTER) study evaluated more than 36,000 pregnancies. There were 32 fetuses (0.09%) with NT ≥ 4.0 mm (the median for the 10 to 13-week interval evaluated runs about 0.8-1.2 mm), and the BEST risk assessment for these pregnancies was 1:7 (ie, 1 in 8). Although some women in the 3 to 4-mm NT group had risk estimates below 1:200, none of those age 35 years or older achieved a risk better than 1:100.

These results are clinically important for those doing NT assessments in their practices, and can save time for patients needing to make decisions about invasive, definitive testing. Some couples with frank cystic hygromas will choose to terminate pregnancies even before the karyotypes are performed because of the risks, but we must emphasize to our patients that these are risk numbers, not diagnoses. Further information collected by Souka et al[1] in the United Kingdom has suggested that those fetuses with elevated NTs and normal karyotypes and normal ultrasounds can still have good outcomes.

J. A. Copel, MD

Reference

1. Souka AP, Von Kaisenberg CS, Hyett JA, Sonek JD, Nicolaides KH. Increased nuchal translucency with normal karyotype. *Am J Obstet Gynecol.* 2005;192: 1005-1021.

Four-dimensional sonographic assessment of fetal facial expression early in the third trimester
Yan F, Dai S-Y, Akther N, et al (Kagawa Univ, Japan)
Int J Gynecol Obstet 94:108-113, 2006   1–7

Objective.—To evaluate the characteristic patterns of facial expression in fetuses aged from 28 to 34 weeks using 4-dimensional (4-D) ultrasonography.

Methods.—The faces of 10 healthy fetuses aged from 28 to 34 weeks were recorded continuously for 15 min with a 4-D ultrasonographic machine performing up to 25 frames per second. The occurrence rates of blinking, mouthing, yawning, tongue expulsion, smiling, scowling, and sucking were evaluated.

Results.—Mouthing was the most frequent facial expression (median, 6.5; range, 2–19) whereas the least frequent were scowling (median, 1;

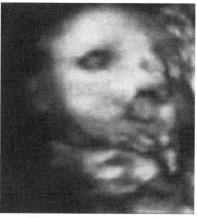

FIGURE 3.—4-D ultrasonographic observation of fetal yawning at 28 weeks. Yawning is a slow, wide, prolonged opening of the jaws followed by quick closure with simultaneous retroflexion of the head. (Courtesy of Yan F, Dai S-Y, Akther N, et al. Four-dimensional sonographic assessment of fetal facial expression early in the third trimester. *Int J Gynecol Obstet.* 2006;94:108-113.)

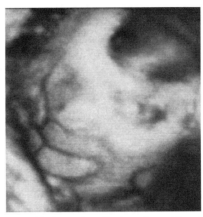

FIGURE 4.—4-D ultrasonographic observation of fetal tongue expulsion at 30 weeks. The mouth is open and the tongue protruding. (Courtesy of Yan F, Dai S-Y, Akther N, et al. Four-dimensional sonographic assessment of fetal facial expression early in the third trimester. *Int J Gynecol Obstet.* 2006;94:108-113.)

range, 0–9) and sucking (median, 1; range, 0–2). Mouthing was evident in all fetuses and significantly more frequent than any other movement ($P<.05$). Yawning (median, 3; range, 0–6), smiling (median, 2; range, 0–9), and blinking (median, 1.5; range, 0–6) were observed in most cases. Tongue expulsion (median, 1.5; range, 0–5), scowling, and sucking were each observed in 6 cases.

Conclusion.—4-D sonography provides a means of evaluating fetal facial expression early in the third trimester. It may be a key to predicting fetal brain function and well-being and an important modality in future fetal neurophysiologic research (Figs 3, 4, and 6).

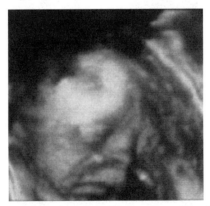

FIGURE 6.—4-D ultrasonographic observation of fetal scowling at 28 weeks. There is a bilateral contraction of the eyebrows accompanied by a bilateral drop of the mouth angles, with curling of the upper or lower lip. (Courtesy of Yan F, Dai S-Y, Akther N, et al. Four-dimensional sonographic assessment of fetal facial expression early in the third trimester. *Int J Gynecol Obstet.* 2006;94:108-113.)

▶ Scoring systems, such as the Neonatal Facial Coding System,[1] have been used to measure the pain response in neonates and to evaluate the response to interventions aimed at reducing stress and pain. The detailed facial images obtained by these authors using 4-D ultrasonography appear able to differentiate between facial movements including yawning (Fig 3), tongue protrusion (Fig 4), and scowling (Fig 6). The authors commented that although 4-D sonography might be useful in the study of fetal behavior, performing these studies is very time demanding and only the quantity of facial movements, not the quality, was currently possible. Nonetheless, one can envision a time, sooner as opposed to later, when images of fetal facial expressions will be used as another marker of fetal well-being.

R. A. Ehrenkranz, MD

Reference

1. Grunau RE, Oberlander T, Holsti L, Whitfield MF. Bedside application of the Neonatal Facial Coding System in pain assessment of premature neonates. *Pain.* 1998;76:277-286.

Imaging the fetal spine using in utero MR: diagnostic accuracy and impact on management
Griffiths PD, Widjaja E, Paley MNJ, et al (Univ of Sheffield, England)
Pediatr Radiol 36:927-933, 2006   1–8

Background.—In-utero MR imaging (iuMR) has entered the clinical arena during the last decade. It is used mainly for imaging fetal brain abnormalities.

Objective.—To report our experience of imaging the fetal spine and spinal cord in fetuses with known or suspected abnormalities diagnosed on US imaging.

Materials and Methods.—Prospective imaging and retrospective analysis of the possible impact on management of 50 consecutive fetuses with spinal abnormalities detected by antenatal US imaging.

Results.—In 40 (80%) of 50 fetuses, iuMR and US imaging were in complete agreement. In the other 10 fetuses (20%), iuMR provided additional information or changed the diagnosis, including 8 fetuses where the iuMR could find no abnormality and was found to be correct by later follow-up.

Conclusion.—IuMR is useful in fetuses with a suspected spinal abnormality. The clinical impact of iuMR may be numerically less than with brain abnormalities, but is still sufficient to warrant its use, especially if there is any uncertainty about the US imaging, and particularly as a relatively high proportion of diagnoses on US imaging are false positives.

▶ Recent advances in technology have made fetal MR imaging available to evaluate the fetal brain and spine. Investigators, thus, have the opportunity to study brain development *in vivo* as well as the ability to easily and early detect congenital anomalies which would not be apparent by prenatal US.[1]

Miller et al[2] were able to confirm that prenatal MR imaging can reliably and accurately delineate and characterize a variety of brain and spine disorders, which is of immense value in planning postnatal management and surgical interventions. They suggested that prenatal multiplanar images "may obviate the need for early postnatal computed tomography or MR imaging."

A. A. Fanaroff, MD

References

1. Glenn OA, Barkovich AJ. Magnetic resonance imaging of the fetal brain and spine: an increasingly important tool in prenatal diagnosis, part 1. *AJNR Am J Neuroradiol.* 2006;27:1604-1611.
2. Miller E, Ben-Sira L, Constantini S, Beni-Adani L. Impact of prenatal magnetic resonance imaging on postnatal neurosurgical treatment. *J Neurosurg.* 2006;105: 203-209.

Incidence, origin, and character of cerebral injury in twin-to-twin transfusion syndrome treated with fetoscopic laser surgery

Lopriore E, van Wezel-Meijler G, Middeldorp JM, et al (Leiden Univ, The Netherlands)

Am J Obstet Gynecol 194:1215-1220, 2006   1–9

Objective.—The objective of the study was to determine the incidence, origin, and character of cerebral lesions in monochorionic twins with twin-to-twin transfusion syndrome treated with fetoscopic laser surgery.

Study Design.—This was a prospective study of monochorionic twins with twin-to-twin transfusion syndrome treated with fetoscopic laser surgery and monochorionic twins without twin-to-twin transfusion syndrome delivered at our center between June 2002 and September 2005, using cranial ultrasonography.

Results.—Incidence of antenatally acquired severe cerebral lesions in the twin-to-twin transfusion syndrome group was 10% (8/84) and 2% (2/108) in the non–twin-to-twin transfusion syndrome group ($P = .02$). Incidence of severe cerebral lesions at discharge was 14% (12/84) in the twin-to-twin transfusion syndrome group and 6% (6/108) in the non–twin-to-twin transfusion syndrome group ($P = .04$). Antenatal injury was responsible for severe cerebral lesions in 67% (8/12) of the twin-to-twin transfusion syndrome group.

Conclusion.—Incidence of severe cerebral lesions in twin-to-twin transfusion syndrome treated with fetoscopic laser surgery is high and results mainly from antenatal injury.

▶ Lopriore et al used prospectively collected data on 108 consecutive monochorionic twin pregnancies managed in their center to examine the relationship between cranial US-detected cerebral injuries, and twin-to-twin transfusion syndrome (TTTS) treated with fetoscopic laser surgery. Forty-eight of the pregnancies had evidence of TTTS and underwent treatment with fetoscopic laser surgery, and 60 pregnancies did not have TTTS and served as a control population. Severe cerebral lesions on cranial US were defined as the "presence of at least 1 of the following findings: IVH grade III, periventricular hemorrhagic infarction, PVL grade II or greater, porencephalic cysts, and ventricular dilatation." In addition, "severe cerebral lesions were considered to be of antenatal onset if present on the first US scan on day 1."

Because the control group lacked evidence of TTTS, infants in that group had a much lower a priori risk of cerebral injury than the infants exposed to fetoscopic laser surgery for TTTS. In addition, the control infants were more mature at birth and decreasing birth weight was found to be the only independent predictor of cerebral injury. Therefore, it is not surprising that infants in the TTTS group were found to have a significantly higher incidence of antenatally acquired severe cerebral lesions.

More importantly, while severe neuroimaging abnormalities are often associated with adverse neurodevelopmental outcomes, they should not be used as surrogates of long-term neurodevelopmental outcomes. The randomized control trial (RCT) by Senat et al[1] reported that fetoscopic laser surgery was a more effective treatment than serial amnioreduction for severe TTTS, and found that infants in the laser group were more likely to be free of neurologic complications at 6 months of age. The NICHD RCT comparing aggressive amnioreduction with selective fetoscopic laser surgery for severe TTTS included a neurodevelopmental assessment at 18 to 22 months' corrected age. However, that trial was stopped early because of poor enrollment and the data have not been reported.[2] Nonetheless, because fetoscopic laser surgery for TTTS has become an "accepted" practice, and because there are limited long-term neurodevelopmental outcome data of survivors of fetoscopic laser surgery for TTTS, clinicians should carefully monitor the developmental outcomes of infants exposed to fetoscopic laser surgery for TTTS.

R. A. Ehrenkranz, MD

References

1. Senat MV, Deprest J, Boulvain M, Paupe A, Winer N, Ville Y. Endoscopic laser surgery versus serial amnioreduction for severe twin-to-twin transfusion syndrome. *N Engl J Med.* 2004;351:136-144.
2. Harkness UF, Crombleholme TM. Twin-to-twin transfusion syndrome: where do we go from here? *Semin Perinatol.* 2005;29:296-304.

Outcome of antenatally suspected congenital cystic adenomatoid malformation of the lung: 10 years' experience 1991–2001
Calvert JK, Boyd PA, Chamberlain PC, et al (John Radcliffe Hosp, Oxford, England; Univ of Oxford, England)
Arch Dis Child 91:26-28, 2006
1–10

Objective.—To determine the outcome of antenatally suspected congenital cystic adenomatoid malformation of the lung (CCAM) over a 10 year period.

Methods.—This is a retrospective study of all babies diagnosed antenatally in the Prenatal Diagnosis Unit and delivered in Oxford between 1991 and 2001. Data were obtained from the Oxford Congenital Anomaly Register, theatre records, and histopathology reports.

Results.—Twenty eight cases of CCAM were diagnosed antenatally. Five pregnancies were terminated. Data are available on all 23 of the pregnancies that continued and resulted in two neonatal deaths and 21 surviving babies. Eleven of the 23 cases (48%) showed some regression of the lesion antenatally, and four of these cases appeared to resolve completely on prenatal ultrasound. Three of the 23 babies (13%) were symptomatic in the early neonatal period, and three developed symptoms shortly afterwards. Seventeen of the 23 babies (74%) were asymptomatic, of whom 12 had abnormalities on chest radiograph or computed tomography scan and had elective surgery. Two babies (8%) had completely normal postnatal imaging, and three had abnormalities which resolved in the first year of life. Seventeen of the 23 babies (74%) had surgery. Histology at surgery was heterogeneous. Of the 23 live births, all 21 survivors (91%) are well at follow up or have been discharged.

Conclusions.—All babies diagnosed antenatally with CCAM require postnatal imaging with computed tomography irrespective of signs of antenatal resolution. In asymptomatic infants, the recommendations are close follow up and elective surgery for persistent lesions within the first year of life. Histology at surgery was heterogeneous, and this should be considered when counselling parents.

▶ This series from Oxford, England adds to the lore of CCAM. The 28 cases, including 5 who were terminated, comprise an experience of greater than a decade. There are no startling revelations, but the authors reaffirm that some lesions resolve before birth; their recommendation for imaging all infants with CT scans is reasonable. The outcome for the group was excellent and confirms the data from Ierullo's series of 34 cases[1] acquired over a 4-year period at St. George's Hospital in London. Of note, too, fetal surgery is a treatment option for fetuses with congenital cystic CCAM of the lung who develop hydrops before 32 weeks of gestation.

In addition to CCAM, intralobar sequestration (ILS), extralobar sequestration (ELS), and lobar emphysema (LE) are other intrathoracic lesions to be considered. Fetal CCAM is a pulmonary developmental anomaly arising from an overgrowth of the terminal respiratory bronchioles, but there may also be an accompanying bronchial atresia. Riedlinger et al[2] prospectively evaluated 47 lung specimens resected over a 4-year period with the clinical impression of ELS (n = 11), ILS (n = 11), CCAM (n = 20), LE (n = 4), and airway esophageal communication (n = 1). Pathologic examination revealed atresia of a lobar, segmental, or subsegmental bronchus in 100% of ELS, 82% of ILS, 70% of CCAM, and 50% of LE. They speculated that as bronchial atresia and CCAM nearly always coexist, they have the same etiology with the anatomical differences modified genetically or by other accompanying insults.

A. A. Fanaroff, MD

References

1. Ierullo AM, Ganapathy R, Crowley S, Craxford L, Bhide A, Thilaganathan B. Neonatal outcome of antenatally diagnosed congenital cystic adenomatoid malformations. *Ultrasound Obstet Gynecol.* 2005;26:150-153.
2. Riedlinger WF, Vargas SO, Jennings RW, et al. Bronchial atresia is common to extralobar sequestration, intralobar sequestration, congenital cystic adenomatoid malformation, and lobar emphysema. *Pediatr Dev Pathol.* 2006;9:361-373.

Doppler Ultrasonography versus Amniocentesis to Predict Fetal Anemia
Oepkes D, for the DIAMOND Study Group (Leiden Univ, the Netherlands; et al)
N Engl J Med 355:156-164, 2006   1–11

Background.—Pregnancies complicated by Rh alloimmunization have been evaluated with the use of serial invasive amniocentesis to determine bilirubin levels by measuring in the amniotic fluid the change in optical density at a wavelength of 450 nm (ΔOD_{450}); however, this procedure carries risks. Noninvasive Doppler ultrasonographic measurement of the peak velocity of systolic blood flow in the middle cerebral artery also predicts severe fetal anemia, but this test has not been rigorously evaluated in comparison with amniotic-fluid ΔOD_{450}.

Methods.—We performed a prospective, international, multicenter study including women with RhD-, Rhc-, RhE-, or Fy^a-alloimmunized pregnancies with indirect antiglobulin titers of at least 1:64 and antigen-positive fetuses to assess whether Doppler ultrasonographic measurement of the peak systolic velocity of blood flow in the middle cerebral artery was at least as sensitive and accurate as measurement of amniotic-fluid ΔOD_{450} for diagnosing severe fetal anemia. The results of the two tests were compared with the incidence of fetal anemia, as determined by measurement of hemoglobin levels in fetal blood.

Results.—Of 165 fetuses, 74 had severe anemia. For the detection of severe fetal anemia, Doppler ultrasonography of the middle cerebral artery had a sensitivity of 88 percent (95 percent confidence interval, 78 to 93 percent), a specificity of 82 percent (95 percent confidence interval, 73 to 89 percent), and an accuracy of 85 percent (95 percent confidence interval, 79 to 90 percent). Amniotic-fluid ΔOD_{450} had a sensitivity of 76 percent (95 percent confidence interval, 65 to 84 percent), a specificity of 77 percent (95 percent confidence interval, 67 to 84 percent), and an accuracy of 76 percent (95 percent confidence interval, 69 to 82 percent). Doppler ultrasonography was more sensitive, by 12 percentage points (95 percent confidence interval, 0.3 to 24.0), and more accurate, by 9 percentage points (95 percent confidence interval, 1.1 to 15.9), than measurement of amniotic-fluid ΔOD_{450} (Fig 2).

Conclusions.—Doppler measurement of the peak velocity of systolic blood flow in the middle cerebral artery can safely replace invasive testing in the management of Rh-alloimmunized pregnancies.

A

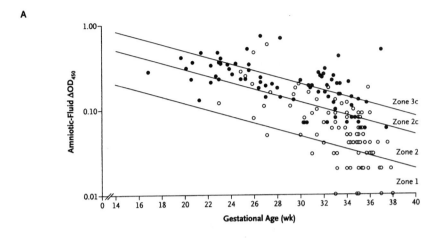

B

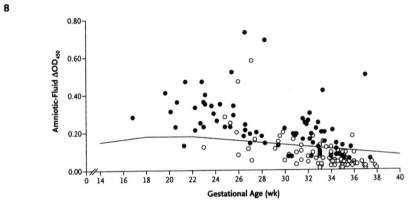

FIGURE 2.—Results of Amniotic Fluid ΔOD_{450} for 165 Fetuses at Risk for Severe Anemia. Panel A shows the results of a modified Liley's chart (Liley AW. Liquor amii analysis in the management of the pregnancy complicated by rhesus sensitization. *Am J Obstet Gynecol*. 1969;82:1359-1370.). Zone 2c is the upper third of Liley's original zone 2. Values above the line separating zone 2 and zone 2c are considered to indicate fetal anemia requiring transfusion. Panel B shows the results plotted on Queenan's chart. The solid line represents the cutoff between zones 1 to 3 and zone 4, adapted from Queenan et al. (Queenan JT, Tomai TP, Ural SH, King JC. Deviation in amniotic fluid optical density at a wavelength of 450 nm in Rh-immunized pregnancies from 14 to 40 weeks' gestation: a proposal for clinical management. *Am J Obstet Gynecol*. 1993;168:1370-1376.); values above this line are considered to indicate a risk of intrauterine death requiring transfusion. (Reprinted by permission from Oepkes D, for the DIAMOND Study Group. Doppler ultrasonography versus amniocentesis to predict fetal anemia. *N Engl J Med*. 365:156-164. Copyright 2006, Massachusetts Medical Society. All rights reserved.)

▶ Over the past 30 years the inner sanctum of the fetus has been invaded and disrupted, and we have witnessed the birth of the field of fetology. A host of medical and surgical interventions are available for the fetus, but questions remain regarding efficacy. The technologic advances have been spectacular, and the ability to open the uterus without immediately interrupting the pregnancy has been almost magical. All in all, the therapies have met with varying degrees of success. True, the surgery is possible, but has the outcome been improved? The ongoing randomized trial of correction of spina bifida in utero will yield the definitive answer.

With regard to the management of erythroblastosis fetalis and the detection of fetal anemia, the pendulum has swung through the whole spectrum, from expectant to invasive and now back again to noninvasive. Initially, perinatologists and neonatologists (were these terms even used then?) stood by and waited until the fetus was delivered and then attempted to treat the anemic, hydropic, jaundiced neonate with exchange transfusions. Then came the use of amniocentesis and the Liley curves which predicted fetal anemia, subsequently treated by intraperitoneal transfusions. With the enhanced imaging ability of ultrasound, the blind needle intraperitoneal needle placement was followed by direct sampling from and transfusion into the umbilical vein. (It is worth noting that the survival for fetuses requiring intrauterine transfusions was in the range of 40%.) The use of Rh immune globulin at 28 weeks' gestation and following delivery dramatically reduced the incidence of Rh alloimmunization and represented a major advance. But despite the introduction of anti-D immune globulin for the prevention of anti-D red-cell alloimmunization, hemolytic disease of the newborn continues to occur, either because of the lack or failure of prophylaxis or because of maternal alloimmunization against other red-cell antigens for which prophylaxis is not available. Therefore, there is an ongoing need to recognize fetal anemia. It is pleasing to learn from Oepkes' data that this can be accomplished in a noninvasive manner by Doppler evaluation of the middle cerebral artery peak systolic velocity, and this methodology is more sensitive and accurate than the amniotic-fluid ΔOD_{450}, which is an indirect measurement of fetal hemoglobin. I appreciated Moise's title of the editorial that accompanied the paper of Oepkes et al—it is time to put the needles away.[1]

A. A. Fanaroff, MD

Reference

1. Moise KJ Jr. Diagnosing hemolytic disease of the fetus—time to put the needles away? *N Engl J Med.* 2006;355:192-194.

Liver, meconium, haemorrhage: the value of T1-weighted images in fetal MRI
Zizka J, Elias P, Hodik K, et al (Charles Univ, Hradec Kralove, Czech Republic; Inst of Clinical and Experimental Medicine, Prague, Czech Republic)
Pediatr Radiol 36:792-801, 2006   1–12

Background.—Ultrafast T2-weighted (T2-W) MRI sequences are currently considered a routine technique for fetal MR imaging. Limited experience exists with fetal T1-weighted (T1-W) imaging techniques.

Objective.—To determine MRI patterns of some fetal abdominal or haemorrhagic disorders with particular respect to the diagnostic value of T1-W images.

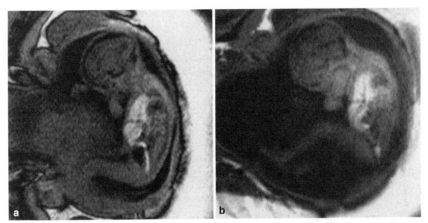

FIGURE 1.—Left-sided diaphragmatic hernia at 23 weeks of gestation, sagittal T1-W images. Although the single-shot TurboFLASH sequence (a) offers overall lower signal-to-noise ratio than multislice FLASH sequence (b), the delineation of hyperintense colon and herniated liver is better on the TurboFLASH image due to the absence of motion artefacts. (Courtesy of Zizka J, Elias P, Hodik K, et al. Liver, meconium, haemorrhage: the value of T1-weighted images in fetal MRI. *Pediatr Radiol.* 2006;36:792-801. Copyright Springer-Verlag.)

Materials and Methods.—In addition to standard T2-W single-shot sequences, T1-W single-shot and/or multislice sequences were employed in 25 MR examinations performed in 23 fetuses between 20 and 36 weeks of gestation for more detailed assessment of liver, meconium-filled digestive tract, haemorrhage, or further characterization of a fetal abdominal mass. Diag-

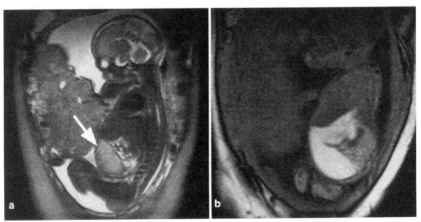

FIGURE 2.—Intestinal perforation with meconium pseudocyst at 31 weeks of gestation. (a) Large, sub-hepatic, moderately T2 hyperintense mass (*arrow*) on sagittal HASTE image. (b) Sagittal TurboFLASH image reveals marked T1 hyperintensity of the pseudocyst lesion, suggesting its meconium nature. (Courtesy of Zizka J, Elias P, Hodik K, et al. Liver, meconium, haemorrhage: the value of T1-weighted images in fetal MRI. *Pediatr Radiol.* 2006;36:792-801. Copyright Springer-Verlag.)

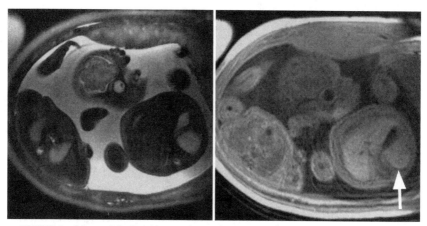

FIGURE 5.—Subacute left adrenal haemorrhage in fetus 'B' in the 35th week of a twin pregnancy. Transverse 12-W HASTE (*left*) and T1-W FLASH (*right*) images of the fetal upper abdomen reveal a sharply delineated and distinctly hyperintense mass posterior to the stomach (*arrow*). (Courtesy of Zizka J, Elias P, Hodik K, et al. Liver, meconium, haemorrhage: the value of T1-weighted images in fetal MRI. *Pediatr Radiol.* 2006;36:792-801. Copyright Springer-Verlag.)

nostic value and presence of motion artefacts on T1-W images was recorded in each case.

Results.—T1-W images enabled superior delineation of fetal liver and large intestine. They provided additional diagnostic information in 9 (39%) of 23 fetuses. One false-positive and one false-negative MRI diagnosis of malrotation anomaly were encountered. Use of single-shot T1-W sequences reduced the occurrence of motion artefacts in 64%.

Conclusion.—Our results suggest that the specific signal properties of methaemoglobin, meconium and liver are sufficiently important for T1-W sequences to become a routine part of fetal MRI protocols when dealing with digestive tract anomalies, diaphragmatic and abdominal wall defects, intraabdominal masses, and fetal haemorrhage (Figs 1, 2, and 5).

▶ Traditional 2-dimensional ultrasonography remains the standard mode to diagnose major structural abnormalities in the fetus, but advances in technology including 3-dimensional US and fetal magnetic resonance imaging (MRI) are altering the "gold standard." The ultrafast MRI sequences provide faster scan time and avoid motion artifacts. It is being widely applied in distinguishing normal from abnormal fetal development in all parts of the fetus. As noted above, Zizka and colleagues accurately defined a number of complex intra-abdominal anomalies with the use of T1-weighted images. Veyrac et al[1] provide additional examples of the application of T1-weighted fat-suppressed 3-dimensional fast low-angle shot sequences to accurately define fetal bowel anomalies. Thirty-two fetuses between 23 and 38 weeks' gestation with abnormal appearance of the GI tract by US underwent MR imaging with T1- and T2-weighted sequences. The MR aspect of intestinal atresia (duodenal atresia, n = 1; small bowel atresia, n = 9) included dilatation of the bowel loops, accurate assessment of the normal bowel distal to the atresia (except in the patient with multiple atresia and apple peel syndrome), and microrectum with decreased T1 signal (except in the patient with duodenal atresia). Megacystis microcolon intestinal hypoperistalsis syndrome (n = 1) was indicated by an abnormal signal of the entire bowel and an abnormal pattern for the urinary tract. Meconium pseudocysts (n = 2) were easily differentiated from enteric cysts (n = 2). High anorectal malformations with or without urinary fistula and cloacal malformation could also be differentiated. In conclusion, Saguintaah et al[2] from the same group has earlier concluded that MRI provided complete visualisation of the fetal GI tract, showed specific signal intensities, identified the level of an obstruction, detected a microcolon, and demonstrated communication between urinary and GI tracts. MRI shows great potential to differentiate gastrointestinal and other anomalies. Incorporating these new imaging modalities into clinical practice should not only improve perinatal outcomes but also definitely enhance patient counseling.

A. A. Fanaroff, MD

References

1. Veyrac C, Couture A, Saguintaah M, Baud C. MRI of fetal GI tract abnormalities. *Abdom Imaging.* 2004;29:411-420.
2. Saguintaah M, Couture A, Veyrac C, Baud C, Quere MP. MRI of the fetal gastrointestinal tract. *Pediatr Radiol.* 2002;32:395-404.

Amniotic fluid cytokine profile in association with fetal hyperechogenic bowel
Oboh AE, Orsi NM, Campbell J (St James's Univ, Leeds, England)
Eur J Obstet Gynecol Reprod Biol 128:86-90, 2006   1–13

Objectives.—Fetal hyperechogenic bowel (FEB) is associated with infection, chromosomal abnormalities and poor fetal outcome. FEB may result from an intrauterine fetal bowel cytokine-mediated inflammatory response. Since alterations in the levels of the cytokines interleukin (IL)-6, IL-8, IL-10, tumour necrosis factor (TNF)-α and interferon (IFN)-γ are associated with pregnancy complications and necrotizing enterocolitis, this study aimed: (i) to determine their involvement in the pathophysiology of FEB and (ii) to identify their role as amniotic fluid markers of this condition.

Study design.—In this prospective case-control study, amniotic fluid was collected by transabdominal amniocentesis from pregnant women with fetuses presenting (n = 10)—or not (n = 30)—with FEB during routine 18–20 week ultrasound scans. Cell-free amniotic fluid samples were analysed for cytokine concentrations by fluid-phase multiplex immunoassay. Data were compared by Mann-Whitney U–tests and Pearson correlations.

Results.—Amniotic fluid IL-8 levels were significantly higher in the FEB group. There was a positive correlation between IL-6 and each of IL-8 and INF-gamma, as well as between IL-8 and IL-10, and TNF-α and INF-γ.

Conclusions.—FEB likely ensues from a fetal inflammatory process involving IL-8 and, possibly, IL-6 and IL-10. This indicates the potential of immunomodulatory therapy in the management of FEB.

▶ Fetal bowel is considered to be hyperechogenic when its echogenicity is broadly similar to, or greater than, that of the surrounding bone. Hyperechogenic fetal bowel is detected in 0.1-1.8% of pregnancies during the second or third trimester.[1] These numbers were derived from a multicenter data analysis and included 682 cases of hyperechogenic fetal bowel. Having established that the bowel is hyperechogenic, recommended investigations should include a detailed scan with Doppler measurements, fetal karyotyping, cystic fibrosis screening, and infectious disease screening; the parents should be made aware of the various possibilities.[1,2] Pregnancy outcome and postnatal follow-up were obtained in 656 of the 682 cases (91%). In 447 cases (65.5%), a normal birth was observed. Multiple malformations were observed in 47 cases (6.9%), a significant chromosomal anomaly was noted in 24 (3.5%), cystic fibrosis in 20 (3%), and viral infection in 19 (2.8%).[1] Remember that intra-amniotic bleeding is another cause of bowel echogenicity.[3] After birth, newborns require careful evaluation because a surgical intervention may be necessary.

A. A. Fanaroff, MD

References

1. Simon-Bouy B, Satre V, Ferec C, et al, for the French Collaborative Group. Hyperechogenic fetal bowel: a large French collaborative study of 682 cases. *Am J Med Genet A*. 2003;121:209-213.
2. Marcus-Soekarman D, Offermans J, Van den Ouweland AM, et al. Hyperechogenic fetal bowel: counseling difficulties. *Eur J Med Genet*. 2005;48:421-425.
3. Petrikovsky B, Smith-Levitin M, Holsten N. Intra-amniotic bleeding and fetal echogenic bowel. *Obstet Gynecol*. 1999;93:684-686.

Fetuses with congenital heart disease demonstrate signs of decreased cerebral impedance
Modena A, Horan C, Visintine J, et al (Thomas Jefferson Univ, Philadelphia; Thammasat Univ, Pathumthani, Thailand)
Am J Obstet Gynecol 195:706-710, 2006   1–14

Objective.—The purpose of this study was to determine whether fetuses with a congenital heart defect demonstrate changes in cerebrovascular impedance.

Study Design.—Fetal echocardiograms from January 2001 to May 2005 were reviewed. Cases had sonographically diagnosed congenital heart defects; control subjects were gestational age–matched fetuses with normal echocardiograms. The pulsatility index in the middle cerebral artery was used to measure impedance to cerebral blood flow. Abnormal middle cerebral artery pulsatility index was defined as less than the 5th percentile. Cases were subgrouped into mixing versus nonmixing lesions.

Results.—Of 142 total fetuses, there were significantly more abnormal middle cerebral artery pulsatility indices in the cases (5/71) than in the control subjects (0/71; $P = .023$); all abnormal middle cerebral artery pulsatility indices occurred in the fetuses with admixing cardiac lesions.

Conclusion.—Fetuses with congenital heart defect are significantly more likely to have decreased cerebrovascular impedance. This may represent a marker of cerebral hypoxemia that is due to intracardiac mixing of oxygenated and deoxygenated blood. Theoretically, this hypoxemia may contribute to the cause of abnormal neurologic development in these infants.

▶ As surgical and intensive care approaches have advanced, survival rates for infants with the most complex congenital cardiac defects have improved substantially. Therefore, there has been increasing concern with respect to brain development and neurodevelopmental outcome among these patients. Magnetic resonance imaging (MRI) evidence of ischemic brain injury, particularly periventricular leukomalacia (PVL), has been reported to be present in greater than 50% of neonates after surgery for congenital heart disease (CHD).[1] Neurodevelopmental outcome studies have shown that delay and impairment are common.[2,3] Even preoperatively, MRI and cranial ultrasound studies suggest that ischemic injury and other abnormalities appear relatively common among infants with CHD.[1,4] The current study by Modena et al is one of very few that investigates cerebral blood flow abnormalities. This demonstrates that fetal cerebrovascular impedance is decreased among those with CHD compared with healthy fetuses, suggesting that the fetus with CHD is attempting to compensate for inadequate or diminished oxygen delivery to the brain. Given evidence for preoperative brain injury, as well as guarded neurodevelopmental outcomes among infants with complex and major CHD, further large-scale longitudinal studies will be crucial to understand the continuum from fetal brain autoregulatory mechanisms, through preoperative and postoperative clinical events and advanced neuroimaging findings, to neurodevelopmental outcomes.

S. R. Hintz, MD, MS

References

1. Mahle WT, Tavani F, Zimmerman RA, et al. An MRI study of neurological injury before and after congenital heart surgery. *Circulation.* 2002;106:I109-I114.
2. Limperopoulos C, Majnemer A, Shevell MI, Rosenblatt B, Rohlicek C, Tchervenkov C. Neurodevelopmental status of newborns and infants with congenital heart defects before and after open heart surgery. *J Pediatr.* 2000;137:638-645.
3. Dittrich H, Bührer C, Grimmer I, Dittrich S, Abdul-Khaliq H, Lange PE. Neurodevelopment at 1 year of age in infants with congenital heart disease. *Heart.* 2003;89:436-441.
4. Te Pas AB, van Wezel-Meijler G, Bökenkamp-Gramann R, Walther FJ. Preoperative cranial ultrasound findings in infants with major congenital heart disease. *Acta Paediatr.* 2005;94:1597-1603.

2 Epidemiology and Pregnancy Complications

Single versus weekly courses of antenatal corticosteroids: Evaluation of safety and efficacy

Wapner RJ, for the National Institute of Child Health and Human Development Maternal Fetal Medicine Units Network (Drexel Univ, Philadelphia; et al)

Am J Obstet Gynecol 195:633-642, 2006   2–1

Objective.—The purpose of this study was to determine if weekly corticosteroids improve neonatal outcome without undue harm.

Study Design.—Women 23 to 32 weeks receiving 1 course of corticosteroids 7 to 10 days prior were randomized to weekly betamethasone or placebo.

Results.—The study was terminated by the independent data and safety monitoring committee with 495 of the anticipated 2400 patients enrolled. There was no significant reduction in the composite primary morbidity outcome (8.0% vs 9.1%, $P = .67$). Repeated courses significantly reduced neonatal surfactant administration ($P = .02$), mechanical ventilation ($P = .004$), CPAP ($P = .05$), pneumothoraces ($P = .03$). There was no significant difference in mean birth weight or head circumference. The repeat group had a reduction in multiples of the birth weight median by gestational age (0.88 vs 0.91) ($P = .01$) and more neonates weighing less than the 10th percentile (23.7 vs 15.3%, $P = .02$). Significant weight reductions occurred for the group receiving ≥ 4 courses.

Conclusion.—Repeat antenatal corticosteroids significantly reduce specific neonatal morbidities but do not improve composite neonatal outcome. This is accompanied by reduction in birth weight and increase in small for gestational age infants.

▶ The 1994 National Institutes of Health (NIH) Consensus Conference on the Effect of Corticosteroids for Fetal Maturation on Perinatal Outcomes recommended the administration of a single course of antenatal corticosteroids to pregnant women between 24 and 34 weeks' gestation who were at risk of preterm delivery within 7 days. That Consensus Conference also noted that the potential risks and benefits of repeated courses of antenatal steroids were unknown and called for clinical trials to resolve that issue.

This randomized, double-masked, placebo-controlled, multicenter clinical trial was performed by the NICHD Maternal-Fetal Medicine Units (MFMU) Network for the purpose of testing the hypothesis that when compared with a single course, weekly courses of antenatal corticosteroids would improve neonatal outcome without causing harm. The primary outcome was a composite endpoint consisting of the presence of any of the following: (1) severe respiratory distress syndrome (RDS), (2) IVH > grade III, (3) periventricular leukomalacia, (4) BPD, or (5) stillbirth or neonatal death. The trial was stopped early because of a tendency toward decreased birth weight in the repeat steroid group without any evident reduction in the primary morbidity outcome and because of poor enrollment.

Interestingly, the MFMU Network trial was initiated shortly after enrollment in a similar multicenter, randomized control trial performed by Guinn et al[1] was terminated early. The trial by Guinn et al[1] also used a composite outcome based on neonatal morbidities; it was stopped early after a total of 502 women had to be randomly assigned because of safety concerns about neurologic complications associated with weekly antenatal steroid therapy and minimal differences of short-term outcomes between the study groups. Anthropometric changes were not observed between the groups.

Of note, the Australasian Collaborative Trial of Repeat Doses of Steroids (ACTORDS)[2] used a similar study design with a primary outcome of occurrence and severity of neonatal respiratory distress syndrome (RDS) and recently reported that fewer infants exposed to repeat courses of antenatal steroids had RDS or severe lung disease. Although some anthropometric differences existed at birth, there were no differences at hospital discharge. If specific infant morbidities described in the Guinn et al and the MFMU Network trials are compared with the ACTORDS trial, similar benefits with respect to severe respiratory distress are noted. Therefore, these data would benefit from a meta-analysis that would evaluate composite outcomes as well as specific infant morbidities. The potential risks and benefits of less frequent repeat courses of antenatal steroid therapy, for example every 14 days instead of weekly or "rescue therapy," have not been evaluated. Thus, weekly courses of antenatal corticosteroids are not routinely administered in the United States.

R. A. Ehrenkranz, MD

References

1. Guinn DA, Atkinson MW, Sullivan L, et al. Single vs weekly courses of antenatal corticosteroids for women at risk of preterm delivery: a randomized controlled trial. *JAMA*. 2001;286:1581-1587.
2. Crowther CA, Haslam RR, Hiller JE, Doyle LW, Robinson JS, for ACTORDS. Neonatal respiratory distress syndrome after repeat exposure to antenatal corticosteroids: a randomized controlled trial. *Lancet*. 2006;367:1913-1919.

Treatment of Periodontal Disease and the Risk of Preterm Birth

Michalowicz BS, for the OPT Study (Univ of Minnesota, Minneapolis; Hennepin County Med Ctr, Minneapolis; Univ of Kentucky, Lexington; et al)
N Engl J Med 355:1885-1894, 2006   2–2

Background.—Maternal periodontal disease has been associated with an increased risk of preterm birth and low birth weight. We studied the effect of nonsurgical periodontal treatment on preterm birth.

Methods.—We randomly assigned women between 13 and 17 weeks of gestation to undergo scaling and root planning either before 21 weeks (413 patients in the treatment group) or after delivery (410 patients in the control group). Patients in the treatment group also underwent monthly tooth polishing and received instruction in oral hygiene. The gestational age at the end of pregnancy was the prespecified primary outcome. Secondary outcomes were birth weight and the proportion of infants who were small for gestational age.

Results.—In the follow-up analysis, preterm birth (before 37 weeks of gestation) occurred in 49 of 407 women (12.0%) in the treatment group (resulting in 44 live births) and in 52 of 405 women (12.8%) in the control group (resulting in 38 live births). Although periodontal treatment improved periodontitis measures (P<0.001), it did not significantly alter the risk of preterm delivery (P=0.70; hazard ratio for treatment group vs. control group, 0.93; 95% confidence interval [CI], 0.63 to 1.37). There were no significant differences between the treatment and control groups in birth weight (3239 g vs. 3258 g, P=0.64) or in the rate of delivery of infants that were small for gestational age (12.7% vs. 12.3%; odds ratio, 1.04; 95% CI, 0.68 to 1.58). There were 5 spontaneous abortions or stillbirths in the treatment group, as compared with 14 in the control group (P=0.08).

Conclusions.—Treatment of periodontitis in pregnant women improves periodontal disease and is safe but does not significantly alter rates of preterm birth, low birth weight, or fetal growth restriction.

▶ Periodontal disease refers to local and systemic inflammation that results from chronic gram-negative anaerobic infection of the periodontium. Direct tissue damage resulting from plaque and bacterial products is combined with indirect damage through host inflammatory and immune responses. The association between periodontal disease and premature onset of labor has been recognized for a decade,[1] and Michalowicz et al was unable to demonstrate that treating periodontal disease reduces preterm birth.

Vergnes and Sixou[2] published a meta-analysis on the topic. Their literature search revealed 17 articles that met the inclusion criteria. Seven thousand one hundred fifty-one women participated in the studies, of whom 1056 delivered preterm and/or low birth weight infants. The overall odds ratio was 2.83 (95% CI, 1.95-4.10; P < .0001). However, the authors commented, "This pooled value needed to be interpreted cautiously because there appeared to be a clear trend for the better quality studies to be of lower association strength." They concluded with the most common and almost invariable ending to an article involving clinical trials: "These findings indicate a likely association, but it needs to be confirmed by large, well designed, multicenter trials."[2] Indeed, as noted by Goldenberg and Culhane[3] in the editorial on the study by Michalowicz et al, 3 ongoing studies[4-6] have enrolled more patients than did Michalowicz et al.

The mechanism of action of periodontitis has been attributed to various possibilities that include translocation of periodontal pathogens to the fetoplacental unit and action of a periodontal reservoir of endotoxin (lipopolysaccharide) on the fetoplacental unit or action of a periodontal reservoir of inflammatory mediators (eg, interleukin-1, interleukin-6, tumor necrosis factor-α, or prostaglandin E2) on the fetoplacental unit, which precipitates preterm labor by increasing the systemic circulation of cytokines. Inflammation and inflammatory products seem to rear their ugly heads in and around preterm labor. The associations are always present, but the ability to deliver a knock-out blow to the pathogens or their inflammatory products remains elusive. Hence, the prevalence of prematurity has increased rather than decreased in the United States.

A. A. Fanaroff, MD

References

1. Offenbacher S, Katz V, Fertik G, et al. Periodontal infection as a possible risk factor for preterm low birth weight. *J Periodontol*. 1996;67:1103-1113.
2. Vergnes JN, Sixou M. Preterm low birth weight and maternal periodontal status: a meta-analysis. *Am J Obstet Gynecol*. 2007;196:135.e1-135.e7.
3. Goldenberg RL, Culhane JF. Preterm birth and periodontal disease. *N Engl J Med*. 2006;355:1925-1927.
4. ClinicalTrials.gov. Prevention of pre-term birth by treatment of periodontal disease. Available at: http://www.clinicaltrials.gov/ct/show/NCT00133926?order=7. Accessed October 12, 2006.
5. ClinicalTrials.gov. MOTOR: Maternal oral therapy to reduce obstetric risk. Available at: http://www.clinicaltrials.gov/ct/show/NCT00097656?order=1. Accessed October 12, 2006.
6. ClinicalTrials.gov. Periodontal infection and prematurity study. Available at: http://www.clinicaltrials.gov/ct/show/NCT00116974?order=1. Accessed October 12, 2006.

Cumulative sum (CUSUM) analysis in the assessment of trainee competence in fetal biometry measurement

Weerasinghe S, Mirghani H, Revel A, et al (United Arab Emirates Univ; Ministry of Health, Al Ain, United Arab Emirates)
Ultrasound Obstet Gynecol 28:199-203, 2006   2–3

Objective.—To determine the value of cumulative sum (CUSUM) analysis in assessing trainee proficiency in fetal biometry measurement.

Methods.—Three primary healthcare doctors with no prior ultrasound training were recruited. Each trainee measured the fetal biparietal diameter (BPD), head circumference (HC), abdominal circumference (AC) and femur length (FL) on 100 consecutive pregnant women. The supervisor repeated the measurements. The CUSUM for each set of trainee measurements was

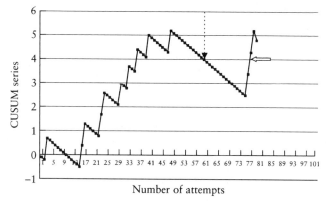

FIGURE 1.—Demonstration of how to interpret a cumulative series (CUSUM) graph. The first half of the graph represents a series of alternating successes (as the graph drops) and failures (as the graph climbs). It is only after 61 attempts (dotted arrow) that the trainee crosses two consecutive boundary lines (CUSUM lines 5 and then 4 on the *y*-axis), indicating that the observed failure rate is lower than the acceptable failure rate, and competence can be declared. At attempt 76 the graph begins an upward slope, crossing the second of two consecutive lines (CUSUM lines 3 and then 4) at attempt number 78 (open arrow); at this point, loss of competence is declared. (Courtesy of Weerasinghe S, Mirghani H, Revel A, et al. Cumulative sum (CUSUM) analysis in the assessment of trainee competence in fetal biometry measurement. *Ultrasound Obstet Gynecol.* 2006;28:199-203. Copyright International Society of Ultrasound in Obstetrics & Gynecology. Reproduced with permission. Permission is granted by John Wiley & Sons LTD on behalf of the ISUOG.)

calculated at a set failure rate of 10%. The point at which the graph fell below two consecutive boundary lines indicated the number of examinations required to achieve competence (Fig 1).

Results.—The CUSUM graphs showed that the rate of learning measurement skills varied among the three trainees. The graph for the CUSUM series for BPD and HC measurement for all trainees fell below two consecutive boundary lines and remained there, indicating competence. The CUSUM series for AC measurement for two of the trainees indicated that competence was achieved; however, for the third trainee, while the graph fell below two consecutive boundary lines, indicating competence, it rose again, crossing two consecutive boundary lines. This indicated a loss of competence and the need for further training. FL measurements for the same trainee never fell below two consecutive boundary lines, indicating failure to achieve competence; the other two achieved competence, but failed to maintain it.

Conclusions.—CUSUM is a useful tool for identifying points of competence and for quantifying the duration of ultrasound training required for each trainee. It provides an early indication of performance, and highlights difficulties in individual performance.

▶ Evidently CUSUM charts are neither intuitive nor simple to operate, but the mathematicians are of the opinion that they are more efficient in detecting small shifts in the mean of a process. I do not pretend to understand the methodology but was intrigued by the fact that trainee competence could be measured both individually and as a group. Granted, this is a very small series, but as we adapt to the 80-hour work week and the demands to document resident competency, we must take advantage of all the help we can get and this appears to be a step in the right direction. At least it is an objective way of determining resident competence in a specific area. Furthermore, it dictates to the residency directors how often a resident must perform a procedure to become competent. As the simulation centers will play a greater role in resident training, this kind of information will be extremely valuable. Clearly we need to be in a position to apply CUSUM to many neonatal procedures.

A. A. Fanaroff, MD

Preeclampsia, gestational hypertension and intrauterine growth restriction, related or independent conditions?
Villar J, for the World Health Organization Antenatal Care Trial Research Group
(World Health Organization, Geneva, Switzerland; et al)
Am J Obstet Gynecol 194:921-931, 2006   2–4

Objective.—Preeclampsia, gestational hypertension, and unexplained intrauterine growth restriction may have similar determinants and consequences. In this study, we compared determinants and perinatal outcomes associated with these obstetric conditions.

Study Design.—We analyzed 39,615 pregnancies (data from the WHO Antenatal Care Trial), of which 2.2% were complicated by preeclampsia, 7.0% by gestational hypertension, and 8.1% by unexplained intrauterine growth restriction (ie, not associated with maternal smoking, maternal undernutrition, preeclampsia, gestational hypertension, or congenital malformations). We compared the risk factors associated with these groups. Fetal death, preterm delivery, and severe neonatal morbidity and mortality were the primary outcomes. Logistic regression analyses were adjusted for study site, socioeconomic status, and (if appropriate) birth weight and gestational age.

Results.—Diabetes, renal or cardiac disease, previous preeclampsia, urinary tract infection, high maternal age, twin pregnancy, and obesity increased the risk of both hypertensive conditions. Previous large-for-age birth, reproductive tract surgery, antepartum hemorrhage and reproductive tract infection increased the risk for gestational hypertension only. Independent of maternal age, primiparity was a risk factor only for preeclampsia. Both preeclampsia and gestational hypertension were associated with increased risk for fetal death and severe neonatal morbidity and mortality (Table 3). Mothers with preeclampsia compared with those with unexplained intrauterine growth restriction were more likely to have a history of diabetes, renal or cardiac disease, chronic hypertension, previous preeclampsia, body mass index more than 30 kg/cm^2, urinary tract infection and extremes of maternal age. Conversely, unexplained intrauterine growth restriction was associated with higher risk of low birth weight in previous pregnancies, but not with previous preeclampsia. Both conditions increased the risk for perinatal outcomes independently but preeclampsia was associated with considerable higher risk (Table 5).

TABLE 3.—Perinatal Outcomes for Preeclampsia and Gestational Hypertension Compared With the Reference Group

Outcome		Preeclampsia	Gestational HTA	Reference Group
Fetal death	n/N (%)	19/874 (2.2)	37/2,745 (1.4)	288/31,183 (0.9)
	Crude OR	2.4 (1.5-3.8)	1.5 (1.0-2.1)	1.0
	Adjusted OR*	2.5 (1.6-4.1)	1.6 (1.1-2.3)	1.0
Preterm delivery	n/N (%)	239/873 (27.4)	301/2,743 (11.0)	2,718/30,927 (8.8)
(< 37 wks)	Crude OR	3.9 (3.4-4.6)	1.3 (1.1-1.5)	1.0
	Adjusted OR*	3.8 (3.3-4.5)	1.2 (1.1-1.4)	1.0
Very early preterm	n/N (%)	42/873 (4.8)	29/2,743 (1.1)	499/30,927 (1.6)
delivery (< 32 wk)	Crude OR	3.1 (2.2-4.3)	0.7 (0.5-1.0)	1.0
	Adjusted OR*	3.0 (2.2-4.2)	0.6 (0.4-0.9)	1.0
NICU stay 7 or	n/N (%)	148/851 (17.4)	181/2,703 (6.7)	1,042/30,849 (3.4)
more days	Crude OR	6.0 (5.0-7.3)	2.1 (1.7-2.4)	1.0
	Adjusted OR†	1.5 (1.2-2.0)	1.2 (1.0-1.5)	1.0
Neonatal death	n/N (%)	20/852 (2.4)	20/2,696 (0.7)	159/30,793 (0.5)
	Crude OR	4.6 (2.9-7.4)	1.4 (0.9-2.3)	1.0
	Adjusted OR‡	0.9 (0.5-1.8)	1.8 (1.0-3.3)	1.0

*Adjusted for site, treatment group of the original trial and socioeconomic status.
†Adjusted for site, treatment group of the original trial, socioeconomic status, and birth weight (linear).
‡Adjusted for site, treatment group of the original trial, socioeconomic status, and birth weight (restricted cubic splines with 3 knots).
(Courtesy of Villar J, for the World Health Organization Antenatal Care Trial Research Group. Preeclampsia, gestational hypertension and intrauterine growth restriction, related or independent conditions? *Am J Obstet Gynecol.* 194:921-931. Copyright 2006 by Elsevier.)

Conclusion.—Preeclampsia and gestational hypertension shared many risk factors, although there are differences that need further evaluation. Both conditions significantly increased morbidity and mortality. Conversely, preeclampsia and unexplained intrauterine growth restriction, often as-

TABLE 5.—Perinatal Outcomes for Preeclampsia and Unexplained IUGR Compared With the Reference Group

Outcome		Preeclampsia	Unexplained IUGR	Reference Group
Fetal death	n/N (%)	19/874 (2.2)	55/3,224 (1.7)	288/31,183 (0.9)
	Crude OR	2.4 (1.5-3.8)	1.9 (1.4-2.5)	1.0
	Adjusted OR*	2.5 (1.6-4.0)	1.8 (1.3-2.4)	1.0
Preterm delivery	n/N (%)	239/873 (27.4)	187/3,224 (5.8)	2,718/30,927 (8.8)
	Crude OR	3.9 (3.4-4.6)	0.6 (0.6-0.8)	1.0
	Adjusted OR†	3.8 (3.2-4.4)	0.7 (0.6-0.8)	1.0
Very early preterm	n/N (%)	42/873 (4.8)	24/3,224 (0.7)	499/30,927 (1.6)
delivery (< 32 wks)	Crude OR	3.1 (2.2-4.3)	0.5 (0.3-0.7)	1.0
	Adjusted OR*	3.0 (2.2-4.2)	0.5 (0.3-0.7)	1.0
NICU stay ≥7 days	n/N (%)	148/851 (17.4)	213/3,164 (6.7)	1,042/30,849 (3.4)
	Crude OR	6.0 (5.0-7.3)	2.1 (1.8-2.4)	1.0
	Adjusted OR*	5.2 (4.3-6.3)	2.9 (2.4-3.3)	1.0
Neonatal death	n/N (%)	20/852 (2.4)	26/3,161 (0.8)	159/30,793 (0.5)
	Crude OR	4.6 (2.9-7.4)	1.6 (1.1-2.4)	1.0
	Adjusted OR*	4.1 (2.5-6.6)	1.8 (1.2-2.8)	1.0

*Adjusted for site, treatment group of the original trial and socioeconomic status.
†Adjusted for site and socioeconomic status.
(Courtesy of Villar J, for the World Health Organization Antenatal Care Trial Research Group. Preeclampsia, gestational hypertension and intrauterine growth restriction, related or independent conditions? *Am J Obstet Gynecol.* 194:921-931. Copyright 2006 by Elsevier.)

sumed to be related to placental insufficiency, seem to be independent biologic entities.

▶ Hypertension complicates approximately 9% of all pregnancies, with preeclampsia-eclampsia a major cause of maternal and perinatal morbidity and mortality worldwide.[1] Intrauterine growth restriction (IUGR), as reflected by small for gestational age, of diverse causes, affects a similar proportion (10% by definition) of newborn infants, especially in developing countries.[2]

It is currently unclear whether preeclampsia and gestational hypertension are separate diseases affecting similar organs systems, or alternatively, different manifestations of single disease entity. Likewise, a similar controversy exists regarding the association between IUGR and preeclampsia. Some forms of IUGR have also been likened to preeclampsia, based on similar placental pathology, which demonstrates shallow trophoblast invasion in both disorders.[3]

The authors performed a secondary analysis of data collected in the WHO Antenatal Care Trial to determine whether preeclampsia, gestational hypertension, and unexplained IUGR have similar determinants and consequences. They analyzed 39,615 pregnancies, of which 2.2% were complicated by preeclampsia, 7.0% by gestational hypertension, and 8.1% by unexplained IUGR.

The major findings included that (1) preeclampsia and gestational hypertension are associated with an increased incidence of preterm delivery, fetal and neonatal morbidity and mortality and NICU stay of more than 7 days compared with unexplained IUGR, (2) the IUGR group had lower rate of preterm delivery, but had higher incidence of fetal and neonatal mortality and NICU stay of more than 7 days compared with the reference group, and (3) mothers with preeclampsia compared with those with unexplained IUGR were more likely to have a history of diabetes, renal or cardiac disease, chronic hypertension, previous preeclampsia, body mass index more than 30 kg/m^2, urinary tract infection, and extremes of maternal age.

The authors conclude that preeclampsia and gestational hypertension share many risk factors, which is not a novel finding. They further concluded that preeclampsia and unexplained IUGR are independent biologic entities. The latter conclusion, as well as the title of this article, are somewhat of an overstatement. Such an epidemiologic study, even a very well-conducted one, at best can provide information about shared risk factors and similarities in outcomes. By its very nature, such a study can provide only modest guidance as to whether 2 diseases are essentially identical or distinct. This study could have been enhanced by collection and analysis of blood and urine specimens in affected subjects, especially with regard to the role of angiogenic factors, which have been shown to play a part in the pathophysiology of preeclampsia, and perhaps, but not yet known, growth restriction.[4]

E. F. Funai, MD

References

1. Axt R, Kordina A, Meyberg R, Reitnauer K, Mink D, Schmidt W. Immunohistochemical evaluation of apoptosis in placentae from normal and intrauterine-growth restricted pregnancies. *Clin Exp Obstet Gynecol.* 1999;26:195-198.

2. Villar J, Say L, Gülmezoglu M, et al. Eclampsia and pre-eclampsia: a worldwide health problem for 2000 years. In: Critchley H, Maclean A, Poston L, Walker J, eds. *Pre-eclampsia.* London: RCOG Press; 2003:189-207.
3. de Onis M, Blössner M, Villar J. Levels and patterns of intrauterine growth retardation in developing countries. *Eur J Clin Nutr.* 1998;52:S5-S15.
4. Widmer M, Villar J, Benigni A, Conde-Agudelo A, Karumanchi SA, Lindheimer M. Mapping the theories of preeclampsia and the role of angiogenic factors: a systematic review. *Obstet Gynecol.* 2007;109:168-180.

Advanced Maternal Age Is an Independent Risk Factor for Intrauterine Growth Restriction

Odibo AO, Nelson D, Stamilio DM, et al (Washington Univ, St Louis; Univ of Pennsylvania, Philadelphia)
Am J Perinatol 23:325-328, 2006   2–5

Reports on the association between advanced maternal age (AMA) and intrauterine growth restriction (IUGR) are conflicting. Our objective was to determine if AMA is an independent risk factor for IUGR. Our case-control study compared cases with IUGR (birthweight < 10th percentile for gestational age) and a control group without IUGR. Gestational ages were all confirmed by ultrasound. The study included only singletons and fetal anomalies were excluded. Both groups were evaluated for maternal demographics and clinical risk factors. AMA was defined as maternal age > 35 years. Univariate and multivariate analyses were used to examine associations. During the study period, there were 824 cases with IUGR meeting the inclusion criteria; these were compared with 1648 controls (no IUGR) randomly selected from the same population during the same study period. The significant factors associated with IUGR multivariate analyses were black race (odds ratio [OR], 22.4; 95% confidence interval [CI], 17.8 to 28); chronic hypertension (OR, 2.2; 95% CI, 1.5 to 3.2); pregestational diabetes (OR, 3.3; 95% CI, 1.6 to 7) illicit drug use (OR, 3.3; 95% CI, 2.2 to 5.2), and AMA (OR, 1.4; 95% CI, 1.1 to 1.8). There was a positive dose-response association between increasing maternal age and increasing risk for IUGR. At maternal age of 40 years or older, the OR and 95% CI for IUGR was 3.2 and 1.9 to 5.4, respectively. AMA is an independent risk factor for IUGR. Our findings suggest that screening for IUGR is indicated in women age 35 years or older.

▶ Over the last 30 years women throughout the United States and much of the world have chosen to delay childbearing. In the United States, there has been an approximately 36% increase in first births among women age 35 to 39 years, and an even greater increase (70%) among women who are 40 to 45 years of age.[1] This shift in maternal demographics may pose new challenges to current paradigms of prenatal care and antenatal testing.

Odibo et al have performed a case-control study that investigates the association between the IUGR (birthweight <10th percentile for gestational age) and AMA (maternal age >35) in singleton gestations and fetuses without any congenital abnormality. They were able to show that IUGR was significantly associated with black race, chronic hypertension, pregestational diabetes mellitus, illicit drug use, and AMA. Furthermore, the association between AMA and IUGR became stronger as maternal age advanced, with mothers at age 40 years and older having the highest risk of IUGR.

In addition to IUGR, compelling evidence suggests that AMA (defined as age ≥ 35 years on the estimated date of delivery) is associated with an increased risk of other complications of pregnancy, including higher rates of preterm labor, gestational diabetes mellitus, gestational hypertension, and placenta previa. AMA may also contribute to excess intrauterine fetal death (IUFD).[2,3] Many of these complications can be attributed to the increasing prevalence of maternal medical disorders with advancing age.

It is clear that AMA creates new challenges for the current prenatal care system. Increased antenatal surveillance may be a solution to overcome these new problems. On the basis of the results of Obido et al, approximately 19 AMA mothers need to be surveyed to find 1 IUGR fetus. Although the number of AMA mothers increase steadily, the absolute number of pregnancies born to AMA mothers are still very low. Therefore, it is probably cost-effective to monitor AMA women with serial US assessments in an effort to identify fetal growth restriction and to reduce the likelihood of adverse pregnancy and neonatal outcomes.

M. O. Bahtiyar, MD

References

1. Heffner LJ. Advanced maternal age—how old is too old? *N Engl J Med.* 2004;351:1927-1929.
2. Bianco A, Stone J, Lynch L, Lapinski R, Berkowitz G, Berkowitz RL. Pregnancy outcome at age 40 and older. *Obstet Gynecol.* 1996;87:917-922.
3. Callaway LK, Lust K, Mcintyre HD. Pregnancy outcomes in women of very advanced maternal age. *Aust N Z J Obstet Gynaecol.* 2005;45:12-16.

Neonatal Outcomes After Prenatal Exposure to Selective Serotonin Reuptake Inhibitor Antidepressants and Maternal Depression Using Population-Based Linked Health Data
Oberlander TF, Warburton W, Misri S, et al (Univ of British Columbia, Vancouver, Canada)
Arch Gen Psychiatry 63:898-906, 2006   2–6

Context.—Prenatal exposure to selective serotonin reuptake inhibitor (SSRI) antidepressants and maternal depression both alter neonatal health, and distinguishing the effects of each influence remains challenging.

Objective.—To determine whether exposure to SSRIs and depression differs from exposure to maternal depression alone.

Design.—Using population health data, records of neonatal birth outcomes were linked to records of maternal health and prenatal maternal prescriptions for SSRIs.

TABLE 3.—Infant Characteristics*

| | Neonatal Outcomes, Mean | | | Outcome Differences | | | |
| | | | | SE-D–DE | | DE–Nonexposed | |
	SE-D	DE	Nonexposed	Difference (95% CI)	P Value	Difference (95% CI)	P Value
Incidence of cesarean section	0.24	0.21	0.19	0.03 (0.01 to 0.05)	.01†	0.01 (0.01 to 0.02)	<.001†
Birth weight, g	3397	3429	3453	−32 (−1 to −64)	.05‡	−24 (−14 to −39)	<.001‡
Gestational age, wk	38.8	39.1	39.2	−0.35 (−0.25 to −0.45)	<.001†	−0.06 (−0.02 to −0.09)	<.001‡
Incidence of preterm birth (<37 wk)	0.090	0.065	0.059	0.02 (0.009 to 0.04)	<.001†	0.006 (0.002 to 0.010)	.007†
Incidence of birth weight <10th percentile for gestational age	0.085	0.081	0.074	0.005 (−0.01 to 0.02)	.51†	0.007 (0.002 to 0.011)	.005†
Length of hospital stay, d	3.31	2.88	2.76	0.43 (0.12 to 0.74)	.007‡	0.12 (0.03 to 0.20)	.006‡
Incidence of hospital stay >3 d	0.23	0.18	0.17	0.05 (0.03 to 0.07)	<.001†	0.01 (0.01 to 0.02)	<.001†
Incidence of hospital stay >3 d, infants born by vaginal birth	0.16	0.12	0.11	0.036 (0.01 to 0.06)	<.001†	0.01 (0.01 to 0.02)	<.001†
Incidence of respiratory distress	0.139	0.078	0.074	0.063 (0.042 to 0.079)	<.001†	0.004 (−0.0004 to 0.009)	.07†
Incidence of feeding problems	0.039	0.024	0.021	0.015 (0.005 to 0.025)	.002†	0.003 (0.0004 to 0.006)	.02†
Incidence of respiratory distress, infants born by vaginal birth	0.132	0.071	0.068	0.058 (0.038 to 0.079)	<.001†	0.006 (0.0004 to 0.011)	.03†
Incidence of jaundice	0.094	0.075	0.079	0.019 (0.003 to 0.034)	.01†	−0.004 (−0.009 to 0.0004)	.08†
Incidence of convulsions	0.0014	0.0009	0.0011	0.0005 (−0.0015 to 0.0025)	.64†	−0.0002 (−0.0008 to 0.0003)	.49†

Abbreviations: CI, confidence interval; DE, depressed mothers not treated with medication; SE-D, depressed mothers treated with selective serotonin reuptake inhibitors.

*Numbers do not always sum because of rounding.

†Two-tailed Fisher exact test.

‡Two-tailed *t* test, without assuming equal variances. Neonatal outcomes after prenatal exposure to selective serotonin reuptake inhibitor antidepressants and maternal depression using population-based linked health data.

(Courtesy of Oberlander TF, Warburton W, Misri S, et al. *Arch Gen Psychiatry.* 63:898-906. Copyright 2006, American Medical Association.)

TABLE 4.—Comparisons Using Propensity Score Matching: Outcomes for SE-D vs DE Neonates

	Outcome Differences, SE-D − DE			
	Unmatched Difference (95% CI)	P Value	Propensity Score Matched* Difference (95% CI)	P Value†
Incidence of cesarean section	0.03 (0.01 to 0.05)	.01‡	−0.009 (−0.050 to 0.036‡)	.69
Birth weight, g	−32 (−1 to −64)	.05†	10 (−43 to 70†)	.72
Gestational age, wk	−0.35 (−0.25 to −0.45)	<.001†	−0.14 (−0.34 to 0.06‡)	.18
Incidence of preterm birth (<37 wk)	0.02 (0.01 to 0.04)	<.001‡	0.007 (−0.019 to 0.034‡)	.61
Incidence of birth weight <10th percentile for gestational age	0.005 (−0.010 to 0.020)	.51‡	0.033 (0.007 to 0.059‡)	.02
Length of hospital stay, d	0.43 (0.12 to 0.74)	.007†	0.055 (−0.610 to 0.410‡)	.83
Incidence of hospital stay >3 d	0.05 (0.03 to 0.07)	<.001‡	0.037 (−0.004 to 0.075‡)	.07
Incidence of hospital stay >3 d, infants born by vaginal birth‡	0.036 (0.014 to 0.059)	<.001‡	0.035 (−0.005 to 0.072‡)	.08
Incidence of respiratory distress	0.063 (0.042 to 0.079)	<.001‡	0.044 (0.013 to 0.077‡)	.006
Incidence of feeding problems	0.015 (0.004 to 0.025)	.002‡	0.011 (−0.009 to 0.030‡)	.28
Incidence of respiratory distress, infants born by vaginal birth‡	0.058 (0.038 to 0.079)	<.001‡	0.049 (0.017 to 0.088‡)	.006
Incidence of jaundice	0.019 (0.003 to 0.034)	.01‡	0.01 (−0.02 or 0.04‡)	.45
Incidence of convulsions	0.0005 (−0.0015 to 0.0025)	.64‡	0.00077 (−0.0010 to 0.0036§)	.30

Abbreviations: CI, confidence interval; DE, depressed mothers not treated with medication; SE-D, depressed mothers treated with selective serotonin reuptake inhibitors.
*For SE-D group, n = 817; DE group, n = 805.
†P values calculated by means of 2-tailed normal distribution and bootstrapped standard errors (500 repetitions).
‡Bootstrapped bias-corrected 95% CIs.
§Calculated from bootstrapped standard errors.

(Courtesy of Oberlander TF, Warburton W, Misri S, et al. Neonatal outcomes after prenatal exposure to selective serotonin reuptake inhibitor antidepressants and maternal depression using population-based linked health data. *Arch Gen Psychiatry.* 63:898-906. Copyright 2006, American Medical Association.)

Setting.—Population of British Columbia, Canada.

Participants.—Mothers and their infants, representing all live births during a 39-month period (N = 119,547) (1998-2001).

Main Outcome Measures.—Outcomes from infants of depressed mothers treated with SSRIs (SE-D) were compared with outcomes from infants of depressed mothers not treated with medication (DE) and nonexposed controls. To control for maternal mental illness severity, propensity score matching was used to identify a comparison group of DE mothers who were similar to the SE-D mothers in characteristics in the year preceding and during pregnancy.

Results.—Fourteen percent of mothers were diagnosed as having depression during their pregnancy, and the incidence of prenatal SSRI exposure increased from 2.3% to 5.0% during a 39-month period (Table 3). Birth weight and gestational age for SE-D infants were significantly less than for DE infants, as was the proportion of infants born at less than 37 weeks (95% confidence interval [CI], -1 to -64, -0.25 to -0.45, and -0.009 to -0.04, respectively), although differences in the incidence of birth weight less than the 10th percentile for gestational age were not significant. An increased proportion of SE-D infants had neonatal respiratory distress (13.9% vs 7.8%), jaundice (9.4% vs 7.5%), and feeding problems (3.9% vs 2.4%) compared with DE infants (95% CI of difference, 0.042-0.079, 0.003-0.334, and 0.005-0.025, respectively). When outcomes were compared between SE-D and propensity score–matched DE neonates, SE-D was associated with increased incidence of birth weight below the 10th percentile and rates of respiratory distress (Table 4).

Conclusion.—With linked population health data and propensity score matching, prenatal SE-D exposure was associated with an increased risk of low birth weight and respiratory distress, even when maternal illness severity was accounted for.

▶ As Oberlander et al acknowledge, it would not be ethically appropriate to study the effects of SSRIs during pregnancy in the absence of psychiatric illness. Therefore, they undertook a population-based study using administrative health data linking maternal health, including mental health diagnosis and prescription records to neonatal data in an effort to determine whether prenatal exposure to SSRIs and depression differs from exposure to depression alone. This approach demonstrated a clear association between *in utero* SSRI exposure and an increased risk of low-birth weight (below the 10th percentile) and respiratory distress when SSRI-exposed infants were compared with infants delivered from untreated depressed women and a nonexposed control group (Table 3), even when the severity of depression was taken into account (Table 4).

These findings raise questions about whether the maternal benefit from SSRI therapy for depression outweighs or balances the risk of adverse neonatal effects from *in utero* SSRI exposure. A recent commentary[1] compared a withdrawal syndrome in adults after an abrupt discontinuation of SSRI therapy with symptoms of poor neonatal adaptation, which have been associated with postdelivery SSRI "withdrawal." Discontinuation of SSRIs during pregnancy can lead to serious maternal morbidity, including an increased risk of suicidal ideation, substance abuse, hypertension, preeclampsia, preterm birth, and postpartum depression. In addition, depression and anxiety during pregnancy are considered 1 of the strongest predictors of postpartum depression. In contrast, the neonatal symptoms, including jitteriness, poor muscle tone, weak or absent cry, respiratory distress, hypoglycemia, and neurobehavioral changes, were transient and were also seen in SSRI unexposed infants. Although respiratory distress was considered a characteristic finding, it was noted to be self-limiting and benign, and only occasionally requiring respiratory support. Therefore, if started before or in early pregnancy, the balance of evidence supports continued maternal SSRI therapy during pregnancy, followed by observation of the newborn infant for several days postpartum.

R. A. Ehrenkranz, MD

Reference

1. Koren G, Matsui D, Einarson A, Knoppert D, Steiner M. Is maternal use of selective serotonin reuptake inhibitors in the third trimester of pregnancy harmful to neonates? *CMAJ.* 2005;172:1457-1459.

The NICHD-MFMU antibiotic treatment of preterm PROM study: Impact of initial amniotic fluid volume on pregnancy outcome
Mercer BM, for the NICHD-MFMU Network (Bethesda, Md; Univ of Alabama, Birmingham; Univ of Chicago; et al)
Am J Obstet Gynecol 194:438-445, 2006   2–7

Objective.—The purpose of this study was to evaluate the associations between measured amniotic fluid volume and outcome after preterm premature rupture of membranes (PROM).

Study Design.—This was a secondary analysis of 290 women, with singleton pregnancies, who participated in a trial of antibiotic therapy for preterm PROM at 24^0 to 32^0 weeks. Each underwent assessment of the 4 quadrant amniotic fluid index (AFI) and a maximum vertical fluid pocket (MVP) before randomization. The impact of low AFI (< 5.0 cm) and low MVP (< 2.0 cm) on latency, amnionitis, neonatal morbidity, and composite morbidity (any of death, RDS, early sepsis, stage 2-3 necrotizing enterocolitis, and/or grade 3-4 intraventricular hemorrhage) was assessed. Logistic regression controlled for confounding factors including gestational age at randomization, GBS carriage, and antibiotic study group.

Results.—Low AFI and low MVP were identified in 67.2% and 46.9% of women, respectively. Delivery occurred by 48 hours, 1 and 2 weeks in 32.4%, 63.5% and 81.7% of pregnancies, respectively. Both low AFI and low MVP were associated with shorter latency ($P < .001$), and with a higher rate of delivery at 48 hours, 1, and 2 weeks ($P = .02$ for each). However, neither test offered significant additional predictive value over the risk in the total population. Low AFI and low MVP were not associated with increased amnionitis. After controlling for other factors, both low MVP and low AFI were associated with shorter latency ($P \leq .002$), increased composite morbidity ($P = .03$), and increased RDS ($P \leq .01$), but not with increased neonatal sepsis ($P = .85$) or pneumonia ($P = .53$). Alternatively, after controlling for fluid volume, gestational age, and GBS carriage, the antibiotic study group had longer latency, and suffered less common primary outcomes and neonatal sepsis.

Conclusion.—Oligohydramnios should not be a consideration in determining which women will be candidates for expectant management or antibiotic treatment when it is identified at initial assessment of preterm PROM remote from term.

► Early delivery and neonatal infectious morbidity have been associated with low residual fluid volume following preterm premature rupture of membranes (PPROM), but the predictive power of US-determined AFI and MVP for these outcomes has not been well studied. This secondary analysis of a multicenter, prospective study of PPROM treatment with antibiotics between 24^0 and 32^0 weeks is valuable in demonstrating that fluid volume immediately after PPROM is not a useful guide for patient management or pregnancy and neonatal outcome prediction.

The authors assessed data from 290 of the original cohort of 585 women with singleton pregnancies and PPROM, including only those who had recorded measurements of both AFI and MVP. That low AFI (<5.0 cm) and low MVP (<2.0 cm) correlated with a shorter interval to delivery and a higher incidence of delivery by 48 hours and 1 and 2 weeks is not surprising. The relative risk of these tests for delivery was not high. Contrary to what has been suggested by others, low AFI and low MVP were not associated with subsequent clinical or histologic chorioamnionitis, neonatal sepsis, or pneumonia. The authors acknowledge that antibiotic treatment may have reduced the impact of low AFI on infection. They speculate that subclinical contractions, leading to loss of fluid, may be responsible for low AFI and a shorter latency. Both tests were associated with increased composite neonatal morbidity (defined as 1 or more of the following: stillbirth, infant death before discharge, RDS, neonatal sepsis within 72 hours of birth, grade 3 or 4 intraventricular hemorrhage, or stage 2 or 3 necrotizing enterocolitis) and RDS. Receiver operating characteristic curve analysis could not identify an optimal point that would predict neonatal composite morbidity. Ultimately, low AFI may be associated with worsened neonatal outcomes because of brief latency and not increased infection.

The fact that half of the women from the original study did not undergo both tests and were excluded is a limitation. However, this data set is large and compelling. The authors' finding that postrupture AFI and MVP, together or individually, is a poor predictor of infection is helpful. Initial US after PPROM should not guide decisions for expectant management or antibiotic treatment.

D. J. Lyell, MD

Midpregnancy genitourinary tract infection with *Chlamydia trachomatis*: Association with subsequent preterm delivery in women with bacterial vaginosis and *Trichomonas vaginalis*

Andrews WW, for the National Institute of Child Health and Human Development Maternal-Fetal Medicine Units Network (Univ of Alabama at Birmingham; Natl Insts of Health, Bethesda, Md; George Washington Univ, Rockville, Md; et al)

Am J Obstet Gynecol 194:493-500, 2006   2–8

Objective.—The objective of the study was to estimate whether midpregnancy genitourinary tract infection with *Chlamydia trachomatis* is associated with an increased risk of subsequent preterm delivery.

Study Design.—Infection with *C. trachomatis* was determined using a ligase chain reaction assay (performed in batch after delivery) of voided urine samples collected at the randomization visit ($16^{0/7}$ to $23^{6/7}$ weeks' gestation) and the follow-up visit ($24^{0/7}$ to $29^{6/7}$ weeks) among 2470 gravide women with bacterial vaginosis or *Trichomonas vaginalis* infection enrolled in 2 multicenter randomized antibiotic treatment trials (metronidazole versus placebo).

Results.—The overall prevalence of genitourinary tract *C. trachomatis* infection at both visits was 10%. Preterm delivery less than 37 weeks' or less than 35 weeks' gestational age was not associated with the presence or absence of *C. trachomatis* infection at either the randomization (less than 37 weeks: 14% versus 13%, $P = .58$; less than 35 weeks: 6.4% versus 5.5%, $P = .55$) or the follow-up visit (less than 37 weeks: 13% versus 11%, $P = .33$; less than 35 weeks: 4.4% versus 3.7, $P = .62$). Treatment with an antibiotic effective against chlamydia infection was not associated with a statistically significant difference in preterm delivery.

Conclusion.—In this secondary analysis, midtrimester chlamydia infection was not associated with an increased risk of preterm birth. Treatment of chlamydia was not associated with a decreased frequency of preterm birth.

▶ This thought-provoking study casts doubt on the belief that infection with *C trachomatis*, the most common sexually transmitted bacterial disease in the United States, is associated with preterm birth. Contrary to a case-control study by many of the same authors,[1] *C trachomatis* infection did not appear to be associated with preterm delivery, regardless of whether it was treated. However, because of the ancillary nature of this study as a part of 2 randomized trials with different goals, the study's findings have several limitations.

The authors combined data from 2 large, concurrently performed placebo-controlled randomized trials of metronidazole treatment of bacterial vaginosis and *T vaginalis* infection during pregnancy. Once diagnosed with these infections, patients were randomly assigned to their respective trials. Prior to treatment and at a follow-up visit, voided urine samples were collected, archived, and analyzed after delivery for *C trachomatis* by ligase chain reaction for the current trial. Screening and treatment protocols for *C trachomatis* varied by center. Patients may have received antibiotics that were effective against *C trachomatis* for other indications. All patients in the study had coinfection with either *T vaginalis* or bacterial vaginosis. *C trachomatis* DNA may be detected in urine after treatment in a patient without clinical infection. No confirmatory culture data are presented nor are data on partner treatment or data on tests of cure. Finally, data on immunoglobulin M status, which may be associated with preterm delivery among women with *C trachomatis* infection, were not available.

The authors' case-control study, suggesting an association between *C trachomatis* and preterm delivery, is more compelling because of its cleaner study design. Regardless, any patient with *C trachomatis* infection merits treatment due to public health concerns.

D. J. Lyell, MD

Reference

1. Andrews WW, Goldenberg RL, Mercer B, et al. The Preterm Prediction Study: association of second-trimester genitourinary tract chlamydia infection with subsequent spontaneous preterm birth. *Am J Obstet Gynecol.* 2000;183:662-668.

Newborns of pre-eclamptic women: a biochemical difference present *in utero*

Ophir E, Dourleshter G, Hirsh Y, et al (Western Galilee Hosp, Nahariya, Israel; Technion Univ, Haifa, Israel)
Acta Obstet Gynecol Scand 85:1172-1178, 2006

2–9

Background.—Offspring exposed to pre-eclampsia *in utero* had higher systolic blood pressure, and were more obese during adolescence. We hypothesized that metabolic changes, a marker of cardiovascular disease, may be affected by intrauterine exposure to pre-eclampsia.

Methods.—Blood samples were collected from cord blood of 36 newborns who were exposed to pre-eclampsia *in utero* and their mothers, and of 35 newborns and their mothers with noncomplicated pregnancies. Serum levels of lipids, homocysteine, and fibrinogen were determined in all samples.

Results.—Fetuses exposed to pre-eclampsia *in utero* had lower birth weight, smaller abdominal circumference ($p < 0.002$; $p < 0.03$ respectively) and higher levels of low-density lipoprotein, homocysteine, and fibrinogen ($p < 0.01$; $p < 0.001$; $p < 0.001$, respectively), compared with fetuses of normotensive, pregnancies. A significant correlation existed between maternal homocysteine concentration and that of newborn infants ($r = 0.539$; $p < 0.001$) and between maternal low-density lipoprotein and newborn homocysteine ($r = 0.36$; $p < 0.03$). Significant negative correlations were found between abdominal circumference of newborns and cord blood concentration of fibrinogen ($r = -0.52$; $p < 0.001$) and low-density lipoprotein ($r = -0.42$; $p < 0.001$). Maternal plasma homocysteine, low-density lipoprotein, and triglyceride were significantly higher, while high-density lipoprotein was significantly lower in pregnancies with pre-eclampsia as compared with the uncomplicated pregnancy group ($p < 0.001$ for all). Cord blood level of low-density lipoprotein and fibrinogen were best predicted by abdominal circumference of newborn, though maternal level of homocysteine was the most powerful independent predictor of cord homocysteine.

Conclusion.—Intrauterine exposure to pre-eclampsia was associated with untoward effects on biochemical risk factor markers for cardiovascular disease. Our findings suggest that the cardiovascular risk of newborns of pre-eclamptic mothers may begin *in utero.*

▶ Here is more evidence that those at risk of adult cardiovascular disease may be doomed even before birth. Along with increased maternal levels of biochemical markers indicative of cardiovascular risk, babies born to preeclamptic mothers also had increased homocysteine, fibrinogen, and LDL in their cord blood. These findings are striking in that they were evident from the analysis of a relatively small sample size. Although the authors did not show the results of their regression analysis of abdominal size and biochemical markers on the control population, they state that the results were similar to those of the pre-eclamptic group. Assuming that this means that abdominal circumference was a strong predictor of fibrinogen and LDL levels in the control population, the implication is that even in women without overt disease, fetal nutrition may be a potential risk factor for adult cardiovascular disease.

It would be important to track how long these biochemical abnormalities persist. If they continued to persist throughout infancy, this would lend further credence to the notion that early programming may indeed be an important component of risk later in life.

H. C. Lee, MD

Female Survivors of Childhood Cancer: Preterm Birth and Low Birth Weight Among Their Children
Signorello LB, Cohen SS, Bosetti C, et al (Internatl Epidemiology Inst, Rockville, Md; Vanderbilt Univ, Nashville, Tenn; Instituto di Ricerche Farmacologiche Mario Negri, Milan, Italy; et al)
J Natl Cancer Inst 98:1453-1461, 2006   2–10

Background.—Improved survival after childhood cancer raises concerns over the possible long-term reproductive health effects of cancer therapies. We investigated whether children of female childhood cancer survivors are at elevated risk of being born preterm or exhibiting restricted fetal growth and evaluated the associations of different cancer treatments on these outcomes.

Methods.—Using data from the Childhood Cancer Survivor Study, a large multicenter cohort of childhood cancer survivors, we studied the singleton live births of female cohort members from 1968 to 2002. Included were 2201 children of 1264 survivors and 1175 children of a comparison group of 601 female siblings. Data from medical records were used to determine cumulative prepregnancy exposures to chemotherapy and radiotherapy. Logistic regression was used to estimate odds ratios (ORs) for the association between quantitative therapy exposures and preterm (<37 weeks) birth, low birth weight (<2.5 kg), and small-for-gestational-age (SGA) (lowest 10th percentile) births. All statistical tests were two-sided.

Results.—Survivors' children were more likely to be born preterm than the siblings' children (21.1% versus 12.6%; OR = 1.9, 95% confidence interval [CI] = 1.4 to 2.4; P<.001). Compared with the children of survivors who did not receive any radiotherapy, the children of survivors treated with high-dose radiotherapy to the uterus (>500 cGy) had increased risks of being born preterm (50.0% versus 19.6%; OR = 3.5, 95% CI = 1.5 to 8.0; P = .003), low birth weight (36.2% versus 7.6%; OR = 6.8, 95% CI = 2.1 to 22.2; P = .001), and SGA (18.2% versus 7.8%; OR = 4.0, 95% CI = 1.6 to 9.8; P = .003). Increased risks were also apparent at lower uterine radiotherapy doses (starting at 50 cGy for preterm birth and at 250 cGy for low birth weight).

Conclusions.—Late effects of treatment for female childhood cancer patients may include restricted fetal growth and early births among their offspring, with risks concentrated among women who receive pelvic irradiation.

▶ Preterm birth has many possible causes, of which most neonatologists are well aware. However, another cause may become important as more successes occur in the treatment of female childhood cancer, especially in those requiring pelvic irradiation. This study demonstrates that the lucky female survivors of childhood cancer may face later maternal risks of preterm birth and low birth weight infants. Not much can be done about this risk unless the approaches to certain childhood cancers are changed and, in particular, pelvic irradiation can be avoided. Now, neonatologists can be added to the list of subspecialists relevant to the management of childhood cancer. However, in the case of neonatology, it is not the childhood cancer survivor who benefits directly but, instead, her offspring.

D. K. Stevenson, MD

Sonographic estimate of birth weight among high-risk patients: Feasibility and factors influencing accuracy
Chauhan SP, Parker D, Shields D, et al (Aurora Health Care, West Allis, Wis; Spartanburg Regional Med Ctr, SC; Univ of Texas, Brownsville)
Am J Obstet Gynecol 195:601-606, 2006   2–11

Objective.—This study was undertaken to determine the feasibility of detecting abnormal fetal growth among patients undergoing biophysical profile (BPP) and to identify the factors those influence the accuracy.

Study Design.—Retrospectively singletons with reliable gestational age (GA) having a BPP were identified. Fetal growth restriction (FGR) and large-for-gestational age (LGA) were based on estimated or actual birth weight 10% or less or 90% or greater for GA, respectively. Likelihood ratio (LR), odds ratio (OR) and 95% CIs were calculated and multivariate predictive models used.

Results.—Among the 1934 consecutive patients that met the inclusion criteria, the LR of detecting FGR was 10.9 and of LGA, 17.4. Multivariate analysis indicates that accurate classification of fetal growth is significantly better with hydramnios (OR 1.78, 95% CI 2.68), if the GA is less than 32 weeks (OR 3.71, 95% CI 1.50-9.16) or GA is between 32.1 and 36.9 weeks (OR 1.43, 95% CI 1.05-1.96).

Conclusion.—It is feasible to accurately identify abnormal growth among high-risk patients and to delineate factors that influence the correct classification of fetal growth.

▶ As noted by these authors, it would be clinically useful to be able to accurately estimate fetal weight (FW). The purposes of this retrospective study were to evaluate the feasibility of accurately estimating FW and of detecting abnormal fetal growth among women undergoing serial biophysical profiles (BPP) and of identifying the factors that affect the accuracy of that estimate. The study population consisted of 1954 consecutive patients who met the study's inclusion criteria: singleton pregnancy; nonanomalous fetus; reliable gestational age (GA) based on clinical history, physical examination, and sonographic examination before 22 weeks; medical or obstetric complications requiring antepartum testing; and delivery at the investigators' hospital within 4 weeks of the last biometric measurements. Correctly classifying a fetus as being growth restricted, appropriate for GA, or large for GA relies on accurate knowledge of the duration of pregnancy and the ability to accurately obtain the measurements required by the regression equation used to calculate estimated FW. Because all study participants supposedly had "reliable GA based on clinical history, physical examination, and sonographic examination before 22 weeks," and because the serial growth measurements performed during the repeated BPP studies were obtained by a small group of trained registered diagnostic medical sonographers, the investigators were able to assess interval FW gain and correctly classify the intrauterine growth of the majority of the infants, meeting their objectives. Unfortunately, the question of generalizability still remains!

R. A. Ehrenkranz, MD

Subclinical Hyperthyroidism and Pregnancy Outcomes
Casey BM, Dashe JS, Wells CE, et al (Univ of Texas, Dallas)
Obstet Gynecol 107:337-341, 2006   2–12

Objective.—Subclinical hyperthyroidism has long-term sequelae that include osteoporosis, cardiovascular morbidity, and progression to overt thyrotoxicosis or thyroid failure. The objective of this study was to evaluate pregnancy outcomes in women with suppressed thyroid-stimulating hormone (TSH) and normal free thyroxine (fT_4) levels.

Methods.—All women who presented to Parkland Hospital for prenatal care between November 1, 2000, and April 14, 2003, underwent thyroid screening by chemiluminescent TSH assay. Women with TSH values at or below the 2.5th percentile for gestational age and whose serum fT_4 levels were 1.75 ng/dL or less were identified to have subclinical hyperthyroidism. Those women screened and delivered of a singleton infant weighing 500 g or more were analyzed. Pregnancy outcomes in women identified with subclinical hyperthyroidism were compared with those in women whose TSH values were between the 5th and 95th percentiles.

Results.—A total of 25,765 women underwent thyroid screening and were delivered of singleton infants. Of these, 433 (1.7%) were considered to have subclinical hyperthyroidism, which occurred more frequently in African-American and/or parous women. Pregnancies in women with subclinical hyperthyroidism were less likely to be complicated by hypertension (adjusted odds ratio 0.66, 95% confidence interval 0.44–0.98). All other pregnancy complications and perinatal morbidity or mortality were not increased in women with subclinical hyperthyroidism.

Conclusion.—Subclinical hyperthyroidism is not associated with adverse pregnancy outcomes. Our results indicate that identification of subclinical hyperthyroidism and treatment during pregnancy is unwarranted.

▶ These investigators performed thyroid screening tests on a large group of pregnant women to establish the prevalence and impact of subclinical hyperthyroidism on pregnancy outcomes. Because thyroid functions are not part of their routine prenatal laboratory tests, excess serum from blood tested for rubella antibody was assayed for TSH and fT_4. Rubella antibody testing is part of the same-day prenatal laboratory testing at Parkland Hospital; samples were obtained from 25,765 women. Subclinical hyperthyroidism was determined by a TSH value less than 2.5th percentile for gestational age with serum fT_4 levels less than 1.75 ng/dL. Pregnancy and neonatal outcomes of the 433 women (1.7%) identified with subclinical hyperthyroidism were compared with the outcomes of the 23,124 normal control women; outcomes of the 93 women identified with overt hyperthyroidism were excluded from the analyses. Because subclinical hyperthyroidism was not associated with any adverse pregnancy or neonatal outcomes, the investigators rightly concluded that universal TSH screening during pregnancy is unwarranted.

R. A. Ehrenkranz, MD

Intrahepatic Cholestasis of Pregnancy and Neonatal Respiratory Distress Syndrome
Zecca E, De Luca D, Marras M, et al (Catholic Univ of the Sacred Heart, Rome)
Pediatrics 117:1669-1672, 2006   2–13

Objectives.—We sought to verify the association between maternal intrahepatic cholestasis of pregnancy (ICP) and neonatal respiratory distress syndrome (RDS) and to determine how bile acids levels alter the risk of developing neonatal RDS.

Methods.—We extracted data from our divisional database about all of the newborns born during the years 2000–2004. We compared 77 neonates born from pregnancies complicated by ICP with 427 neonates in the same range of gestational age born from noncomplicated pregnancies. We studied maternal bile acids levels immediately before delivery in mothers with ICP and measured bile acid levels during the first 24 hours of life in their newborns.

Results.—The incidence of RDS in newborns from cholestatic pregnancies was twice that the reference population (28.6% vs 14%). The multivariate analysis showed that the risk of RDS in these newborns was ~2.5 times higher than in control infants. Within the ICP group, maternal and neonatal bile acid levels of infants affected by RDS were not significantly higher than those of healthy infants. The multivariate analysis showed that a low gestational age was the most important risk factor, but the probability of respiratory distress syndrome also increased by $2\%_{o}$ for every additional micromole of the interaction term "neonatal by maternal bile acids level."

Conclusions.—Maternal ICP is significantly associated with the occurrence of RDS in the newborn. We hypothesize that bile acids can produce surfactant depletion in the alveoli reverting the reaction of phospholipase A2. This hypothesis could potentially be confirmed by bronchoalveolar lavage study.

▶ ICP is defined as pruritus and elevated bile acid serum concentrations in late pregnancy. Other causes of cholestasis, such as oligosymptomatic choledocolithiasis, viral hepatitis, and other underlying liver disorders, such as primary biliary cirrhosis, should be ruled out. This disorder was mysterious for many years, but recent reports have described splicing mutations in the multidrug resistance p glycoprotein 3 (MDR3, ABCB4) gene in up to 20% of ICP women. In addition, mutations in the aminophospholipid transporter ATP8B1 and the bile salt export pump (BSEP, ABCB11) have been found in patients diagnosed with ICP.[1,2] Schneider et al reported that splicing mutations in the MDR3 gene can cause ICP with normal gamma GT and may be associated with stillbirths and gallstone disease.[1] Treatment with ursodeoxycholic acid (UDCA) is partially effective in ameliorating the cholestasis and improving liver function.

Zecca et al describe the association between ICP and respiratory distress presumably caused by surfactant dysfunction. This series of 77 patients with ICP follows the 3 patients that they initially reported in 2004,[3] wherein they titled the report "Bile Acid Pneumonia: A "New" Form of Neonatal Respiratory Distress Syndrome?" Adult RDS is an integral part of liver failure and we now are aware of the link between ICP and RDS in neonates.

A. A. Fanaroff, MD

References

1. Schneider G, Paus TC, Kullak-Ublick GA, et al. Linkage between a new splicing site mutation in the MDR3 alias ABCB4 gene and intrahepatic cholestasis of pregnancy. *Hepatology.* 2007;45:150-158.
2. Arrese M. Cholestasis during pregnancy: rare hepatic diseases unmasked by pregnancy. *Ann Hepatol.* 2006;5:216-218.
3. Zecca E, Costa S, Lauriola V, Vento G, Papacci P, Romagnoli C. Bile acid pneumonia: a "new" form of neonatal respiratory distress syndrome? *Pediatrics.* 2004;114:269-272.

Pregnancy, delivery, and neonatal complications after treatment with antiepileptic drugs

Pilo C, Wide K, Winbladh B (Karolinska Institutet Stockholm; Karolinska Univ, Huddinge, Sweden)
Acta Obstet Gynecol Scand 85:643-646, 2006   2–14

Aim.—To study the risk for complications during pregnancy, delivery, and neonatal period after the use of antiepileptic drugs (AEDs) during pregnancy.

Methods.—Women treated with AEDs during pregnancy and with singleton deliveries were identified from the Swedish Medical Birth Registry during the period July 1, 1995 to and including 2001 (*n* = 1350). Risk estimates were made using the Mantel-Haenszel procedure and comparisons with all singleton births in Sweden during this period (*n* = 559,491). Stratification was made for year of birth, maternal age, parity, and smoking habits.

Results.—Most of the women (*n* = 1207, 89%) used AEDs in monotherapy. Carbamazepine was the most commonly used drug (*n* = 683), followed by valproic acid (*n* = 255). The rate of caesarean sections was significantly increased (OR = 1.64, 95% CI 1.43–1.89), but it was not possible to differentiate between elective and emergency sections. The risk for preeclampsia (OR = 1.66, 95% CI 1.32–2.08) and for hemorrhage after vaginal delivery was increased (OR = 1.29, 95% CI 1.02–1.63). The neonates showed an increased risk for respiratory distress (OR = 2.06, 95% CI 1.62–2.63).

Conclusion.—The study demonstrates a slightly increased risk only for preeclampsia, vaginal hemorrhage after delivery, and respiratory distress in the newborn after the use of AEDs during pregnancy.

In utero antiepileptic drug exposure: Fetal death and malformations

Meador KJ, for the NEAD Study Group (Univ of Florida, Gainesville; et al)
Neurology 67:407-412, 2006   2–15

Background.—Pregnancy outcomes following in utero exposure to antiepileptic drugs (AEDs) are uncertain, limiting an evidenced-based approach.

Objective.—To determine if fetal outcomes vary as a function of different in utero AED exposures.

Methods.—This ongoing prospective observational study across 25 epilepsy centers in the USA and UK enrolled pregnant women with epilepsy from October 1999 to February 2004 to determine if differential long-term cognitive and behavioral neurodevelopmental effects exist across the four most commonly used AEDs. This initial report focuses on the incidence of serious adverse outcomes including major congenital malformations (which could be attributable to AEDs) or fetal death. A total of 333 mother/child pairs were analyzed for monotherapy exposures: carbamazepine (n = 110), lamotrigine (n = 98), phenytoin (n = 56), and valproate (n = 69).

Results.—Response frequencies of pregnancies resulting in serious adverse outcomes for each AED were as follows: carbamazepine 8.2%, lamotrigine 1.0%, phenytoin 10.7%, and valproate 20.3%. Distribution of serious adverse outcomes differed significantly across AEDs and was not explained by factors other than in utero AED exposure. Valproate exhibited a dose-dependent effect.

Conclusions.—More adverse outcomes were observed in pregnancies with in utero valproate exposure vs the other antiepileptic drugs (AEDs). These results combined with several recent studies provide strong evidence that valproate poses the highest risk to the fetus. For women who fail other AEDs and require valproate, the dose should be limited if possible.

▶ Population-based studies provide the best estimates of event frequencies. Therefore, this "population-based register study of pregnancy and delivery complications and neonatal diagnoses after maternal use of antiepileptic drugs (AEDs) in early pregnancy" is interesting. For the Pilo et al report (Abstract 2–14), the use of AEDs in early pregnancy was taken as a proxy for AED use at delivery, because, in the authors' experience, it was associated with AED use throughout the pregnancy. Carbamazepine and valporic acid were the most commonly used AEDs recorded in the Swedish Medical Birth Registry between 1995 and 2001; of the 1207 women reporting AED monotherapy, 938 (78%) used 1 of those 2 medications. Although the rate of cesarean section delivery was significantly higher in women receiving AED therapy, the registry did not differentiate between elective or emergency cesarean section deliveries. The risks of preeclampsia and of vaginal hemorrhage after delivery were also significantly increased in women receiving AEDs. In neonates, maternal AED treatment was associated with a significantly increased risk of respiratory distress and a significantly decreased risk of hyperbilirubinemia. Unfortunately, the investigators did not comment about any association between maternal AED therapy and the rate of congenital malformations and definitions of "respiratory distress" and "icterus" were not provided. While this report met its objective of providing data about pregnancy and delivery complications, it falls short with respect to neonatal outcomes.

However, the report by Meador et al (Abstract 2–15) does describe the AED-associated risks of major congenital malformations or fetal death. This report is part of Neurodevelopmental Effects of Antiepileptic Drugs (NEAD) Study, an ongoing prospective observational investigation that enrolls "mother/child pairs during pregnancy across 25 centers in the USA and UK. The primary aim of the study is to determine the long-term effects of AED monotherapy on the children's neurodevelopmental outcomes." The data displayed in Tables 2 and 4 of the original article support the authors' conclusion that valproate "not be used as the AED of first choice for women of child-bearing potential, and, when used, its dose should be limited, if possible."

R. A. Ehrenkranz, MD

Pregnancy outcome in women who use opiates
Fajemirokun-Odudeyi O, Sinha C, Tutty S, et al (Women & Children's Hosp, Hull, England; SSMS, Hull, England)
Eur J Obstet Gynecol Reprod Biol 126:170-175, 2006   2–16

Background.—Opiate use in pregnancy is on the increase. There are a number of complications associated with this problem but current data from UK centres are sparse.

Design.—A retrospective study.

Setting.—A North of England Hospital.

Methods.—Maternal and neonatal case records were studied and a standard data set completed.

Main Outcome Measures.—Maternal and neonatal outcomes were classified by the woman's drug usage at the end of pregnancy.

Results.—One hundred and ten babies born to 108 women were studied and 41% had evidence of previous exposure to the hepatitis C virus. Women who took heroin in later pregnancy were significantly more likely than women who were stabilised on methadone to have a baby who needed morphine (40% versus 19%), had higher mean maximum neonatal abstinence scores (NAS) (5.8 versus 4.7) and stayed in the neonatal unit significantly longer (mean 17.2 days versus 11.8 days). There were two neonatal deaths and the overall rate of prematurity was 29%.

Conclusions.—The outcome for pregnancy in women who use opiates is complicated by high rates of prematurity and neonatal death. Women who used heroin in later pregnancy had babies who developed more severe NAS and needed a longer hospital stay than women who used only methadone.

▶ Illicit drug use during pregnancy is common and probably underestimated in the majority of published studies. Women who use cocaine or opiates during pregnancy are at increased risk of a number of high-risk conditions and behaviors. Data collected at 4 clinical centers in the United States indicate that, compared with women who were not exposed to these substances during pregnancy, those who used them were more likely to be infected with syphilis, gonorrhea, hepatitis, or HIV; to have psychiatric or emotional disorders, and to have experienced pregnancy-related bleeding. These women also were significantly more likely than others to have used tobacco, alcohol, or marijuana while pregnant.[1] At least half of the women who are dependent on opiates suffer anemia, heart disease, diabetes, pneumonia, or hepatitis during pregnancy and childbirth. These women also experience more: spontaneous abortions, breech deliveries, cesarean sections, premature births, still births, and neonatal deaths. The infant exposed to opiates or other drugs of dependency during intrauterine development is at risk for postnatal withdrawal as well as to long-term problems that are associated with drug effects combined with adverse social circumstances.[2]

It has become fashionable to test meconium to document fetal drug exposure. Montgomery et al[3] reveal that the cord is just as effective in assessing fetal drug exposure to amphetamines, opiates, cocaine, and cannabinoids. Also, the cord is immediately available permitting a more rapid turn around than meconium, especially, when there is some delay in the passage of meconium.

A. A. Fanaroff, MD

References

1. Bauer CR, Shankaran S, Bada HS, et al. The Maternal Lifestyle Study: drug exposure during pregnancy and short-term maternal outcomes. *Am J Obstet Gynecol.* 2002;186:487-495.
2. Oei J, Lui K. Management of the newborn infant affected by maternal opiates and other drugs of dependency. *J Paediatr Child Health.* 2007;43:9-18.
3. Montgomery D, Plate C, Alder SC, Jones M, Jones J, Christensen RD. Testing for fetal exposure to illicit drugs using umbilical cord tissue vs meconium. *J Perinatol.* 2006;26:11-14.

Seroepidemiological profile of pregnant women after inadvertent rubella vaccination in the state of Rio de Janeiro, Brazil, 2001–2002
da Silva e Sá GR, Gamacho LAB, Siqueria MM, et al (Centro de Vigiîncia Epidemioloógica, Rio de Janeiro, Brazil; Fundação Oswaldo Cruz, Rio de Janeiro, Brazil)
Rev Panam Salud Publica 19:371-377, 2006   2–17

Objectives.—To analyze postvaccination serological status in pregnant women inadvertently vaccinated against rubella in the state of Rio de Janeiro, Brazil.

Methods.—This was a cross-sectional study of pregnant women 15 to 29 years old, vaccinated against rubella and measles from November 2001 to March 2002, who were unaware of their pregnancy at the time of vaccination or who became pregnant within 30 days thereafter. They were tested for rubella-specific immunoglobulin M (IgM) and G (IgG) and classified as immune (IgM-negative, IgG-positive, tested within 30 days after vaccination), susceptible (IgM-positive after vaccination) or indeterminate (IgM-negative, IgG-positive, vaccination–serological testing interval greater than 30 days).

Results.—Of 2 292 women, 288 (12.6%) were susceptible, 316 (13.8%) immune, 1 576 (68.8%) indeterminate, 8 (0.3%) ineligible, and 104 (4.5%) lost to follow-up. IgM seropositivity by vaccination–serological testing interval was 16.1% (≤ 30 days), 15.4% (30–60 days), and 14.2% (61–90 days). Considering the campaign's target age, the 20-to-24-year age group had the largest proportion of individuals susceptible to rubella (14.8%) and represented 42.4% (122/288) of all susceptible women. In 75% of susceptible pregnant women, gestational age was 5 weeks or less at the time of vaccination.

Conclusions.—Mass immunization of childbearing-age women was justified on the basis of epidemiological and serological data. Follow-up of vaccinated pregnant women revealed no cases of congenital rubella syndrome due to rubella vaccination. However, the observed rate of congenital infection supports the recommendation to avoid vaccinating pregnant women, and to avoid conception for up to 1 month following rubella vaccination.

▶ It has been well described that pregnant women infected with the rubella virus are at risk of developing congenital rubella syndrome (CRS) in their fetuses, especially during the first trimester. CRS is a devastating disease characterized by congenital heart disease, cataracts, and deafness.[1] A live-attenuated rubella virus vaccine has been available for use since 1969, either alone or in combination with measles (MR) or with both measles and mumps (MMR). Approximately 99% of persons who are susceptible to rubella develop measurable antibody after vaccination; 1 dose of vaccine is approximately 90% efficacious in preventing rubella disease.[2] It is recommended that rubella vaccine be offered to all rubella susceptible women of childbearing age to prevent CRS.[3]

In the United States the vaccination program has been exceptionably successful. In 2005, the Centers for Disease Control (CDC) convened an expert panel that concluded that rubella is no longer endemic in the United States.[4] Nonetheless, the disease has not been completely eradicated. The continuing occurrence of rubella among women of childbearing age indicates the need for continuing vaccination of susceptible adolescent and adult women of childbearing age. As with other live vaccines, vaccination of pregnant women with rubella vaccine is contraindicated—a precaution based mostly on the theoretical risk of fetal infection. However, data from the United States indicate that immunization during pregnancy does not seem to lead to adverse outcomes— CDC collected data on 275 rubella-susceptible women in the United States who inadvertently received rubella vaccine while pregnant and found that 83% delivered living infants, all 229 of whom were free of defects associated with CRS.[5]

This cross-sectional study conducted by da Silva et al evaluated the postvaccination serologic status of women in Brazil who, inadvertently, received the rubella vaccine while pregnant. The authors evaluated women age 15 to 19 years and performed rubella-specific immunoglobulin at certain intervals to document the serologic status of these women. Although limited by the fact that they did not have access to serologic status of the women before immunization, that the study was not truly population based, and that follow-up was not ensured, the study provides interesting data on susceptibility to rubella in young women in Brazil. The authors were able to show that the highest proportion of susceptible women were those age 20 to 24 years, a group that had not been the target in the area and, similar to the experience in the United States, concluded that their mass vaccination program posed no risk to the mothers or their infants. This study also provided an interesting look into Brazil's vaccine strategy to control the persisting circulation of the virus among childbearing-aged women and CRS. Mass immunization campaigns, although challenging, can be beneficial to populations and to individuals.

M. Vázquez, MD

References

1. Gregg NM. Congenital cataract following German measles in the mother. *Trans Ophthalmol Soc Aust.* 1941;3:35-46.
2. Orenstein WA, Bart KJ, Hinman AR, et al. The opportunity and obligation to eliminate rubella from the United States. *JAMA.* 1984;251:1988-1994.
3. Centers for Disease Control. Rubella vaccine: recommendation of the Immunization Practices Advisory Committee (ACIP). *MMWR.* 1978;27:451-459.
4. Centers for Disease Control. Achievements in public health: elimination of rubella and congenital rubella syndrome—United States, 1969-2004. *MMWR.* 2005;54:279-282.
5. Centers for Disease Control. Rubella and congenital rubella syndrome—US, 1994-1997. *MMWR.* 1997;46:350-354.

Neonatal Effects of Maternal Hypothyroxinemia During Early Pregnancy

Kooistra L, Crawford S, van Baar AL, et al (Univ of Calgary, Alta, Canada; Alberta Children's Hosp, Calgary, Canada; Univ of Tilburg, The Netherlands)

Pediatrics 117:161-167, 2006   2–18

Objective.—We sought to examine the neurobehavioral profile of neonates who are born to women with hypothyroxinemia during early pregnancy.

Methods.—Examined were 108 neonates who were born to mothers with low maternal free thyroid hormone (fT4 concentrations; <10th percentile) at 12 weeks' gestation (case patients) and 96 neonates who were born to women whose fT4 values were between the 50th and 90th percentiles, matched for parity and gravidity (control subjects). Newborn development was assessed at 3 weeks of age using the Neonatal Behavioral Assessment Scale. Maternal thyroid function (fT4 and thyrotropin hormone) was assessed at 12, 24, and 32 weeks' gestation.

Results.—Infants of women with hypothyroxinemia at 12 weeks' gestation had significantly lower scores on the Neonatal Behavioral Assessment Scale orientation index compared with subjects. Regression analysis showed that first-trimester maternal fT4 but not maternal TSH or fT4 later in gestation was a significant predictor of orientation scores.

Conclusions.—This study confirms that maternal hypothyroxinemia constitutes a serious risk factor for neurodevelopmental difficulties that can be identified in neonates as young as 3 weeks of age.

▶ Hypothyroxinemia, common in pregnancy, is a state in which maternal fT4 is decreased along with normal thyrotropin hormone concentrations. This has been implicated as a potential risk for developmental delay in the newborn if found during early pregnancy. The authors found that early hypothyroxinemia was associated with differences in a behavioral scale at 3 weeks of age. The Neonatal Behavioral Assessment Scale, which was used in this study, is lacking in normative data, and the implications for long-term outcomes are unknown. Furthermore, there was a significant difference found in only 1 of 7 indexes. Nevertheless, the finding that some effect was seen on behavior so soon after birth would help to minimize effects of the postnatal environment and add to the literature regarding this issue. More studies will need to be performed to assess the value of testing for this condition, looking at long-term outcomes and the potential utility of treatment. It is also notable that this study was performed in The Netherlands, with a 100% white, homogenous population. As such, it is yet too early to call for universal screening of maternal fT4.

H. C. Lee, MD

Moderate to severe thrombocytopenia during pregnancy
Parnas M, Sheiner E, Shoham-Vardi I, et al (Ben Gurion Univ of the Negev, Be'er-Sheva, Israel)
Eur J Obstet Gynecol Reprod Biol 128:163-168, 2006   2–19

Objective.—The objective was to investigate obstetric risk factors, complications, and outcomes of pregnancies complicated by moderate to severe thrombocytopenia.

Materials and Methods.—A retrospective case-control study comparing 199 pregnant women with moderate to severe thrombocytopenia (platelet count below $100 \times 10^9/l$) with 201 pregnant women without thrombocytopenia, who delivered between January 2003 to April 2004. Stratified analysis, using the Mantel–Haenszel procedure was performed in order to control for confounders.

Results.—The main causes of thrombocytopenia were gestational thrombocytopenia (GT) (59.3%), immune thrombocytopenic purpura (ITP) (11.05%), preeclampsia (10.05%), and HELLP (Hemolysis, elevated liver enzymes and low platelet count) syndrome (12.06%). Women with thrombocytopenia were significantly older (30.7 ± 5.9 versus 28.7 ± 5.7; $p = 0.001$) compared with patients without thrombocytopenia, and had higher rates of labor induction (OR = 4.0, 95% CI = 2.2–7.6, $p < 0.001$) and preterm deliveries (OR = 3.5, 95% CI = 1.9–6.5, $p < 0.001$). Even after controlling for labor induction, using the Mantel–Haenszel technique, thrombocytopenia was significantly associated with preterm delivery (weighted OR = 3.14, 95% CI = 1.7–6.0, $p < 0.001$). Higher rates of placental abruption were found in pregnant women with thrombocytopenia (OR = 6.2, 95% CI = 1.7–33.2, $p = 0.001$). In a comparison of perinatal outcomes, higher rates of Apgar scores <7 at 5 min were noted in infants of mothers with thrombocytopenia (OR = 6.3, 95% CI = 1.8–33.8, $p = 0.001$), intrauterine growth restriction (IUGR; OR = 4.6, 95% CI = 1.5–19.1, $p = 0.003$), and stillbirth (65/1000 versus 0 $p < 0.001$). These adverse perinatal outcomes were found in rare causes of thrombocytopenia such as disseminated intravascular coagulation (DIC), familial thrombotic thrombocytopenic purpura (TTP), anti-phospholipid antibodies (APLA) syndrome, and myeloproliferative disease, and not among patients with GT.

Conclusions.—Moderate to severe maternal thrombocytopenia points to a higher degree of severity of the primary disease, which increases perinatal complications. However, the adverse outcome is specifically attributed to preeclampsia, HELLP syndrome, and rare causes, while the perinatal outcome of GT and ITP is basically favorable. Special attention should be given to patients with thrombocytopenia due to preeclampsia, HELLP syndrome, and rarer causes during pregnancy.

▶ This study investigates obstetric risk factors and outcomes of pregnancies complicated by moderate (<100 × 10⁹ platelets/L) or severe (<50 × 10⁹ platelets/L) thrombocytopenia compared with those in healthy women with normal pregnancies. They also compare the outcomes of different causes of maternal thrombocytopenia.

Thrombocytopenia, defined as a platelet count of less than 150×10^9/L, occurs in 10% to 12% of all pregnant women. GT accounts for 75% of these cases and is a benign condition. Most cases of GT are mild: platelet counts range between 110 and 150×10^9/L.

Of 17,499 deliveries that occurred during the 15-month study period, 199 pregnant women (1.14%) were found to have moderate to severe thrombocytopenia. The control group consisted of consecutive patients without low platelet counts or hypertensive disorders.

Even in the moderate to severe category, GT figured prominently (58.2%), and these obstetric and perinatal outcomes were uniformly good. Likewise, the mothers with ITP (11%) fared well. IUGR was more common in preeclampsia/ HELLP syndrome compared with other causes. Placental abruption, still births, and low Apgar scores (<7 at 1 and 5 minutes) were more common among the 15 patients carrying the diagnoses of DIC, familial TTP, APLA syndrome, and myeloproliferative disease.

Interestingly, only 7 infants born to those mothers with low platelet counts had thrombocytopenia, and no bleeding complications occurred in these babies. Of course, many cases of severe neonatal thrombocytopenia are unrelated to maternal platelet counts, for example, in alloimmune thrombocytopenia, neonatal sepsis syndrome, or congenital TORCH (toxoplasmosis, other [*Treponema pallidum*, varicella-zoster virus, parvovirus B19], rubella virus, cytomegalovirus, and herpes simplex virus) infections. While this was not the focus of this study, I could not help but wonder how many thrombocytopenic infants were born to mothers with normal platelet counts among the 17,499 births reviewed for this study.

The authors conclude that thrombocytopenia in this study cohort served as a severity marker for the mothers' underlying disease rather than a direct cause of perinatal morbidity in affected mothers and their babies. The more severe the underlying disease is in the mother, the higher the rate of maternal and perinatal complications.

E. K. Stork, MD

3 Genetics and Teratology

Survival and major neonatal complications in infants born between 22 0/7 and 24 6/7 weeks of gestation (1999-2003)
Herber-Jonat S, Schulze A, Kribs A, et al (Univ of Munich; Univ of Cologne, Germany; Univ of Ulm, Germany)
Am J Obstet Gynecol 195:16-22, 2006   3–1

Objective.—This study was undertaken to compare survival and morbidity until discharge in infants born after 22-23 versus 24 weeks' gestational age (GA).

Study Design.—Cohort study of all infants 25 weeks or less, born in 3 tertiary perinatal centers (1999-2003).

Results.—Of a total of 336 infants, 133 (40%) died before or immediately after birth without the provision of life support, 203 (60%) received active neonatal treatment. Infants with life support (n = 82 at 22 to 23 weeks, n = 121 at 24 weeks) differed with respect to antenatal steroid prophylaxis

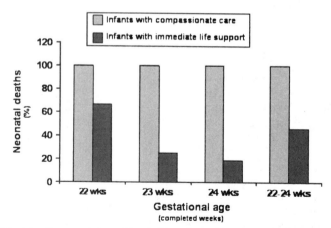

FIGURE.—Mortality among infants with and without the provision of immediate life support after birth. Total number of infants at each GA interval and the subset of infants with immediate life support, respectively: 22 weeks, n = 83/15; 23 weeks, n = 115/67; 24 weeks, n = 138/121. (Courtesy of Herber-Jonat S, Schulze A, Kribs A, et al. Survival and major neonatal complications in infants born between 22 0/7 and 24 0/7 weeks of gestation (1999-2003). *Am J Obstet Gynecol.* 195:16-22. Copyright 2006 by Elsevier.)

TABLE 4.—Results of Logistic Regression Analyses (Univariate and Multivariate) of Factors Associated with Survival to Discharge

	Univariate		Multivariate	
	OR (95% CI)	P	OR (95% CI)	P
Antenatal steroids	4.22 (1.97-9.05)	<.0001	4.1 (1.63-10.3)	.003
Complete course	2.95 (1.51-5.80)	.002		
Incomplete course	0.89 (0.44-1.84)	.76		
GA 24 wk	2.37 (1.44-3.89)	.001	4.44 (1.24-15.54)	.02
Multiple gestation	0.43 (0.22-0.86)	.017		
Chorioamnionitis	1.52 (0.79-2.90)	.21		
PROM	1.25 (0.65-2.41)	.5		
Cesarean section	1.11 (0.58-2.17)	.74		
Female gender	1.0 (0.52-1.91)	>.99		

OR, Odds ratio.
Courtesy of Herber-Jonat S, Schulze A, Kribs A, et al. Survival and major neonatal complications in infants born between 22 0/7 and 24 0/7 weeks of gestation (1999-2003). Am J Obstet Gynecol. 195:16-22. Copyright 2006 by Elsevier.

(44% vs 62%) and cesarean section rate (51% vs 71%). Survival was 67% compared with 82% (*P* = .016). The incidence of intraventricular hemorrhage III or greater or periventricular leukomalacia (15/15%), severe retinopathy of prematurity (18/15%), and chronic lung disease (40/47%) was similar in both GA groups.

Conclusions.—The provision of life support for extremely preterm infants increases their chance of survival without more neonatal morbidity (Figure and Table 4).

▶ The results of this study of infants born at the limits of viability in Germany during the years 1999 to 2003 indicate the degree to which survival can be attained with aggressive delivery room life support. The authors note that current management recommendations in Germany mandate a proactive management for all imminent deliveries from 24 weeks' gestation onward, including life support immediately after delivery. According to the guidelines, intensive treatment is optional at 22 to 23 weeks if parents request life support "after obstetric and neonatal counseling." Although "life support" is not defined in the article, one presumes that this includes endotracheal intubation and assisted ventilation.

According to these guidelines, for proactive management after birth, 67% of 22- to 23-week gestation infants and 82% of 24-week gestation infants survived to discharge. It is of interest that the high rates of neonatal complications did not differ between surviving infants born at 23 weeks and those born at 24 weeks' gestation; at 22-23 versus 24 weeks' gestation, 40% and 47%, respectively had chronic lung disease; 18% and 15% required laser therapy for severe retinopathy of prematurity; 15% in each group had grade III or more intraventricular bleeding or periventricular leukomalacia (PVL); and 30% and 12%, respectively, had necrotizing enterocolitis. Infants of 23 weeks 6 days are very similar to those of 24 weeks 1 day because reliability of measuring gestational age is within a few days. The lack of difference in neonatal morbidity at 23 and 24 weeks' gestation is thus not surprising.

Nonsurviving infants (ie, those who died before discharge) were more likely to have severe intraventricular bleeding or periventricular leukomalacia. It is not clear to what extent life support therapy in such infants was withdrawn, or whether the infants died "naturally" while receiving assisted ventilation. With the very high survival rates described for these very immature infants, I doubt whether treatment was withdrawn in many instances.

The authors note that their results suggest revisiting existing guidelines. However, any revision of the guidelines would be unwise without longer term follow-up of postdischarge mortality rates and early childhood morbidity and neurodevelopmental outcomes.

M. Hack, MD

Smoking Habits, Nicotine Use, and Congenital Malformations
Morales-Suárez-Varela MM, Bille C, Christensen K, et al (Univ of Valencia, Spain; Dr Peset Univ, Valencia, Spain; Univ of Southern Denmark, Odense; et al)
Obstet Gynecol 107:51-57, 2006   3–2

Objective.—We examined whether maternal smoking and use of nicotine substitutes during the first 12 weeks of pregnancy increased the prevalence of congenital malformations in general and of certain congenital malformations in particular.

Methods.—In the Danish National Birth Cohort (1997–2003) we identified 76,768 pregnancies (and their subsequent singleton births); 20,603 were exposed to tobacco smoking during the first 12 weeks of pregnancy. Birth outcomes were collected by linkage to the Central Population Register, the National Patients Register, and the National Birth Register. We identified congenital malformations from the Hospital Medical Birth Registry as they were recorded at birth or in the first year of follow-up.

Results.—Smoking mothers were younger, weighed less, consumed more alcohol, and had received less education. Children exposed to prenatal tobacco smoking had no increase in congenital malformations prevalence compared with the nonexposed children in both crude and adjusted analyses. Children born to nonsmokers, but who used nicotine substitutes, had a slightly increased relative congenital malformations prevalence ratio; relative prevalence rate ratio was 1.61 (95% confidence interval 1.01–2.58), which represents a 60% increased risk. When the analysis was restricted to musculoskeletal malformations, the relative prevalence rate ratio was 2.63 (95% confidence interval 1.53–4.52).

Conclusion.—Our results showed no increase in congenital malformations related to prenatal tobacco smoking. However, we identified an increase of malformations risk in nonsmokers using nicotine substitutes. This finding needs to be replicated in other data sources.

▶ This study reports 2 interesting findings: (1) smoking at any level during the first trimester was not associated with congenital malformations, and (2) the use of nicotine substitutes was associated with congenital malformations, particularly musculoskeletal malformations. The results suggest that the use of nicotine substitutes poses a risk to the developing fetus. I wish to make 2 comments about this study.

1. The study was remarkable for the large cohort studied, that of the Danish National Birth Cohort. In this cohort, 78,500 pregnant women were enrolled. However, the cohort lacked collection of biomarkers by which exposure could be confirmed. In our previous study,[1] cord blood cotinine levels used as biomarkers for maternal smoking were occasionally elevated in women who denied smoking. A biomarker for the exposure in this cohort would be extremely useful. Additionally, a biomarker would indicate whether women who reported no smoking were exposed to significant levels of environmental tobacco smoke. It may be that no difference in congenital malformations was found because the nonexposed group was misclassified. The National Children's Study, now being implemented in the United States, plans to enroll 100,000 infants preconceptually and collect numerous biological samples for biomarker measurements. The National Children's Study will be able to refute or confirm the findings reported in this article.

2. It is extremely interesting and provocative that the authors found an association between nicotine substitutes and congenital malformations. One would expect that replacing a single exposure (nicotine) from a multitude of exposures, including nicotine, would lessen the risk. However, the authors have ignored that nicotine substitutes also come with other exposures, that is, the chemicals used to render the nicotine absorbable in patches, gum, and other substitutes. These chemicals are called vehicles or inert ingredients but may exert biological effects. Hence, the nicotine substitutes may constitute an exposure other than nicotine and should be further investigated.

C. F. Bearer, MD, PhD

Reference

1. Bearer C, Emerson RK, O'Riordan MA, Roitman E, Shackleton C. Maternal tobacco smoke exposure and persistent pulmonary hypertension of the newborn. *Environ Health Perspect.* 1997;105:202-206.

Malformation risks of antiepileptic drugs in pregnancy: a prospective study from the UK Epilepsy and Pregnancy Register

Morrow J, Russell A, Guthrie E, et al (Royal Group of Hosps, Belfast, Ireland; Southern Gen Hosp, Glasgow, Scotland; Glasgow, Scotland; et al)
J Neurol Neurosurg Psychiatry 77:193-198, 2006   3–3

Objective.—To assess the relative risk of major congenital malformation (MCM) from in utero exposure to antiepileptic drug (AEDs).

Methods.—Prospective data collected by the UK Epilepsy and Pregnancy Register were analysed. The presence of MCMs recorded within the first three months of life was the main outcome measure.

Results.—Full outcome data were collected on 3607 cases. The overall MCM rate for all AED exposed cases was 4.2% (95% confidence interval (CI), 3.6% to 5.0%). The MCM rate was higher for polytherapy (6.0%) (n = 770) than for monotherapy (3.7%) (n = 2598) (crude odds ratio (OR) = 1.63 (p = 0.010), adjusted OR = 1.83 (p = 0.002)). The MCM rate for women with epilepsy who had not taken AEDs during pregnancy (n = 239) was 3.5% (1.8% to 6.8%). The MCM rate was greater for pregnancies exposed only to valproate (6.2% (95% CI, 4.6% to 8.2%) than only to carbamazepine (2.2% (1.4% to 3.4%) (OR = 2.78 (p<0.001); adjusted OR = 2.97 (p<0.001)). There were fewer MCMs for pregnancies exposed only to lamotrigine than only to valproate. A positive dose response for MCMs was found for lamotrigine (p = 0.006). Polytherapy combinations containing valproate carried a higher risk of MCM than combinations not containing valproate (OR = 2.49 (1.31 to 4.70)).

Conclusions.—Only 4.2% of live births to women with epilepsy had an MCM. The MCM rate for polytherapy exposure was greater than for monotherapy exposure. Polytherapy regimens containing valproate had significantly more MCMs than those not containing valproate. For monotherapy exposures, carbamazepine was associated with the lowest risk of MCM (Table 3).

▶ This article describes a study using a large database on the MCMs associated with the use of AEDs. The overall data are relatively reassuring: 96% of infants born to women with epilepsy did not have a major malformation. Which antiepileptics are used and whether they are used in combination appear to be a reason for concern. In addition, what is notable about this article is what is not mentioned. Here is a teratogenic exposure for which timing and dose are readily available and for which some idea of the mechanism of toxicity exists (ie, effects on folate metabolism), yet our knowledge seems rudimentary at best. Nonetheless, no data are presented on folate levels in these women nor are the frequencies of the known genetic polymorphisms in folate metabolism given. Clearly, a preconceptual prospective longitudinal study of children exposed to antiepileptics in utero is needed to further understand the risks of an MCM. Maternal and fetal polymorphisms in folate and other pathways could be studied, and maternal folate, B6, and B12 levels could be followed during the early stages of pregnancy. Only in such a study could the multitude of risk

TABLE 3.—Types of Major Congenital Malformation by Antiepileptic Drug

Drug	Cases (n)	NTD	Facial Cleft	Cardiac	Hypospadias/GUT	GIT	Skeletal	Other
Carbamazepine	900	2 (0.2%)	4 (0.4%)	6 (0.7%)	2 (0.2%)	2 (0.2%)	3 (0.3%)	1 (0.1%)
Valproate	715	7 (1.0%)	11 (1.5%)	5 (0.7%)	9 (1.3%)	2 (0.3%)	8 (1.1%)	2 (0.3%)
Lamotrigine	647	1 (0.2%)	1 (0.2%)	4 (0.6%)	6 (0.9%)	3 (0.5%)	2 (0.3%)	4 (0.6%)
Phenytoin	82	0 (0.0%)	1 (1.2%)	1 (1.2%)	0 (0.0%)	1 (1.2%)	0 (0.0%)	0 (0.0%)

GIT, gastrointestinal tract defects; GUT, genitourinary tract defects; NTD, neural tube defects.
(Courtesy of Morrow J, Russell A, Guthrie E, et al. Malformation risks of antiepileptic drugs in pregnancy: a prospective study from the UK Epilepsy and Pregnancy Register. *J Neurol Neurosurg Psychiatry.* 2006;77:193-198. Reproduced with permission from the BMJ Publishing Group.)

factors be ascertained, and potentially rational nutritional interventions could then be put in place. The National Children's Study is such a study. Currently just getting under way, the National Children's Study will enroll 100,000 children preconceptually and follow them up to age 21. It is hoped that the impact of antiepileptics will be a focus in the early stages of this study.

C. F. Bearer, MD, PhD

Major Congenital Malformations after First-Trimester Exposure to ACE Inhibitors

Cooper WO, Hernandez-Diaz S, Arbogast PG, et al (Vanderbilt Univ, Nashville, Tenn; Boston Univ)
N Engl J Med 354:2443-2451, 2006   3–4

Background.—Use of angiotensin-converting–enzyme (ACE) inhibitors during the second and third trimesters of pregnancy is contraindicated because of their association with an increased risk of fetopathy. In contrast, first-trimester use of ACE inhibitors has not been linked to adverse fetal outcomes. We conducted a study to assess the association between exposure to ACE inhibitors during the first trimester of pregnancy only and the risk of congenital malformations.

Methods.—We studied a cohort of 29,507 infants enrolled in Tennessee Medicaid and born between 1985 and 2000 for whom there was no evidence of maternal diabetes. We identified 209 infants with exposure to ACE inhibitors in the first trimester alone, 202 infants with exposure to other antihypertensive medications in the first trimester alone, and 29,096 infants with no exposure to antihypertensive drugs at any time during gestation. Major congenital malformations were identified from linked vital records and hospitalization claims during the first year of life and confirmed by review of medical records.

Results.—Infants with only first-trimester exposure to ACE inhibitors had an increased risk of major congenital malformations (risk ratio, 2.71; 95 percent confidence interval, 1.72 to 4.27) as compared with infants who had no exposure to antihypertensive medications. In contrast, fetal exposure to other antihypertensive medications during only the first trimester did not confer an increased risk (risk ratio, 0.66; 95 percent confidence interval, 0.25 to 1.75). Infants exposed to ACE inhibitors were at increased risk for malformations of the cardiovascular system (risk ratio, 3.72; 95 percent confidence interval, 1.89 to 7.30) and the central nervous system (risk ratio, 4.39; 95 percent confidence interval, 1.37 to 14.02).

Conclusions.—Exposure to ACE inhibitors during the first trimester cannot be considered safe and should be avoided.

▶ The process for approving drugs by the Food and Drug Administration does not usually include studies of drug safety among pregnant populations. Indeed, research into the possible associations of drugs used in pregnancy and their increased risk of birth defects is a very difficult undertaking, fraught with uncertainty and with a long history of either delayed recognition of real effects (eg, thalidomide) or the erroneous labeling of teratogenicity (eg, bendectin). The recent report by Cooper et al of an association between ACE inhibitors and congenital malformations comes almost a quarter of a century after widespread use of ACE inhibitors, and of prior reports suggesting that these drugs were not teratogenic.[1] Is the current report credible and does it document causality?

The Tennessee Medicaid database in which this study was conducted is one of the premier resources for postmarketing surveillance of drug safety, and the investigators have previously documented several important validity criteria.[2] However, even the best designed studies may not be able to control for all the biases that plague this area of research. Foremost is whether the drug of interest, or the condition which it is treating, is responsible for the observed association (called "indication bias"). This study attempts to control this by comparing other drugs in the same class used to treat hypertension. However, this may not fully rule out residual confounding because the drug of interest may be used in more severe cases ("severity bias"), or used when other drugs have failed ("selection bias"). It is also possible that in this special population of Medicaid patients, ACE inhibitors are differentially used in subsets of the population at higher risk. Also of concern is whether other conditions, especially obesity and diabetes, confound the association. Persons with diabetes are at higher risk for birth defects and for using the drug.[3] The investigators are well aware of this risk and took several steps to address it,[3] but concern remains that unmeasured and unrecorded diabetes in the study population may persist. Other limitations to accepting causality are that the associations are generally small (relative risks in the order of 2-3), the number of exposed infants is few (<20); and there is no analysis of a dose response.

What are the implications of continuing uncertainty about the association of ACE inhibitors and birth defects? From a research perspective, there is clearly a need for replication. Other existing databases where this might be done are the General Practice Research Database (GPRD) in the United Kingdom[4] and the large linked databases in Denmark, Sweden, and Norway. Some of these databases have the same methodologic problems as the Tennessee database but consistency in observing risk across other studies would be very reassuring that this was a real association. For the clinician, the important statistic from the current research is the "number needed to harm," which can be estimated as 22 from the current study. That is, 1 in 22 exposed women may deliver a child with a major malformation owing to use of the drug. This risk is large enough to consider switching a patient who is on an ACE inhibitor to another drug. However, as warned in the editorial accompanying this article, even less may be known about the risk of congenital malformations from using alternative antihypertensive therapies and untreated hypertension in pregnancy is itself of major concern.[5] Unfortunately, the most appropriate clinical management of patients in this situation is not yet fully informed by high-quality evidence.

M. B. Bracken, PhD, MPH

References

1. Schaefer C. Angiotensin II-receptor-antagonists: further evidence of fetotoxicity but not teratogenicity. *Birth Defects Res A Clin Mol Teratol.* 2003;67:591-594.
2. Ray WA, Griffin MR. Use of Medicaid data for pharmacoepidemiology. *Am J Epidemiol.* 1989;129:837-849.
3. Scialli AR, Lione A. ACE inhibitors and major congenital malformations. *N Engl J Med.* 2006;355:1280; author reply 1281.
4. Hardy JR, Holford TR, Hall GC, Bracken MB. Strategies for identifying pregnancies in the automated medical records of the General Practice Research Database. *Pharmacoepidemiol Drug Saf.* 2004;13:749-759.
5. Friedman JM. ACE inhibitors and congenital anomalies. *N Engl J Med.* 2006;354:2498-2500.

Genetic Polymorphisms of Hemostasis Genes and Primary Outcome of Very Low Birth Weight Infants

Härtel C, König I, Köster S, et al (Univ at Lübeck, Germany; Kinderklinik auf der Bult, Hannover, Germany; Olgahospital, Stuttgart, Germany; et al)
Pediatrics 118:683-689, 2006   3–5

Background.—Recent investigations have reported an influence of thrombophilic mutations and antithrombotic risk factors with development of intraventricular hemorrhage. It was our objective for this study to investigate the impact of genetic polymorphisms of hemostasis genes on the primary outcome measures of sepsis, bronchopulmonary dysplasia, intraventricular hemorrhage, and periventricular leukomalacia in a large cohort of very low birth weight infants.

Methods.—There were 586 very low birth weight infants enrolled prospectively in a multicenter trial between September 2003 and July 2005, and an additional 595 very low birth weight infants, who had been recruited in a previous prospective trial, were studied. DNA samples were taken by buccal swab, and genotypes of factor V Leiden mutation, prothrombin G20210A mutation, the factor VII-323 del/ins polymorphism, and the factor XIII-Val34Leu polymorphisms were determined by polymerase chain reaction and restriction enzyme digestion.

Results.—In contrast to data published previously, the frequency of intraventricular hemorrhage or periventricular leukomalacia was not significantly influenced by any of the genetic variants tested. Carriers of the factor XIII-Val34Leu polymorphism, however, had a higher sepsis rate and a longer period of hospital care compared with noncarriers. The factor VII-323 del/ins polymorphism was found to be a potential protective factor against bronchopulmonary dysplasia.

Conclusions.—We could not confirm previously reported associations of hemostasis gene variants and development of intraventricular hemorrhage in very low birth weight infants. To better understand gene-disease associations in very low birth weight infants, the prospective development of large-scale cohorts with well-defined phenotypes and corresponding DNA samples is essential.

▶ The decrease in frequency of grade III-IV intravascular hemorrhage (IVH) between 1987 and 1993 from 18% to 11% in very low birth weight infants is mostly attributed to improvements in neonatal fluid resuscitation, blood pressure management, and indocin prophylaxis.[1] But since 1993 the frequency seems to be unchanged, perhaps reflecting maximization of benefits from tweaking clinical protocols. The authors of this paper and others[2] hypothesize that in addition to significant environmental effects—fluid resuscitation, for example—susceptibility to IVH may be conferred by genetic factors. Although the frequency is considerably lower, similar arguments can be made for periventricular leukomalacia (PVL).

Using a candidate gene approach these authors previously reported association of increased PVL with the factor XIII Val34Leu polymorphism in 40 cases and 491 controls.[3] If indeed thrombostasis plays a role in IVH or PVL, factors of the coagulation cascade would be reasonable candidates to interrogate. But this latest report of 27 very low birth weight babies with PVL and 737 controls does not replicate the PVL association and confirms no association with IVH. Even with a relatively strong genotypic relative risk of 2.0 and maximizing the genetic model, there would only be approximately 70% power to detect an allele with frequency of 0.15 or greater for a study of this size.[4]

Recently, using meta-analyses of published studies Trikalinos et al[5] examined the frequency that genetic association is replicated in follow-up studies. The results are disheartening; approximately half of initial genetic association studies, even those with strong effects (odds ratio greater than 2.0) or with low P values (<.001), are not replicated. The reasons include population admixture (unmatched cases and controls), phenotypic heterogeneity (inclusion of both genetic and nongenetic cases) and, commonly, underpowered studies (not enough subjects). With a total of 63 cases in their first report (468 controls) and 132 cases in this report (633 controls), both studies of factor XIII Val34Leu are adequately powered for IVH (all IVH grades I to IV). But with only 40 PVL cases (491 controls) in their first report and 27 cases in this report (737 controls), both studies are underpowered for PVL. It is no surprise then that the PVL association could not be replicated. Regarding the new findings of association between the factor XIII Val34Leu polymorphism with sepsis, and between the factor VII 323del/ins polymorphism with bronchopulmonary dysplasia, these appear to be polymorphisms in search of diseases.

Kudos to the authors and to the editors of *Pediatrics* for publishing negative data. While formal heritability studies showing that IVH or PVL have quantifiable genetic contributions to the variance are lacking, it is still likely that genetic factors figure prominently in both disorders. These studies and similar candidate gene approaches confirm how little we understand about the involved complex metabolic pathways. I believe that the components of these pathways will only be revealed by adequately powered genome-wide association studies that by design are not hindered by preconceptions of untested genetic components; until completed, the prospects for further understanding the basic mechanisms of IVH and PVL remain guarded.

J. R. Gruen, MD

References

1. Fanaroff AA, Hack M, Walsh MC. The NICHD neonatal research network: changes in practice and outcomes during the first 15 years. *Semin Perinatol.* 2003;27:281-287.
2. Bhandari V, Bizzarro MJ, Shetty A, et al. Familial and genetic susceptibility to major neonatal morbidities in preterm twins. *Pediatrics.* 2006;117:1901-1906.
3. Göpel W, Kattner E, Seidenberg J, Kohlmann T, Segerer H, Möller J, for the Genetic Factors in Neonatology Study Group. The effect of the Val34Leu polymorphism in the factor XIII gene in infants with a birth weight below 1500 g. *J Pediatr.* 2002;140:688-692.
4. Purcell S, Cherny SS, Sham PC. Genetic Power Calculator: design of linkage and association genetic mapping studies of complex traits. *Bioinformatics.* 2003;19:149-150.
5. Trikalinos TA, Ntzani EE, Contopoulos-Ioannidis DG, Ioannidis JP. Establishment of genetic associations for complex diseases is independent of early study findings. *Eur J Hum Genet.* 2004;12:762-769.

Genetic Variation in the Sodium-dependent Vitamin C Transporters, *SLC23A1*, and *SLC23A2* and Risk for Preterm Delivery

Erichsen HC, Mulherin Engel SA, Eck PK, et al (Natl Cancer Inst, Bethesda, Md; Mount Sinai School of Medicine, New York; NIH, Bethesda, Md; et al)
Am J Epidemiol 163:245-254, 2006   3–6

Vitamin C has been the focus of epidemiologic investigation in preterm delivery (<37 weeks' gestation), which is a leading cause of neonatal mortality and birth-related morbidity. There are two sodium-dependent membrane transporters encoded by *SLC23A1* and *SLC23A2*, which have key roles in human vitamin C metabolism and which control dietary uptake, reabsorption, and tissue distribution of vitamin C. Using maternal DNA, the authors evaluated common single-nucleotide polymorphisms (SNPs) in *SLC23A1* and *SLC23A2* in a nested case-control analysis of the Pregnancy, Infection, and Nutrition Study (1995–2000) cohort. Of the associations observed for both haplotypes in *SLC23A1* and individual SNPs in *SLC23A2*, the most robust finding is with an intron 2 variant in *SLC23A2*. Heterozygotes and homozygotes for this variant had a 1.7-fold (95% confidence interval: 0.9, 3.3) and a 2.7-fold (95% confidence interval: 1.2, 6.3) elevation in the risk of spontaneous preterm birth, respectively. Semi-Bayesian hierarchical regression analysis, which simultaneously adjusted for multiple SNPs within the same gene, gave comparable results. The authors' findings link genetic variants in the vitamin C transporters to spontaneous preterm birth, which may explain previous dietary associations. If the findings from this study are confirmed, they may serve as the foundation for genetic risk assessment of nutritional pathways in preterm birth.

▶ Vitamin C is an essential cofactor for 8 mammalian enzymes and quenches reactive oxygen species. Vitamin C also plays an important role in embryogenesis and fetal growth as well as in the progression of pregnancy and delivery. Therefore, it is important to understand the mechanism that mediates its transport to the fetus as well as the possible influences by endogenous and exogenous substances on its placental uptake. As noted above, sodium-dependent vitamin C transport is mediated by two transporters, SVCT 1 and SVCT 2, encoded by *SLC23A1* and *SLC23A2*. Eck et al[1] characterized the genomic structures of *SLC23A1* and *SLC23A2* and determined that for *SLC23A1*, the majority of single nucleotide polymorphisms (SNPs) are population specific in either African Americans or Caucasians, including 3 of 4 nonsynonymous SNPs. In contrast, most SNPs in *SLC23A2* are shared between African Americans and Caucasians, and there are no nonsynonymous SNPs in *SLC23A2*. Erichsen et al have detected that variants of *SLC23A2* are associated with an increased risk of preterm birth. This presents an important link between nutrition and preterm birth.

A. A. Fanaroff, MD

Reference

1. Eck P, Erichsen HC, Taylor JG, et al. Comparison of the genomic structure and variation in the two human sodium-dependent vitamin C transporters, *SLC23A1* and *SLC23A2*. *Hum Genet*. 2004;115:285-294.

Hospitalizations of Newborns With Folate-Sensitive Birth Defects Before and After Fortification of Foods With Folic Acid
Robbins JM, Tilford JM, Bird TM, et al (Univ of Arkansas for Med Sciences, Little Rock; Arkansas Children's Hosp, Little Rock)
Pediatrics 118:906-915, 2006   3–7

Context.—The prevalence of neural tube defects is reduced in populations of women who receive folic acid supplementation. Since 1998, grain products in the United States have been fortified with folic acid. Fortification may have additional benefits by reducing the national prevalence of newborn hospitalizations for other folate-sensitive birth defects.

Objective.—Our purpose with this work was to compare rates of hospitalizations of newborns with folate-sensitive birth defects before and after implementation of fortification of grains.

Method.—National hospital discharge data from the Healthcare Cost and Utilization Project were used to compute rates of newborn hospitalizations for selected birth defects per 10,000 live births in the United States. Newborn hospitalization rates involving congenital anomalies recognizable at birth were analyzed for 5 years before fortification of grains and 5 years after fortification. Additional analyses compared changes in newborn hospitalization rates for birth defects by race/ethnicity, income, insurance status, and region of the country.

Results.—Newborn hospitalization rates for spina bifida decreased 21% from 1993–1997 to 1998–2002. Newborn hospitalization rates also decreased for anencephaly (20%) and limb-reduction defects (4%). Decline in hospitalizations for spina bifida occurred more often among Hispanic newborns (33%) than among white (13%) or black (21%) newborns. Decline in limb-reduction defects was seen primarily among blacks (11%). Findings using hospitalization data were similar to recent reports using birth defect surveillance systems with the exception of findings for orofacial clefts and conotruncal heart defects. No reductions were noted in newborn hospitalizations for these anomalies.

Conclusions.—Results from this ecological study fail to demonstrate substantial declines in newborn hospitalizations beyond those anticipated from a reduction in neural tube defects. The society-wide impact of the fortification program on birth defects and other health conditions should continue to be monitored.

▶ Although this study failed to demonstrate a substantial decline in newborn hospitalizations for cleft palate, cleft lip, and Down syndrome, this negative finding does not lessen the importance or impact of the folic acid fortification program in the United States, which is justified largely by the anticipated society-wide reductions in the prevalence and concomitant reductions in newborn hospitalizations and other health care resource use of infants born with neural tube defects. The current fortification level required by the US Food and Drug Administration is 140 µg per 100 g of grain. This has definitely led to an increase in serum and red cell folate levels in Americans. What is currently being debated is whether the amount of folic acid supplementation currently recommended should be increased because of the possibility of a further reduction in neural tube defects without an adverse impact on the population. Although targeted education of the public might be another way to ensure better folic acid status, increasing the fortification level some more would also help. International experience is supportive in this latter regard, but the decision must be made in consideration of our societal complexities and potential risks, although the risks are not likely to be great with a modest increase in fortification. At the very least, such a strategy should be studied by the Food and Drug Administration. Opportunities that have the potential for such a great benefit to individuals and the public are few.

D. K. Stevenson, MD

4 Labor and Delivery

Survival Advantage Associated With Cesarean Delivery in Very Low Birth Weight Vertex Neonates

Lee HC, Gould JB (Stanford Univ, Palo Alto, Calif)
Obstet Gynecol 107:97-105, 2006   4–1

Objective.—To identify the indications for and any survival advantage associated with very low birth weight (VLBW) neonates delivered by cesarean.

Methods.—Maternal and infant data from the National Center for Health Statistics linked birth/death data set for 1999 to 2000 were analyzed. Maternal conditions associated with cesarean delivery were compared among birth weight groups for vertex neonates. Birth weight–specific 28-

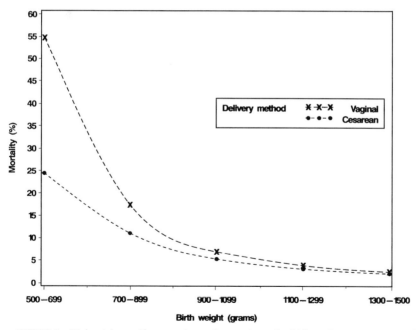

FIGURE 2.—Birth weight–specific neonatal mortality rates by mode of delivery. Data source: National Center for Health Statistics. 1999, 2000 Birth Cohort Linked Birth and Infant Death Data Set. (Courtesy of: Lee HC, Gould JB. Survival advantage associated with cesarean delivery in very low birth weight vertex neonates. *Obstet Gynecol.* 2006;107:97-105. Reprinted with permission from Lippincott William & Wilkins at http://lww.com.)

day mortality rates and relative risks were calculated with 95% confidence intervals. Multivariate logistic regression was performed to adjust for other factors that may be associated with survival.

Results.—Cesarean delivery occurred frequently, more than 40% in most VLBW birth weight groups. Conditions associated with cesarean delivery in VLBW vertex neonates differed from those seen in non-VLBW vertex neonates. A survival advantage was associated with cesarean delivery in the birth weight analysis up to 1,300 g ($P < .05$). This decreased mortality for VLBW neonates delivered by cesarean persisted after adjusting for other factors associated with mortality.

Conclusion.—Very low birth weight vertex neonates are often born by cesarean delivery and have different maternal risk profiles from non-VLBW vertex neonates born by this route. Neonatal mortality was decreased in VLBW neonates delivered by cesarean. Further study is warranted to determine whether this may be a causal relationship or a marker of quality of care (Fig 2).

▶ The most optimal route of delivery for preterm low birth weight (LBW) infants will continue to be debated, despite this article demonstrating a survival advantage with operative deliveries. The data are derived from the huge national birth certificate database but, as noted by the authors, "has limitations with respect to both the depth and accuracy of the clinical information available for analysis," and is devoid of morbidity and long-term outcome information. Nonetheless, this is probably as good as it gets, and it is most unlikely that a randomized trial will address this issue. Of note, the survival advantage from cesarean delivery is most prominent in the smallest neonates, a fact that may merely reflect decisions by the health care team in conjunction with the parents to be more aggressive at the borders of viability. In light of Lee and Gould's data, operative delivery must be given serious consideration for extremely immature and LBW infants.

Remarkably, the debate on cesarean section is not confined to the preterm infants. Lavender et al,[1] in a Cochrane review of cesarean section for nonmedical reasons at term noted, "There is no evidence from randomized controlled trials, upon which to base any practice recommendations regarding planned caesarean section for nonmedical reasons at term. In the absence of trial data, there is an urgent need for a systematic review of observational studies and a synthesis of qualitative data to better assess the short- and long-term effects of caesarean section and vaginal birth."

A. A. Fanaroff, MD

Reference

1. Lavender T, Hofmeyr GJ, Neilson JP, Kingdon C, Gyte GM. Caesarean section for non-medical reasons at term. *Cochrane Database Syst Rev.* 2006;3:CD004660.

Caesarean before labour between 34 and 37 weeks: What are the risk factors of severe neonatal respiratory distress?
Le Ray C, Boithias C, Castaigne-Meary V, et al (Maternity of Antoine Béclère Hosp (APHP), Clamart, Cedex, France)
Eur J Obstet Gynecol Reprod Biol 127:56-60, 2006   4–2

Objective.—To assess the frequency of severe neonatal respiratory distress and identify its risk factors in caesarean deliveries before labour between 34 and 37 weeks' gestation.

Study Design.—Retrospective study of children born by caesarean delivery before labour between 34 and 37 weeks, between 1999 and 2003 in a level 3 maternity unit. The frequencies of severe and mild neonatal respiratory distress were calculated. Univariate and multivariate analyses studied the factors potentially associated with severe respiratory distress: gestational age, type of pregnancy (singleton or multiple), condition of membranes, maternal diabetes, indication for caesarean, antenatal corticosteroid therapy, intrauterine growth retardation, infant's sex and birth weight.

Results.—The 189 study subjects included 107 singletons and 82 twins: 28% required intensive care for severe respiratory distress and 30.2% developed mild respiratory distress. Gestational age was a significant risk factor ($p = 0.01$), especially before 36 weeks (adjusted OR = 2.1; 95% CI: 1.0–4.4). The multivariate analysis indicated that singleton pregnancies (adjusted OR = 3.2; 95% CI: 1.5–6.7) and caesareans for fetal indications (adjusted OR = 2.7; 95% CI: 1.2–5.7) are also risk factors and that premature rupture of the membranes is a "protective" factor against respiratory complications (adjusted OR = 0.2; 95% CI: 0.1–0.8).

Conclusion.—More than a quarter of the infants delivered by caesarean before labour between 34 and 37 weeks' gestation in our level 3 maternity unit had severe respiratory distress. Although our population may not be typical of the general population, this finding and the risk factors associated with it should be taken into account in determining the best time and place for delivery of each patient.

▶ The problems, care, and management of late preterm infants, those preterm infants between 34 and 37 weeks' gestation, have tended to be minimized when compared with similar concerns for preterm infants less than 30 weeks' gestation. In fact, in many hospitals, infants greater than 2000 g birthweight and older than 35 weeks' gestation are discharged home with their mothers several days after delivery. The impetus for this retrospective study was to provide information that could be taken into consideration when discussions about delivery location for late preterm infants were held. Specifically, should a woman who had been transferred to a level 3 referral maternity unit and who had reached 34 weeks' gestation be transferred back to a level 2 maternity unit for delivery? Therefore, this study sought to determine the frequency of severe respiratory distress in late preterm infants delivered by caesarean section without labor and to identify possible risk factors. Severe respiratory distress was defined as the need for resuscitation, followed by admission to the NICU and treatment with assisted ventilation or treatment with nasal continuous positive airway pressure (NCPAP) with oxygen for at least 2 hours. Although the conclusions would have been enhanced if this study had been performed at a level 2 maternity unit that was a member of a perinatal care network rather than a level 3 referral maternity center, the results should not be ignored.

R. A. Ehrenkranz, MD

Recurrent of spontaneous versus medically indicated preterm birth
Ananth CV, Getahun D, Peltier MR, et al (Univ of Medicine and Dentistry of New Jersey, New Brunswick)
Am J Obstet Gynecol 195:643-650, 2006   4–3

Objective.—Despite the increased tendency of preterm birth to recur, little is known with regard to recurrence risks for spontaneous and medically indicated preterm birth as well as recurrence risks in relation to severity of preterm birth. We examined the recurrence of spontaneous and medically indicated preterm birth.

Study Design.—A population-based, retrospective cohort study of births in Missouri (1989 to 1997) was carried out with analyses restricted to women who delivered their first 2 consecutive singleton live births (n = 154,809). Women who experienced spontaneous onset of labor and subsequently delivered preterm (less than 35 weeks) were classified as spontaneous preterm birth. Medically indicated preterm birth included women who delivered preterm through a labor induction or a prelabor cesarean delivery. Risk and odds ratio of preterm birth recurrence were derived from fitting multivariate conditional logistic regression models after adjusting for potential confounders.

Results.—If the first pregnancy resulted in a spontaneous preterm birth, then affected women were more likely to deliver preterm spontaneously (adjusted odds ratio 3.6, 95% confidence interval 3.2, 4.0) and also as a medically indicated preterm birth (odds ratio 2.5, 95% confidence interval 2.1, 3.0) in the second birth. Similarly, if the first pregnancy resulted in a medically indicated preterm birth, affected women were 10.6-fold (95% confidence interval 10.1, 12.4) more likely to deliver preterm because of medical indications in the second pregnancy as well as preterm spontaneously (odds ratio 1.6, 95% confidence interval 1.3, 2.1). The greatest risk of recurrence of preterm birth in the second pregnancy tended to occur around the same gestational age as preterm birth in the first pregnancy, regardless of the clinical subtype.

Conclusion.—The observation that spontaneous preterm birth is not only associated with increased recurrence of spontaneous but also medically indicated preterm birth and vice versa, suggests that the 2 clinical subtypes may share common etiologies.

▶ Preterm birth (PTB) remains a common event (12.7% of all births in the United States in 2005[1]) and a major cause of perinatal morbidity and mortality. A detailed obstetric history is a routine part of prenatal care to estimate, among other risks, the likelihood that the current pregnancy too will deliver prematurely. It has long been known that PTB tend to recur. Indeed, a prior spontaneous PTB is the single strongest historic predictor of preterm delivery in the index pregnancy.[2,3] However, approximately 20% of all PTB are iatrogenic (medically indicated) and performed for maternal and/or fetal indications. Whether a prior medically indicated PTB is also associated with an increased risk of PTB in a subsequent pregnancy has not previously been systematically examined.

To further investigate this issue, Ananth et al carried out a population-based, retrospective cohort study of all women who delivered their first 2 consecutive singleton live births in the state of Missouri between January 1, 1989 and December 31, 1997 (n = 154,809). Women whose first pregnancy resulted in a spontaneous PTB <35 weeks were more likely to have a recurrent spontaneous PTB (OR, 3.6; 95% CI, 3.2-4.0) or medically indicated PTB (OR, 2.5; 95% CI, 2.1-3.0) in the second pregnancy. Similarly, if the first pregnancy ended in a medically indicated PTB, the second pregnancy was more likely to end in a recurrent medically indicated PTB (OR, 10.6; 95% CI, 10.1-12.4) or spontaneous PTB (OR, 1.6; 95% CI, 1.3-2.1). Interestingly, and consistent with prior publications,[4-6] the greatest risk of recurrence was in women who had their first PTB remote from term (<28 weeks' gestation), and recurrent PTB in a second pregnancy tended to occur around the same gestational age as the PTB in the first pregnancy, regardless of the clinical subtype. Although not specifically addressed in this study, prior publications have shown that black women are at increased risk of a first PTB compared with white women[5-8] and, perhaps more importantly, are at significantly increased risk of recurrent PTB.[2]

These epidemiologic observations are interesting, but what is their clinical significance? The data suggest that a history of a prior PTB should be regarded as significant regardless of the cause. However, this is unlikely to alter clinical management since it is well known that reliance on historic risk factors alone will fail to identify more than 60% of women who deliver preterm and, of those who screen positive, the vast majority will go on to deliver at term.[9,10] Perhaps more importantly, the study may give some insight into the pathophysiology of PTB. As the authors themselves conclude, the observation that spontaneous PTB is associated with an increased risk of both recurrent spontaneous PTB and medically indicated PTB in a subsequent pregnancy (and vice versa), suggests that these 2 clinical subtypes may share common causes. An equally plausible explanation is that they share a common genetic predisposition. Familial clustering,[2,3] racial disparities,[5-8] and the high incidence of recurrent preterm birth[4] all suggest a critical role for maternal genetic factors in the timing of labor. Moreover, early horse-donkey (ass) crossbreeding experiments resulted in a gestational length intermediate between that of horses (365 days) and that of donkeys (340 days),[11] suggesting a role also for the fetal genotype in the timing of labor. A significant role for genetic or gene-environment factors may explain why, although obstetric care providers are getting better at identifying women at high risk of PTB, most interventions designed to prevent preterm delivery have proven ineffective.

E. R. Norwitz, MD, PhD

References

1. Hamilton BE, Minio AM, Martin JA, Kochanek KD, Strobino DM, Guyer B. Annual summary of vital statistics: 2005. *Pediatrics.* 2007;119:345-360.
2. Iams JD, Goldenberg RL, Mercer BM, et al. The Preterm Prediction Study: recurrence risk of spontaneous preterm birth. National Institute of Child Health and Human Development Maternal-Fetal Medicine Units Network. *Am J Obstet Gynecol.* 1998;178:1035-1040.
3. Winkvist A, Mogren I, Högberg U. Familial patterns in birth characteristics: impact on individual and population risks. *Int J Epidemiol.* 1998;27:248-254.
4. Mercer BM, Goldenberg RL, Moawad AH, et al. The Preterm Prediction Study: effect of gestational age and cause of preterm birth on subsequent obstetric outcome. National Institute of Child Health and Human Development Maternal-Fetal Medicine Units Network. *Am J Obstet Gynecol.* 1999;181:1216-1221.
5. Carmichael SL, Iyasu S, Hatfield-Timajchy K. Cause-specific trends in neonatal mortality among black and white infants, United States, 1980-1995. *Matern Child Health J.* 1998;2:67-76.
6. Ekwo E, Moawad A. The risk for recurrence of premature births to African-American and white women. *J Assoc Acad Minor Phys.* 1998;9:16-21.
7. Blackmore CA, Ferré CD, Rowley DL, Hogue CJ, Gaiter J, Atrash H. Is race a risk factor or a risk marker for preterm delivery? *Ethn Dis.* 1993;3:372-377.
8. Blackmore-Prince C, Kieke B Jr, Kugaraj KA, et al. Racial differences in the patterns of singleton preterm delivery in the 1988 National Maternal and Infant Health Survey. *Matern Child Health J.* 1999;3:189-197.
9. American College of Obstetricians and Gynecologists. ACOG Practice Bulletin. Assessment of risk for preterm birth. Clinical management guidelines for obstetrician-gynecologists. Number 31, October 2001. *Obstet Gynecol.* 2001;98:709-716.
10. Mercer BM, Goldenberg RL, Das A, et al. The preterm prediction study: a clinical risk assessment system. *Am J Obstet Gynecol.* 1996;174:1885-1893.
11. Liggins GC. Initiation of labour. *Biol Neonate.* 1989;55:366-375.

Use and Efficacy of Endotracheal Versus Intravenous Epinephrine During Neonatal Cardiopulmonary Resuscitation in the Delivery Room
Barber CA, Wyckoff MH (Univ of Texas, Dallas)
Pediatrics 118:1028-1034, 2006   4–4

Objective.—Given the paucity of information regarding endotracheal epinephrine for newborn resuscitation, the objectives of this study were: (1) to determine the frequency of endotracheal epinephrine use in newborns in the delivery room, and (2) to determine whether the previously recommended dose of 0.01 to 0.03 mg/kg of endotracheal epinephrine is effective in establishing a return of spontaneous circulation.

Patients and Methods.—A retrospective review was conducted for all neonates who received ≥1 dose of epinephrine in the delivery room between January 1999 and December 2004. Infants who received ≥1 dose of endotracheal epinephrine in the delivery room during resuscitation were included in the study population whether or not they survived to be admitted to the NICU. Exclusion criteria included lethal congenital anomalies, delivery outside the hospital, and missing medical charts.

Results.—Of 93,656 infants, 52 neonates (0.06%) received epinephrine in the delivery room, 5 of whom met exclusion criteria. Of the remaining 47 infants, 44 (94%) received the first dose via the endotracheal tube. Only 14 (32%) of 44 achieved return of spontaneous circulation after endotracheal tube administration of epinephrine. Of the 30 remaining infants, 23 (77%) had return of spontaneous circulation with intravenous epinephrine after initially failing endotracheal tube epinephrine. There were no differences in clinical characteristics between newborns who responded to endotracheal tube versus intravenous epinephrine except for a lower blood glucose on NICU admission (52 vs 113 mg%).

Conclusions.—Endotracheal epinephrine is frequently used when intensive resuscitation is required in the delivery room. The previously recommended endotracheal epinephrine dose of 0.01 to 0.03 mg/kg is often ineffective. Higher endotracheal doses will likely be needed to improve efficacy. A prospective study is needed to determine the best endotracheal epinephrine dosing regimen. Until such information is available, intravenous administration should be the preferred route of delivery.

▶ The 5th edition of the Neonatal Resuscitation Program's (NRP) *Textbook of Neonatal Resuscitation*[1] published in 2006 recommended that, if epinephrine treatment was indicated during delivery room (DR) resuscitation, it "should be given intravenously, although administration may be delayed by the time required to establish intravenous access." This was a major change from earlier editions of the *Textbook of Neonatal Resuscitation* that recommended "epinephrine should be given by the most accessible route that will deliver drug to the heart muscle;" either via an endotracheal tube or via a catheter inserted into the umbilical vein. In addition, the current NRP guidelines recommend that higher doses of epinephrine be administered if delivered via endotracheal tube. Specifically, instead of the previously recommended dose of 0.1 to 0.3 mL/kg of a 1:10,000 solution (0.01-0.03 mg/kg), a dose of 0.3 to 1.0 mL/kg (0.03-0.1 mg/kg) should be given endotracheally.

This article provides some of the supporting data for the current NRP recommendation. Although the study is retrospective, the authors provide clear evidence that the lower endotracheal epinephrine dose is often ineffective and suggested that a higher dose will likely be needed to stimulate heart rate and achieve a return of spontaneous circulation. The safety and efficacy of the higher endotracheal epinephrine dose suggested by the NRP guidelines has not been established. Given the consent issues associated with performing random control trials in emergency situations, it is unlikely that a safe and efficacious endotracheal epinephrine dose will be established in a clinical trial, and that animal studies will be required.

R. A. Ehrenkranz, MD

Reference

1. Kattwinkle J, Short J, eds. *Textbook of Neonatal Resuscitation.* 5th ed. Elk Grove Village, IL: American Academy of Pediatrics; 2006.

Delayed Cord Clamping in Very Preterm Infants Reduces the Incidence of Intraventricular Hemorrhage and Late-Onset Sepsis: A Randomized, Controlled Trial
Mercer JS, Vohr BR, McGrath MM, et al (Univ of Rhode Island, Kingston; Brown Med School, Providence, RI)
Pediatrics 117:1235-1242, 2006   4–5

Objective.—This study compared the effects of immediate (ICC) and delayed (DCC) cord clamping on very low birth weight (VLBW) infants on 2 primary variables: bronchopulmonary dysplasia (BPD) and suspected necrotizing enterocolitis (SNEC). Other outcome variables were late-onset sepsis (LOS) and intraventricular hemorrhage (IVH).

Study Design.—This was a randomized, controlled unmasked trial in which women in labor with singleton fetuses <32 weeks' gestation were randomly assigned to ICC (cord clamped at 5–10 seconds) or DCC (30–45 seconds) groups. Women were excluded for the following reasons: their obstetrician refused to participate, major congenital anomalies, multiple gestations, intent to withhold care, severe maternal illnesses, placenta abruption or previa, or rapid delivery after admission.

Results.—Seventy-two mother/infant pairs were randomized. Infants in the ICC and DCC groups weighed 1151 and 1175 g, and mean gestational ages were 28.2 and 28.3 weeks, respectively. Analyses revealed no difference in maternal and infant demographic, clinical, and safety variables. There were no differences in the incidence of our primary outcomes (BPD and suspected NEC). However, significant differences were found between the ICC and DCC groups in the rates of IVH and LOS. Two of the 23 male infants in the DCC group had IVH versus 8 of the 19 in the ICC group. No cases of sepsis occurred in the 23 boys in the DCC group, whereas 6 of the 19 boys in the ICC group had confirmed sepsis. There was a trend toward higher initial hematocrit in the infants in the DCC group.

Conclusions.—Delayed cord clamping seems to protect VLBW infants from IVH and LOS, especially for male infants.

▶ Despite the fact that mankind has been clamping the umbilical cord for thousands of years, there remains uncertainty as to the optimal time to clamp the cord. Concerns about polycythemia and increased hyperbilirubinemia appear to have been unfounded, and a summary of the prevailing theme from the modern literature is that delayed cord clamping reduces anemia in term infants and decreases intraventricular hemorrhage (IVH) and LOS in preterm infants.

After a review of 40 years of articles, van Rheenen et al[1] found "that delayed cord clamping in a group that contains both AGA and SGA infants was associated with higher hemoglobin levels at 2 to 3 months of age in term infants and a reduction in the number of blood transfusions needed in the 1st 4 to 6 weeks of life in preterm infants. No reliable conclusions could be drawn about the potential adverse effects of DCC." Chaparro et al (Abstract 11–12) confirm that a delay in cord clamping of 2 minutes could help prevent iron deficiency from developing before 6 months of age, when iron- fortified complementary foods could be introduced.[2] Ceriani et al[3] randomly assigned infants to cord clamping within the first 15 seconds (group 1), at 1 minute (group 2), or at 3 minutes after birth (group 3). The infants' venous hematocrit value was measured 6 hours after birth. They, too, found that DCC at birth increases neonatal mean venous hematocrit within a physiologic range. Neither significant differences nor harmful effects were observed among groups. Aladangady and colleagues[4] used a tripronged approach to promote placental blood transfer at preterm delivery. They delayed clamping of the cord 30 seconds, kept the infant below the placenta, and administered oxytocics. Although the blood volume was, on average, increased in the DCC group for both vaginal and cesarean deliveries, euvolemia was not attained with the third-stage management methods outlined above. The Cochrane Review, led by Rabe et al[5] also concluded that DCC reduced the need for blood transfusions and was associated with less IVH. There is still much work to be done to change obstetrical behavior and convince the obstetricians not to rush to clamp the cords in preterm infants.

A. A. Fanaroff, MD

References

1. van Rheenen PF, Gruschke S, Brabin BJ. Delayed umbilical cord clamping for reducing anaemia in low birthweight infants: implications for developing countries. *Ann Trop Paediatr.* 2006;26:157-167.
2. Chaparro CM, Neufeld LM, Tena Alavez G, Eguia-Líz Cedillo R, Dewey KG. Effect of timing of umbilical cord clamping on iron status in Mexican infants: a randomised controlled trial. *Lancet.* 2004;367:1997-2004.
3. Ceriani-Cernadas JM, Carroli G, Pellegrini L, et al. The effect of timing of cord clamping on neonatal venous hematocrit values and clinical outcome at term: a randomized, controlled trial. *Pediatrics.* 2006;11:779-786.
4. Aladangady N, McHugh S, Aitchison TC, Wardrop CA, Holland BM. Infants' blood volume in a controlled trial of placental transfusion at preterm delivery. *Pediatrics.* 2006;117:93-98.
5. Rabe H, Reynolds G, Diaz-Rossello J. Early versus delayed umbilical cord clamping in preterm infants. *Cochrane Database Syst Rev.* 2004;4:CD003248.

Fetal growth and onset of delivery: A nationwide population-based study of preterm infants
Morken N-H, Källen K, Jacobsson B (Telemark Hosp, Skien, Norway; Univ of Lund, Sweden; Sahlgrenska Academy, Göteborg, Sweden; et al)
Am J Obstet Gynecol 195:154-161, 2006   4–6

Objective.—This study was undertaken to assess whether deviations from normal fetal growth are associated with spontaneous preterm delivery.

Study design.—A population-based study was performed, using Swedish Medical Birth Register data from 1991 through 2001. The total population comprised 1,007,648 singleton births. Intrauterine-derived growth standards were used to identify individual standard deviation (SD) from expected birth weight. Spontaneous preterm infants were compared with infants born after spontaneous labor at term. Results were obtained by using multiple logistic regression analysis.

Results.—Associations between smaller than population mean and spontaneous preterm birth were evident for all gestational age groups. The largest risk was found at 28 to 31 gestational weeks and birth weight less than −3 SD (OR: 13.3; 95% CI: 10.3-17.2). Spontaneous preterm infants born at 34 to 36 gestational weeks weighed 1 to 1.9 SD (OR: 1.1; 95% CI: 1.1-1.2) or 2 to 2.9 SD (OR: 1.6; 95% CI: 1.5-1.7) above the expected mean more often (Tables 3 and 4).

Conclusion.—Deviation of fetal growth from the expected mean is associated with spontaneous preterm delivery.

TABLE 3.—Odds Ratio, with 95% CI, for SD Classes (< -3, -3 to -2.1, -2 to -1.1, 1 to 1.9, and 2 to 2.9) Versus Appropriate for Gestational Age (-1 SD to 0.99 SD) Among Infants Born After Spontaneous Preterm Labor, Compared with Term Infants (Born Spontaneously After at Least 37 Weeks of Pregnancy)*

SD Classes	<28 wks (95% CI)	28-31 wks (95% CI)	32-33 wks (95% CI)	34-36 wks (95% CI)
<-3	9.3 (6.2-13.8)	13.3 (10.3-17.2)	5.9 (4.4-7.9)	3.1 (2.6-3.6)
-3 to -2.1	2.6 (2.0-3.3)	3.2 (2.7-3.8)	1.9 (1.6-2.2)	1.2 (1.1-1.3)
-2 to -1.1	1.8 (1.6-2.1)	2.0 (1.8-2.2)	1.3 (1.2-1.5)	1.0 (1.0-1.0)
1 to 1.9	0.6 (0.5-0.7)	0.5 (0.5-0.6)	0.7 (0.7-0.8)	1.1 (1.1-1.2)
2 to 2.9	0.4 (0.2-0.7)	0.4 (0.2-0.6)	0.8 (0.6-1.0)	1.6 (1.5-1.7)

Results were obtained from 5 multiple logistic regression analyses, each with one of the 5 SD classes as the dependent variable, and gestational age (class variables as specified) as independent variables. Adjustments were made for year of birth (continuous independent variable), maternal age and (maternal age [Goldenberg RL, Nelson KG, Koski JF, Cutter GR. Low birth weight, intrauterine growth retardation, and preterm delivery. Am J Obstet Gynecol. 1985;142:980-984.]) (continuous 5-year classes), parity (class variables 1, 2, 3, 4+), and maternal smoking (0, 1-10, ≥10—as continuous independent variable).
*Intrauterine-derived growth standards.
(Courtesy of Morken N-H, Källen K, Jacobsson B. Fetal growth and onset of delivery: a nationwide population-based study of preterm infants. Am J Obstet Gynecol. 195:154-161. Copyright 2006 by Elsevier.)

TABLE 4.—Association Between SGA (< −2 SD) and Preterm Birth, According to Gestational Age and Mode of Onset of Labor*

	SGA† (%)	Total Births	OR (95% CI)
<28 wks, Total	382 (22.5)	1,697	10.7 (9.5-12.0)
Iatrogenic preterm birth	284 (64.5)	440	73.0 (59.7-89.1)
Spontaneous preterm birth	98 (7.8)	1,257	3.0 (2.4-3.7)
28-31 wks, Total	1,179 (30.2)	3,905	16.0 (14.9-17.2)
Iatrogenic preterm birth	962 (57.7)	1,667	53.2 (48.1-58.9)
Spontaneous preterm birth	217 (9.7)	2,238	3.8 (3.3-4.4)
32-33 wks, Total	933 (17.7)	5,260	7.7 (7.2-8.3)
Iatrogenic preterm birth	731 (38.6)	1,892	23.9 (21.7-26.4)
Spontaneous preterm birth	202 (6.0)	3,368	2.2 (1.9-2.5)
34-36 wks, Total	2,687 (7.6)	35,363	3.0 (2.9-3.2)
Iatrogenic preterm birth	1,730 (20.8)	8,322	10.5 (9.9-11.1)
Spontaneous preterm birth	957 (3.5)	27,041	1.3 (1.2-1.4)
Preterm, <37 wks Total	5,181 (11.2)	46,225	4.6 (4.5-4.8)
Iatrogenic preterm birth	3,707 (30.1)	12,321	16.4 (15.9-17.0)
Spontaneous preterm birth	1,474 (4.3)	33,904	1.6 (1.5-1.7)
Term, 37+, Total	27,044 (2.8)	961,423	
Induced labor or elective CS	7,045 (5.6)	126,665	2.4 (2.3-2.5)
Spontaneous onset	19,999 (2.4)	834,758	References
Total births	32,225 (3.2)	1,007,648	

Results were obtained from a multiple logistic regression analysis, with SGA (<2 SD below expected birth weight according to gestational length) as the dependent variable, and gestational age (class variables as specified) as independent variables. Adjustments were made for year of birth (continuous independent variable), maternal age and (maternal age [Goldenberg RL, Nelson KG, Koski JF, Cutter GR. Low birth weight, intrauterine growth retardation, and preterm delivery. *Am J Obstet Gynecol.* 1985;142:980-984.]) (continuous 5-year classes), parity (class variables 1, 2, 3, 4+), and maternal smoking (0, 1-10, ≥10—as continuous independent variable). CS, Cesarean section.

*OR with 95% CI, after stratification for year of birth, maternal age, parity, and smoking. Multiple gestations, congenital malformations, and antenatal deaths were excluded Sweden, 1991-2001.

†<2 SD below expected birth weight, according to intrauterine-derived growth standards.

(Courtesy of Morken N-H, Källen K, Jacobsson B. Fetal growth and onset of delivery: a nationwide population-based study of preterm infants. *Am J Obstet Gynecol.* 2006;195:154-161. Copyright 2006 by Elsevier.)

▶ The preterm birth rate (births before 37 completed weeks of gestation) has been increasing in the United States, largely driven by an increase in infants delivered between 34 and 36 weeks, often called near-term, but preferably referred to as late preterm. In 2004, the preterm birth rate was 12.5%, the highest rate since the National Center for Health Statistics began tracking such data.[1] The factors that place a woman at higher risk for premature labor include a previous preterm birth, multiple gestations, infections such as bacterial vaginosis and trichomoniasis, and a short cervix. Progesterone supplementation may reduce preterm birth in a woman who has had a previous preterm infant,[2] but the treatment of infections has been ineffective in reducing prematurity.

Known risk factors for fetal growth restriction include genetic conditions or environmental exposures. Maternal disorders including hypertension and sickle cell disease may influence fetal growth. The major risk factors for fetal growth restriction include tobacco use during pregnancy, low pre-pregnancy weight, and poor weight gain during pregnancy. Alcohol and drug use will also significantly restrict fetal growth.

There have been many discussions with regard to the disproportionate number of small for gestational age infants among a cohort of infants with birth weight less than 1500 g. This huge national database representing over a decade of data collection sheds some light on this matter. The association between smaller than population mean and spontaneous preterm birth was strongest at 28 to 31 weeks' gestation, which would translate into a birth weight of less than 1500 g. Surprisingly, at 34 to 36 weeks the weight of the infants was above the mean. These are the late preterm infants who masquerade as term infants, but need close observation and are more likely to experience drops in temperature, hypoglycemia, respiratory distress, and jaundice.

A. A. Fanaroff, MD

References

1. Raju TN. Epidemiology of late preterm (near-term) births. *Clin Perinatol.* 2006;33:751-763.
2. Meis PJ, Klebanoff M, Dombrowski MP, et al. Does progesterone treatment influence risk factors for recurrent preterm delivery? *Obstet Gynecol.* 2005;106: 557-561.

Birth weight at high altitudes in Peru
Hartinger S, Tapia V, Carrillo C, et al (Universidad Peruana Cayetano Heredia, Peru)
Int J Gynecol Obstet 93:275-281, 2006   4–7

Objective.—To determine whether birth weights are lower at high altitudes, and whether gestational age at birth and a population's length of residence mitigate the effect of high altitude.

Methods.—The birth weights of 84,173 neonates recorded in the Peruvian Perinatal Information System Database were analyzed between 1995 and 2002 for the cities of Lima (150 m), Huancayo (3280 m), Cuzco (3400 m), and Juliaca (3800 m).

Results.—Birth weight was lower at high altitude, but there was no linear relation between altitude of residence and birth weight. Mean birth weight was higher in Juliaca than in Huancayo. There were no significant differences between the 4 cities regarding birth weights of infants born between 28 and 35 weeks of gestation. However, for infants born between 36 and 42 weeks, birth weight was lower at higher altitudes. This may be due to inadequate maternal oxygenation later in pregnancy at high altitude. In the multivariate analysis, after controlling for maternal age, marital status, parity, body mass index, pre-eclampsia or hemorrhage during pregnancy, and education, as well as sex of the newborn and gestational age at birth, birth weight was lower in all cities located at a higher altitude than Lima. Yet, longer residence at high altitudes may play a protective role. Juliaca (3800 m), where the population has resided the longest, had the lowest reduction in birth weight compared with Lima (150 m); Cuzco had intermediate values; and Huancayo (3280 m), where the population has resided the shortest, had the highest reduction in birth weight.

Conclusions.—Birth weight reduction, which is independent of socioeconomic factors, occurs only in births at term and may be less severe in populations that have resided longer at high altitudes.

► This study by Hartinger et al confirms the effect of high altitude on the birthweight of infants born at term. However, with the use of the Peruvian Perinatal Information System Database, knowledge of the historical background of the populations inhabiting 4 Peruvian cities, and multivariate analysis, the investigators report that the influence of altitude on term birthweight is lessened in populations who have resided at high altitudes for multiple generations. This important observation was found to be independent of socioeconomic and nutritional factors and to be consistent with the known physiologic adaptation to prolonged residence at high altitude.

Does the mobile society in the United States account for the linear relationship between the extent of birthweight reduction at term and altitude that has been observed in Colorado?[1] In that report, investigators found that birthweight declined 121 g for every 1000-m gain in elevation when the influence of altitude was considered alone, or 102 g when adjusted for other independent variables, such as gestation, parity, smoking, and pregnancy-induced hypertension, and concluded that high altitude acts independently, and additively with other risk factors that effect birthweight at all altitudes.

Therefore, as part of assessing the risk that high altitude has on birthweight, perhaps the prenatal history should include questions about how long a pregnant woman and her family has lived at high altitude.

R. A. Ehrenkranz, MD

Reference

1. Jensen GM, Moore LG. The effect of high altitude and other risk factors on birthweight: independent or interactive effects? *Am J Public Health.* 1997;87:1003-1007.

Effect of Labor Epidural Analgesia with and without Fentanyl on Infant Breast-feeding: A Prospective, Randomized, Double-blind Study
Beilin Y, Bodian CA, Weiser J, et al (New York Univ)
Anesthesiology 103:1211-1217, 2005   4–8

Background.—The influence of labor epidural fentanyl on the neonate is controversial. The purpose of this study was to determine whether epidural fentanyl has an impact on breast-feeding.

Methods.—Women who previously breast-fed a child and who requested labor epidural analgesia were randomly assigned in a double-blinded manner to one of three groups: (1) no fentanyl group, (2) intermediate-dose fentanyl group (intent to administer between 1 and 150 μg epidural fentanyl), or (3) high-dose epidural fentanyl group (intent to administer > 150 μg epi-dural fentanyl). On postpartum day 1, the mother and a lactation consultant separately assessed whether the infant was experiencing difficulty breast-feeding, and a pediatrician assessed infant neurobehavior. All women were contacted 6 weeks postpartum to determine whether they were still breast-feeding.

Results.—Sixty women were randomly assigned to receive no fentanyl, 59 were randomly assigned to receive an intermediate dose, and 58 were ran-domly assigned to receive high-dose fentanyl. On postpartum day 1, women who were randomly assigned to receive high-dose fentanyl reported diffi-culty breast-feeding (n = 12, 21%) more often than women who were ran-domly assigned to receive an intermediate fentanyl dose (n = 6, 10%), or no fentanyl (n = 6, 10%), although this did not reach statistical significance (*P* = 0.09). There was also no significant difference among groups in breast-feeding difficulty based on the lactation consultant's evaluation (40% diffi-culty in each group; *P* = 1.0). Neurobehavior scores were lowest in the in-fants of women who were randomly assigned to receive more than 150 μg fentanyl (*P* = 0.03). At 6 weeks postpartum, more women who were ran-domly assigned to high-dose epidural fentanyl were not breast-feeding (n = 10, 17%) than women who were randomly assigned to receive either an in-termediate fentanyl dose (n = 3, 5%) or no fentanyl (n = 1, 2%) (*P* = 0.005).

Conclusions.—Among women who breast-fed previously, those who were randomly assigned to receive high-dose labor epidural fentanyl were more likely to have stopped breast-feeding 6 weeks postpartum than woman who were randomly assigned to receive less fentanyl or no fentanyl.

▶ Some, but not all, previous studies have shown an association of epidural labor analgesia with reduced breast-feeding (BF) duration.[1,2] A large recent prospective cohort study (n = 1280) found, after controlling for confounding factors, that women who received epidural analgesia were less likely to exclu-sively breast-feed in the first week and were more likely to stop BF in the first 24 weeks.[3] Mechanisms for this possible effect on BF include (1) selection ef-fect, that is, mothers who choose or need epidural analgesia are experiencing labor stress that inhibits lactogenesis II ("milk coming in"); or (2) pharmaco-logic inhibition of lactogenesis II that is caused by one or more epidural medi-cations; or (3) infant alertness, which is associated with BF behavior, is im-paired by either epidural medications or labor stress.[4,5] It will be critical to identify which, if any, of these factors is operative because management im-plications differ. Daily postpartum evaluation of BF through the first week of life using objective measures such as test weighing, and neurobehavioral as-sessment of the infant using a validated measure, will help clarify this di-lemma.[6] The results of Beilin et al's study should not be ignored or wished away. Future research should include the strong study design of this trial, but with more detailed and objective follow-up of BF outcomes for a longer period of time.

L. M. Furman, MD

References

1. Henderson JJ, Dickinson JE, Evans SF, McDonald SJ, Paech MJ. Impact of intrapartum epidural analgesia on breast feeding duration. *Aust N Z J Obstet Gynaecol.* 2003;43:372-377.
2. Chang ZM, Heaman MI. Epidural analgesia during labor and delivery: effects on the initiation and continuation of effective breastfeeding. *J Hum Lact.* 2005;21:305-314.
3. Torvaldsen S, Roberts CL, Simpson JM, Thompson JF, Ellwood DA. Intrapartum epidural analgesia and breastfeeding: a prospective cohort study. *Int Breastfeed J.* 2006;1:24.
4. Chen DC, Nommsen-Rivers L, Dewey KG, Lönnerdal B. Stress during labor and delivery and early lactation performance. *Am J Clin Nutr.* 1998;68:335-344.
5. Radzyminski S. Neurobehavioral functioning and breastfeeding behavior in the newborn. *J Obstet Gynecol Neonatal Nurs.* 2005;34:335-341.
6. Meier PP, Engstrom JL. Test weighing for term and premature infants is an accurate procedure. *Arch Dis Child Fetal Neonatal Ed.* 2007;92:F155-F156.

5 Infectious Disease and Immunology

Neonatal-Onset Multisystem Inflammatory Disease Responsive to Interleukin-1β Inhibition
Goldbach-Mansky R, Dailey NJ, Canna SW, et al (NIH, Bethesda, Md; Univ of North Carolina, Chapel Hill; Univ of Michigan, Ann Arbor; et al)
N Engl J Med 355:581-592, 2006   5–1

Background.—Neonatal-onset multisystem inflammatory disease is characterized by fever, urticarial rash, aseptic meningitis, deforming arthropathy, hearing loss, and mental retardation. Many patients have mutations in the cold-induced autoinflammatory syndrome 1 (*CIAS1*) gene, encoding cryopyrin, a protein that regulates inflammation.

Methods.—We selected 18 patients with neonatal-onset multisystem inflammatory disease (12 with identifiable *CIAS1* mutations) to receive anakinra, an interleukin-1–receptor antagonist (1 to 2 mg per kilogram of body weight per day subcutaneously). In 11 patients, anakinra was withdrawn at three months until a flare occurred. The primary end points included changes in scores in a daily diary of symptoms, serum levels of amyloid A and C-reactive protein, and the erythrocyte sedimentation rate from baseline to month 3 and from month 3 until a disease flare.

Results.—All 18 patients had a rapid response to anakinra, with disappearance of rash. Diary scores improved (P<0.001) and serum amyloid A (from a median of 174 mg to 8 mg per liter), C-reactive protein (from a median of 5.29 mg to 0.34 mg per deciliter), and the erythrocyte sedimentation rate decreased at month 3 (all P<0.001), and remained low at month 6. Magnetic resonance imaging showed improvement in cochlear and leptomeningeal lesions as compared with baseline. Withdrawal of anakinra uniformly resulted in relapse within days; retreatment led to rapid improvement. There were no drug-related serious adverse events.

Conclusions.—Daily injections of anakinra markedly improved clinical and laboratory manifestations in patients with neonatal-onset multisystem inflammatory disease, with or without *CIAS1* mutations.

▶ I must admit that, prior to the publication of this series, I was not familiar with neonatal-onset multisystem inflammatory disease, evidently also known as chronic infantile neurologic cutaneous articular syndrome, but then again the usual onset is the first 6 weeks of life and neonatologists are more focused only on the first 28 days of life. The manifestations appear to be fairly characteristic and identifiable and include, according to Goldbach-Mansky et al, the development of an urticarial rash within the first 6 weeks of life and a characteristic bony overgrowth predominantly involving the knees. CNS manifestations include chronic aseptic meningitis, increased intracranial pressure, cerebral atrophy, ventriculomegaly, and chronic papilledema, with associated optic nerve atrophy and loss of vision, mental retardation, seizures, and sensorineural hearing loss. Other manifestations include short stature, hepatosplenomegaly, leukocytosis, and elevations in serum levels of amyloid A and C-reactive protein and the erythrocyte sedimentation rate. It is intriguing that therapy based on the understanding of the underlying pathogenesis was successful and independent of the presence of the genetic mutation. Furthermore, when the therapy was withdrawn, the symptoms recurred. The duration of therapy was insufficient, however, to determine whether long-term treatment will prevent the onset of systemic amyloidosis.

A. A. Fanaroff, MD

The Adenosine System Selectively Inhibits TLR-Mediated TNF-α Production in the Human Newborn

Levy O, Coughlin M, Cronstein BN, et al (Children's Hosp, Boston; Harvard Med School; New York Univ)
J Immunol 177:1956-1966, 2006   5–2

Human newborns are susceptible to microbial infection and mount poor vaccine responses, yet the mechanisms underlying their susceptibility are incompletely defined. We have previously reported that despite normal basal expression of TLRs and associated signaling intermediates, human neonatal cord blood monocytes demonstrate severe impairment in TNF-α production in response to triacylated (TLR 2/1) and diacylated (TLR 2/6) bacterial lipopeptides (BLPs). We now demonstrate that in marked contrast, BLP-induced synthesis of IL-6, a cytokine with anti-inflammatory and Th2-polarizing properties, is actually greater in neonates than adults. Remarkably, newborn blood plasma confers substantially reduced BLP-induced monocyte synthesis of TNF-α, while preserving IL-6 synthesis, reflecting the presence in neonatal blood plasma of a soluble, low molecular mass inhibitory factor (<10 kDa) that we identify as adenosine, an endogenous purine metabolite with immunomodulatory properties. The neonatal adenosine system also inhibits TNF-α production in response to whole microbial particles known to express TLR2 agonist activity, including *Listeria monocytogenes*, *Escherichia coli* (that express BLPs), and zymosan particles. Selective inhibition of neonatal TNF-α production is due to the distinct neonatal adenosine system, including relatively high adenosine concentrations in neonatal blood plasma and heightened sensitivity of neonatal mononuclear cells to adenosine A3 receptor-mediated accumulation of cAMP, a second messenger that inhibits TLR-mediated TNF-α synthesis but preserves IL-6 production. We conclude that the distinct adenosine system of newborns polarizes TLR-mediated cytokine production during the perinatal period and may thereby modulate their innate and adaptive immune responses.

▶ Human newborns are susceptible to microbial infection and mount poor vaccine responses, yet the mechanisms underlying their susceptibility are incompletely defined. We have previously reported that despite normal basal expression of toll-like receptors (TLRs) and associated signaling intermediates, human neonatal cord blood monocytes demonstrate severe impairment in TNF-α production in response to triacylated (TLR 2/1) and diacylated (TLR 2/6) bacterial lipopeptides (BLPs). We now demonstrate that in marked contrast, BLP-induced synthesis of IL-6, a cytokine with anti-inflammatory and Th2 polarizing properties, is actually greater in neonates than in adults. Remarkably, newborn blood plasma confers substantially reduced BLP-induced monocyte synthesis of TNF-α, while preserving IL-6 synthesis, reflecting the presence in neonatal blood plasma of a soluble, low molecular mass inhibitory factor (<10 kDa) that we identify as adenosine, an endogenous purine metabolite with immunomodulatory properties. The neonatal adenosine system also inhibits TNF-α production in response to whole microbial particles known to express TLR2 agonist activity, including *Listeria monocytogenes*, *Escherichia coli* (that express BLPs), and zymosan particles. Selective inhibition of neonatal TNF-α production is due to the distinct neonatal adenosine system, including relatively high adenosine concentrations in neonatal blood plasma and heightened sensitivity of neonatal mononuclear cells to adenosine A3 receptor-mediated accumulation of cyclic adenosine monophosphate (cAMP), a second messenger that inhibits TLR-mediated TNF-α synthesis but preserves IL-6 production. We conclude that the distinct adenosine system of newborns polarizes TLR-mediated cytokine production during the perinatal period and may thereby modulate their innate and adaptive immune responses.

The adenosine system plays a vital role in situations of high energy consumption by cells and tissues. Endogenous adenosine may be pharmacologically affected by blocking cell receptors with methylxanthines (caffeine and theophylline) for the treatment of apnea of prematurity. Exogenous adenosine is used mainly in neonates to break supraventricular tachycardia, but may also be indicated to induce controlled and stable hypotension during anesthesia, to reduce after load in various forms of low cardiac output states, to cause platelet preservation during cardiopulmonary bypass. Levy et al add to our knowledge of the adenosine system and define its role in inhibiting TNF-α production, adding to the database as to why neonates are vulnerable to microbial infections.

A. A. Fanaroff, MD

Risk Factors for Invasive, Early-Onset *Escherichia coli* in the Era of Widespread Intrapartum Antibiotic Use

Schrag SJ, Hadler JL, Arnold KE, et al (Natl Ctr for Infectious Diseases, Atlanta, Ga; Connecticut Dept of Public Health, Hartford; Georgia Dept of Human Resources, Atlanta; et al)

Pediatrics 118:570-576, 2006   5–3

Objective.—The goal was to evaluate risk factors for invasive *Escherichia coli* infections in the first week of life (early onset), focusing on the role of intrapartum antibiotic use.

Methods.—We conducted a retrospective case-control study. Between 1997 and 2001, case infants, defined as infants <7 days of age with *E coli* isolated from blood or cerebrospinal fluid, were identified in selected counties of California, Georgia, and Connecticut by the Active Bacterial Core Surveillance/Emerging Infections Program Network. Control infants (N = 1212) were identified from a labor and delivery record review of a stratified random sample of live births at the same hospitals in 1998 and 1999.

Results.—Surveillance identified 132 *E coli* cases, including 68 ampicillin-resistant cases. The case fatality rate was 16% (21 of 132 cases). Two thirds of case infants were preterm, and 49% (64 of 132 infants) were born at ≤33 weeks of gestation. Fifty-three percent of case mothers (70 of 132 mothers) received intrapartum antibiotic therapy; 70% of those received ampicillin or penicillin. Low gestational age (≤33 weeks), intrapartum fever, and membrane rupture of ≥18 hours were associated with increased odds of early-onset *E coli* infection. Results were similar when case subjects were limited to those infected with ampicillin-resistant strains. Exposure to any intrapartum antibiotic treatment, β-lactam antibiotic treatment, or ≥4 hours of intrapartum antibiotic therapy was associated with increased odds of *E coli* infection and ampicillin-resistant infection in univariate analyses. Among preterm infants, intrapartum antibiotic exposure did not remain associated with either outcome in multivariable models. Among term infants, exposure to ≥4 hours of intrapartum antibiotic therapy was associated with decreased odds of early-onset *E coli* infection.

Conclusions.—Exposure to intrapartum antibiotic therapy did not increase the odds of invasive, early-onset *E coli* infection. Intrapartum antibiotic therapy was effective in preventing *E coli* infection only among term infants.

▶ The debate over the potential adverse effects of intrapartum antibiotic exposure to the neonate has been waged since the near-universal adoption of intrapartum antibiotic prophylaxis (IAP) to treat Group B streptococcal (GBS) disease in the late 1990s. Much of this attention has focused on a possible increase in early-onset *Escherichia coli* sepsis in substitution for a decline in early-onset GBS sepsis. In fact, several reports documented this increase in both *E coli* early-onset sepsis (EOS)[1,2] and in ampicillin-resistance among pathogenic strains of *E coli*[3-5] in the era of widespread IAP, particularly in very low birthweight (VBLW; BW <1500 g) neonates.

In this retrospective, multicenter, case-control study, the authors add to this body of literature by evaluating the use of intrapartum antibiotics as a potential risk factor for invasive and/or ampicillin-resistant neonatal *E coli* infections in the first week of life. Cases of *E coli* bacteremia and meningitis were identified and compared with unmatched, noninfected controls. In a separate analysis, ampicillin-resistant cases of *E coli* infection were identified and compared with cases of ampicillin-sensitive *E coli* (Table 2 of the original article). Intrapartum antibiotic exposure did not increase the odds of invasive, *E coli* infection in the first week of life nor did it increase the odds of infection with a resistant strain of *E coli* in either the term or preterm (<37 weeks' gestation) population (Table 3 of the original article).

Despite these findings, the controversy regarding the possible adverse effect of intrapartum antibiotic exposure on the VLBW neonate continues. Previous studies have focused on the rise of *E coli* EOS,[1,2] the prevalence of ampicillin-resistant *E coli*,[1,5] and an association between IAP and ampicillin-resistance exclusively in this population,[2] particularly in the first 3 days of life. Unfortunately, given discrepancies in the definition of "early-onset" and the absence of a separate analysis of VLBW neonates, we are unable to compare previous findings with those from the current study.

As many as 65% of women with threatened preterm delivery may be exposed to intrapartum antibiotics[6] and therefore continued prospective surveillance as to the possible impact of these practices on the organisms responsible for invasive neonatal infection and their antibiotic resistance patterns are warranted. Despite conflicting data as to the effect of intrapartum antibiotic exposure on infection in the preterm population, particular attention should be paid to the indication for, choice of, and duration of use of IAP for threatened preterm delivery.

M. J. Bizzarro, MD

References

1. Stoll BJ, Hansen NI, Higgins RD, et al. Very low birth weight preterm infants with early onset neonatal sepsis: the predominance of gram-negative infections continues in the National Institute of Child Health and Human Development Neonatal Research Network, 2002-2003. *Pediatr Infect Dis J.* 2005;24:635-639.
2. Stoll BJ, Hansen N, Fanaroff AA, et al. Changes in the pathogens causing early-onset sepsis in very-low-birth-weight infants. *N Engl J Med.* 2002;347:240-247.
3. Alarcon A, Peña P, Salas S, Sancha M, Omeñaca F. Neonatal early onset *Escherichia coli* sepsis: trends in the incidence and antimicrobial resistance in the era of intrapartum antimicrobial prophylaxis. *Pediatr Infect Dis J.* 2004;23:295-299.
4. Hyde TB, Hilger TM, Reingold A, et al. Trends in incidence and antimicrobial resistance of early-onset sepsis: population-based surveillance in San Francisco and Atlanta. *Pediatrics.* 2002;110:690-695.
5. Cordero L, Rau R, Taylor D, Ayers LW. Enteric gram-negative bacilli bloodstream infections: 17 years' experience in a neonatal intensive care unit. *Am J Infect Control.* 2004;32:189-195.
6. Stoll BJ, Hansen N. Infections in VLBW infants: studies from the NICHD neonatal research network. *Semin Perinatol.* 2003;27:293-301.

Impact of Staffing on Bloodstream Injections in the Neonatal Intensive Care Unit

Cimiotti JP, Haas J, Saiman L, et al (Univ of Pennsylvania, Philadelphia; Columbia Univ, New York)
Arch Pediatr Adolesc Med 160:832-836, 2006   5–4

Objective.—To examine the association between registered nurse staffing and healthcare-associated bloodstream infections in infants in the neonatal intensive care unit (NICU).

Design.—Prospective cohort study.

Setting.—Two level III-IV NICUs in New York, NY, from March 1, 2001, through January 31, 2003.

Participants.—A total of 2675 infants admitted to the NICUs for more than 48 hours and all registered nurses who worked in the same NICUs during the study period.

Intervention.—Hours of care provided by registered nurses.

Main Outcome Measure.—Time to first episode of healthcare-associated bloodstream infection.

Results.—A total of 224 infants had an infection that met the study definition of healthcare-associated bloodstream infection. In a multivariate analysis, after controlling for infants' intrinsic and extrinsic risk factors, a greater number of hours of care provided by registered nurses in NICU 2 was associated with a decreased risk of bloodstream infection in these infants (hazard ratio, 0.21; 95% confidence interval, 0.06-0.79).

Conclusion.—Our findings suggest that registered nurse staffing is associated with the risk of bloodstream infection in infants in the NICU.

▶ Healthcare-associated infections (HAI) are estimated to account for approximately 90,000 deaths and 2 million infections per year, worldwide. In addition, approximately $45 billion dollars in excess healthcare are spent per year as a result of HAI.[1] Among other causes, understaffing caused by a national nursing shortage, and the subsequent increased workload on employed registered nurses can increase this burden.[2]

The NICU population is at extremely high risk of HAI. Preterm neonates are at particular risk secondary to immaturity of the immune system, an ineffective skin barrier, prolonged hospitalization, and the use and prolonged need for invasive support apparatus. In this study, the authors investigated the impact of registered nurse staffing on healthcare-associated bacteremia in 2 high-volume and acuity NICUs. This was the first prospective study of its kind performed in the setting of the NICU. After controlling for several other major risk factors for neonatal infection, the authors observed that, in 1 NICU, appropriate staffing (ie, a higher number of hours of care provided by registered nurses) was associated with a decreased risk of healthcare-associated bloodstream infections.

The emergence of HAI in hospitalized patients is a multifactorial process. In preterm neonates, there are several intrinsic and extrinsic factors involved, some of which (ie, prematurity) are beyond the control of the caregiver. It is therefore important to identify those contributory practices at our individual institutions that can be improved on. Although the shortage of registered nurses continues to be a major healthcare dilemma, efforts should be directed not only at increasing this workforce, but at minimizing the impact of HAI through the improved education of the current staff (ie, regarding proper hand hygiene techniques) and improvements in the working environment.

M. J. Bizzarro, MD

References

1. Weinstein RA. Nosocomial infection update. *Emerg Infect Dis.* 1998;4:416-420.
2. Stone PW, Clarke SP, Cimiotti J, Correa-de-Araujo. Nurses' working conditions: implications for infectious disease. *Emerg Infect Dis.* 2004;10:1984-1989.

Community-Acquired *Staphylococcus aureus* Infections in Term and Near-Term Previously Healthy Neonates
Fortunov RM, Hulten KG, Hammerman WA, et al (Baylor College of Medicine, Houston)
Pediatrics 118:874-881, 2006

5–5

Background.—Community-acquired, methicillin-resistant *Staphylococcus aureus* infections are increasing among children.

Objective.—Our goal is to describe the clinical presentation of neonatal community-acquired *S aureus* disease and provide molecular analyses of the infecting isolates.

Patients and Methods.—We retrospectively reviewed the demographics and hospital course of term and near-term previously healthy neonates, ≤30 days of age, with community-acquired *S aureus* infections presenting after nursery discharge between August 2001 and March 2005 at Texas Children's Hospital. Prospectively collected isolates were characterized by pulsed-field gel electrophoresis, staphylococcal cassette chromosome *mec* type, and the presence of PVL genes.

Results.—Of 89 *S aureus* infections, 61 were methicillin-resistant *S aureus*; *S aureus* infections increased each year. Methicillin-resistant *S aureus* infections increased from 10 of 20 to 30 of 36 infections from 2002 to 2004. Most subjects, 65 of 89, were male. Symptoms began at 7 to 12 days of age for 26 of 45 male infants with methicillin-resistant *S aureus*. Most infections, 77 of 89, involved skin and soft tissue; 28 of 61 methicillin-resistant *S aureus* versus 7 of 28 methicillin-susceptible *S aureus* infections required drainage. Invasive manifestations included shock, musculoskeletal and urinary tract infection, perinephric abscess, bacteremia, empyema/lung abscess, and a death. Maternal *S aureus* or skin-infection history occurred with 13 of 61 methicillin-resistant *S aureus* versus 1 of 28 methicillin-susceptible *S aureus* infections. The predominant community clone, USA300 (PVL genes +), accounted for 55 of 57 methicillin-resistant *S aureus* and 3 of 25 methicillin-susceptible *S aureus* isolates.

Conclusions.—Community-acquired methicillin-resistant *S aureus* is a substantial and increasing proportion of *S aureus* infections in previously healthy neonates. Male infants 7 to 12 days of age are affected most often. Neonatal community-acquired *S aureus* infection may be associated with concurrent maternal infection. USA300 is the predominant clone among these neonatal isolates in our region.

▶ I have worried about community-acquired methicillin-resistant *S aureus* for almost 9 years. For the first years, I was an observer of an evolving epidemic. I eagerly read every report from different parts of the country. There were cases of children dying in Minnesota and South Dakota. There were reports of skin and soft tissue infections from Texas, Chicago, and Los Angeles. I knew it would eventually come to Cleveland, but when? In the months preceding the epidemic's arrival in Cleveland, I was like a crazy fortune-teller, announcing to anyone that would listen that this strain would come here; but nobody seemed interested. I gave a talk in 2003 to general pediatricians in Cleveland about emerging resistance. The comments were consistent regarding the community-acquired methicillin-resistant *S aureus* section of the talk. I was told this was "not relevant to my practice" and "why worry about Texas." Then it finally arrived, first noted by local surgeons, including my husband, describing "spider bites that had to be drained." The pockets of pus and pockets of patients grew, first from the southwestern and eastern areas of Cleveland, and now from all areas. First, it was contact with returning soldiers or athletes . . . now it's anyone, anytime. Even the smallest patients are affected. The circle is complete. The last group of patients are reported on in this *Pediatrics* article: healthy, newborn babies, relatively untouched by medicine, except for some, by the hands of health care workers. No longer are there any risk groups for this infection. Some of the moms had infections, but many did not. In 2007, it can be any patient, anytime. What will we do about it? We will remind ourselves to wash our hands when caring for patients. We will try to answer some of the questions that this study poses, such as why little boys are affected more than little girls. This study has given us more pieces of this ever-enlarging puzzle, coaxing us to find their places.

C. Hoyen, MD

Methicillin-Resistant *Staphylococcus aureus* Colonization and Its Association with Infection Among Infants Hospitalized in Neonatal Intensive Care Units
Huang Y-C, Chou Y-H, Su L-H, et al (Chang Gung Univ, Kweishan, Taiwan)
Pediatrics 118:469-474, 2006   5–6

Objectives.—We conducted this study to assess the rate of methicillin-resistant *Staphylococcus aureus* colonization and its association with infection among infants hospitalized in methicillin-resistant *S aureus*–endemic NICUs.

Methods.—Between March 2003 and February 2004, surveillance culture specimens from the nares, postauricular areas, axillae, and umbilicus of infants admitted to the NICUs at a children's hospital in Taiwan were obtained weekly for the detection of methicillin-resistant *S aureus*. All colonized and clinical isolates from each study infant with methicillin-resistant *S aureus* infection were genotyped with pulsed-field gel electrophoresis, with *Sma*1 digestion, and compared.

Results.—A total of 783 infants were included in this study. Methicillin-resistant *S aureus* colonization was detected for 323 infants during their NICU stays, with detection with the first 2 samples for 89%. Nares and umbilicus were the 2 most common sites of initial colonization. Methicillin-resistant *S aureus* colonization was associated significantly with premature birth (≤28 weeks) and low birth weight (≤1500 g), and infants with colonization had a significantly higher rate of methicillin-resistant *S aureus* infection, compared with those without colonization (26% vs 2%). Methicillin-resistant *S aureus* colonization was noted for 84 of 92 infants with methicillin-resistant *S aureus* infections. Of the 68 episodes with previous colonization and isolates available for genotyping analysis, colonized and clinical isolates were indistinguishable in 63 episodes, highly related in 2 episodes, and distinct in 3 episodes.

Conclusions.—More than 40% of the hospitalized infants were colonized with methicillin-resistant *S aureus* during their stay in methicillin-resistant *S aureus*–endemic NICUs; this was associated significantly with methicillin-resistant *S aureus* infection. Most infants with methicillin-resistant *S aureus* infections had previous colonization with an indistinguishable strain.

▶ Seek and ye shall find, if you are looking for methicillin-resistant *S aureus* (MRSA) colonization of premature infants in NICUs in Taiwan. That 41% of all their babies were colonized some time in their NICU stay is remarkable by most United States standards and seems to be higher than their local community colonization rate. Based on their surveillance of health care workers, it seems that little, if any, of this "epidemic" is attributable to the strains carried by the health care workers themselves. As the authors point out, some early colonization may be coming from exposure during delivery, but unless the perineal colonization rate is exceedingly high, then it is likely that most of the colonization comes from cross-contamination within the NICU environment. It is not surprising that the highest rates of colonization occur in the smaller, more premature and, presumably, more immunocompromised babies. It would be interesting to study the association of other clinical factors, such as the duration of central catheters or breast-feeding, with colonization and infection rates. As expected, a markedly higher MRSA infection rate was seen in those babies who were colonized, although only 20% of the positive clinical isolates were blood samples. More than half of the clinical isolates used to define infection were sputum/endotracheal tube aspirates, which many would not even sample or accept as markers of pneumonia or infection. In any case, it remains to be seen whether routine surveillance and determination of colonization status leads to any treatment strategies (eg, cohorting or decolonizing with mupirocin or other drug therapy) that lower the rate of subsequent MRSA infections.

W. D. Rhine, MD

Multicenter Study to Assess Safety and Efficacy of INH-A21, a Donor-Selected Human Staphylococcal Immunoglobulin, for Prevention of Nosocomial Infections in Very Low Birth Weight Infants
Bloom B, for the INH-A21 Phase II Study Team (Wesley Med Ctr, Wichita, Kan; et al)
Pediatr Infect Dis J 24:858-866, 2005   5–7

Background.—Prophylactic administration of intravenous immunoglobulin has been inconsistent in reducing the risk of sepsis in very low birth weight (VLBW) infants presumably because of varying titers of organism specific IgG antibodies. INH-A21 is an intravenous immunoglobulin from donors with high titers of antistaphylococcal antibodies. This dose-ranging study explored safety and preliminary activity of INH-A21 for prevention of staphylococcal sepsis in VLBW infants.

Methods.—This was a multicenter, double blind, group-sequential study. Infants with birth weights 500–1250 g were randomized to receive up to 4 doses of placebo, 250 mg/kg, 500 mg/kg or 750 mg/kg INH-A21. Safety and frequencies of sepsis were compared across treatment groups.

Results.—All treatment groups had similar mean gestational age, birth weight, Apgar score and maternal use of antibiotics. Randomizations to 250 mg/kg (N = 94) and 500 mg/kg (N = 96) doses were terminated after interim analyses demonstrated a low probability of finding a difference when compared with placebo. Infants randomized to the INH-A21 750 mg/kg group (N = 157) had fewer episodes of *Staphylococcus aureus* sepsis [relative risk (RR), 0.37; 95% confidence interval (CI), 0.12–1.12; $P = 0.14$], candidemia (RR 0.34; 95% CI 0.09–1.22; $P = 0.09$) and mortality (RR 0.64; 95% CI 0.25–1.61; $P = 0.27$) when compared with the placebo-treated cohort (N = 158). No dose-related trends were observed for adverse events or morbidities associated with prematurity.

Conclusions.—INH-A21 750 mg/kg demonstrated potential to reduce sepsis caused by *S. aureus*, candidemia and mortality in VLBW infants. Although statistical significance was not reached, based on the magnitude of the estimated differences, the efficacy and safety of INH-A21 750 mg/kg should be evaluated in an adequately powered, well-controlled study.

▶ Neonatal sepsis is a significant problem in low-birth-weight and very-low-birth-weight infants. The Neonatal Research Network estimates that about 21% of premature infants will have blood culture–positive sepsis, with gram-positive organisms being the most common cause.[1] Previous studies of intravenous immunoglobulin (IVIG) have failed to show a consistent reduction in the risk of sepsis or improvement of neonatal outcomes. This multicenter, placebo-controlled study examines the effect of INH A21, an immunoglobulin product containing high polyclonal antibody titers against staphylococcal fibrinogen-binding proteins thought to have activity against both *Staphylococcus aureus* and coagulase-negative staphylococci. This study fails to demonstrate a significant reduction in staphylococcal or other nosocomial infections, or in the occurrence of other morbidities, the length of stay in the neonatal ICU, or the mortality rate.

It seems intuitive that providing high titers of antibodies against staphylococcal organisms should prevent infection. Monthly infusions of standard gammaglobulin (IVIG) products have been very effective in preventing serious bacterial infections in patients with antibody deficiency syndromes. A small but significant reduction of 3% to 4% in neonatal sepsis was demonstrated in a meta-analysis of studies of prophylactic IVIG, but the mortality rate was not reduced.[2] Thus, the benefit is marginal in this population. Hyperimmune globulins containing high titers of antibody against a particular pathogen have been effective in preventing infections with varicella and hepatitis B, but their effectiveness is less robust with other pathogens such as respiratory syncytial virus (RSV) and cytomegalovirus. A therapeutic effect with high-titer IVIG for infections with *Haemophilus influenzae* required antibody titers 100 to 1000 times higher than that given to prevent infection.[3] The level of antibody required to prevent infections with bacterial pathogens such as staphylococci and *E coli* is not known.

Monoclonal antibody preparations against RSV have been very effective in reducing the rate of infection, but polyclonal hyperimmune globulins may have some advantages over monoclonal antibodies. They may contain a more diverse population of antibodies capable of recognizing different microbial epitopes. The lack of effect with the polyclonal antistaphylococcal IgG in this study may be attributed to several possible mechanisms. Although pharmacokinetic studies showed similar titers of IgG compared with other IVIG products, the dosing used in this study may not deliver enough antigen-specific antibody, or the antibody may be cleared too rapidly from the circulation to provide a sustained benefit. Specific antibody against other surface molecules may be more critical in host defenses against staphylococci. Last, the antibody affinity for the staphylococcal antigens may not be high enough to provide for effective clearance of the organism from the circulation.

This study provides additional evidence that passive antibody protection is not likely to be the magic bullet to prevent neonatal sepsis. However, the increasing prevalence of MRSA and other antibiotic-resistant strains of bacteria underscore the importance of refining antibody-based therapies.

L. Kobrynski, MD, MPH

References

1. Stoll BJ, Hansen N, Fanaroff AA, et al. Late-onset sepsis in very low birth weight neonates: The experience of the NICHD Neonatal Research Network. *Pediatrics.* 2002;110:285-291.
2. Ohlsson A, Lacy JB. Intravenous immunoglobulin for preventing infection in preterm and/or low-birth-weight infants. *Cochrane Database Syst Rev.* 2004;1: CD000361.

3. Casadevall A. Antibody-based therapy for emerging infectious disease. *Emerg Infect Dis.* 1996;2:200-208.

Neonatal Candidiasis Among Extremely Low Birth Weight Infants: Risk Factors, Mortality Rates, and Neurodevelopmental Outcomes at 18 to 22 Months

Benjamin DK Jr, for the National Institute of Child Health and Human Development Neonatal Research Network (Duke Clinical Research Inst, Durham, NC; et al)
Pediatrics 117:84-92, 2006   5–8

Background.—Neonatal candidiasis is associated with substantial morbidity and mortality rates. Neurodevelopmental follow-up data for a large multicenter cohort have not been reported.

Methods.—Data were collected prospectively for neonates born at <1000 g at National Institute of Child Health and Human Development-sponsored Neonatal Research Network sites between September 1, 1998, and December 31, 2001. Uniform follow-up evaluations, including assessments of mental and motor development with the Bayley Scales of Infant Development II, were completed for all survivors at corrected ages of 18 to 22 months. We evaluated risk factors for the development of neonatal candidiasis, responses to antifungal therapy, and the association between candidiasis and subsequent morbidity and death.

Results.—The cohort consisted of 4579 infants; 320 of 4579 (7%) developed candidiasis; 307 of 320 had *Candida* isolated from blood, 27 of 320 had *Candida* isolated from cerebrospinal fluid, and 13 (48%) of 27 of those with meningitis had negative blood cultures. In multivariate analysis of risk factors on day of life 3, birth weight, cephalosporins, gender, and lack of enteral feeding were associated with development of candidiasis. After diagnosis, most neonates had multiple positive cultures despite antifungal therapy, and 10% of neonates had candidemia for $\geq$14 days. Death or neurodevelopmental impairment (NDI) was observed for 73% of extremely low birth weight infants who developed candidiasis. Death and NDI rates were greater for infants who had delayed removal or replacement of central catheters (>1 day after initiation of antifungal therapy), compared with infants whose catheters were removed or replaced promptly.

Conclusions.—Blood cultures were negative for approximately one half of the infants with *Candida* meningitis. Persistent candidiasis was common. Delayed catheter removal was associated with increased death and NDI rates.

▶ The National Institute of Child Health and Human Development–sponsored Neonatal Network sites provide a wealth of data regarding a host of neonatal disorders. This study addresses an important cause of nosocomial infection in neonates born at less than 1000 g. A total of 320 (7%) of 4579 infants prospectively enrolled in a database between 1998 and 2001 contracted systemic candidiasis. The peak age of infection was between 11 and 20 days, although some were infected as early as 3 days and as late as 3 months of age. The authors acknowledge that they underestimated the rate of infection because fungal cultures are relatively insensitive, urine culture data were not included, and indirect evidence of fungal infection (eg, abnormal ophthalmoscopic examination and results of echocardiograms) were not considered.

The bloodstream was the predominant site of infection (96%), but 27 neonates had *Candida* isolated from cerebrospinal fluid. Interestingly, almost half of those with *Candida* meningitis had negative blood cultures. *Candida albicans* (~50%) and *C. parapsilosis* (~42%) were the most common species isolated. Although infection eventually was microbiologically eradicated in most infants, the mean duration of positive blood cultures was 3 days, and 10% of infants had candidemia persisting for more than 14 days. Death or long-term NDI occurred in 73% of the infected cohort. Adverse outcomes were greater for infants who had delayed removal of central catheters after beginning antifungal therapy compared with those who had prompt removal of catheters.

The authors appropriately emphasize the substantial morbidity and mortality rates of neonatal fungal infections, underscoring the need for improved strategies for prevention, enhanced diagnostics, and improved therapeutics.

C. G. Prober, MD

Hyperglycaemia as a possible marker of invasive fungal infection in preterm neonates

Manzoni P, Castagnola E, Mostert M, et al (Ospedale S Anna, Turin, Italy; "G Gaslini" Children's Hosp, Genoa, Italy; Univ of Turin, Italy)
Acta Paediatr 95:486-493, 2006   5–9

Aim.—The incidence of invasive fungal infection in preterm newborns is rising steadily. Early recognition and treatment are imperative, but diagnosis is difficult as data from microbiological investigations are often poor, and clinical and laboratory signs do not help in differentiating bacterial from fungal infections. We evaluated whether glucose intolerance could represent a possible surrogate marker predictor of invasive fungal infection in preterm neonates.

Methods.—We performed a case-control study on neonates with birthweight less than 1250 g admitted to our tertiary-level unit during the years 1998–2004 ($n = 383$), comparing those with invasive fungal infection ($n = 45$, group A) to matched controls with late-onset sepsis caused by bacterial agents ($n = 46$, group B). We investigated in both groups the occurrence of hyperglycaemia (serum glycaemia > 215 mg/dl, i.e. 12 mmol/l) in the first month of life, and its temporal relationship with the episodes of sepsis.

Results.—Hyperglycaemia occurred significantly more often in group A (21/45, 46.6%) than in group B neonates (11/46, 23.9%) (OR 1.95, 95% CI 1.235–4.432, $p = 0.008$). Moreover, in 19 of 21 (90.4%) neonates with hyperglycaemia in group A, the carbohydrate intolerance episode typically

occurred 72 h prior to the onset of invasive fungal infection; in contrast, no temporal relationship was found in neonates with bacterial sepsis ($p = 0.002$). Correction of hyperglycaemia was successfully achieved in all neonates of both groups, with no significant differences in the number of days of insulin treatment needed to normalize glycaemia ($p = 0.15$).

Conclusions.—Hyperglycaemia is significantly more frequent in neonates who subsequently develop fungal rather than bacterial late-onset sepsis, with a typical 3-d interval. We suggest that a preterm neonate whose birthweight is less than 1250 g in its first month of life should be carefully evaluated for systemic fungal infection whenever signs of carbohydrate intolerance occur.

▶ This case-control study supports the association between invasive fungal infection (IFI) and hyperglycemia in neonates with birth weight less than 1250 g. Compared with matched controls with late-onset sepsis caused by bacterial agents, the neonates with IFI had significantly higher rates of hyperglycemia, which occurred within the first month of life. Another interesting finding is that the carbohydrate intolerance typically occurred 3 days before the IFI, suggesting that hyperglycemia might be a factor contributing to IFI, perhaps because of the importance of glucose in yeast growth and nutrition. Because of the study design, this conclusion remains speculative but nonetheless provocative. If it could be achieved, better glucose control might contribute to a decreased incidence of IFI. This study has other difficulties as well, not different from other investigations of IFI. For example, the definition of IFI, although reasonable, probably contributes to underestimation of the incidence because yeast has a tropism for tissues and it is a low load condition in bodily fluids. Therefore, ascertainment of IFI by culturing from various sites, including blood, urine, CSF, or intravascular catheter tip, could be insufficient in some proportion of cases. Improved diagnostic technologies are required to improve ascertainment of cases. Nonetheless, hyperglycemia could be used as a clue that, in a deteriorating infant, IFI might be present. Whether the association represents some manner of causation or consequence of the condition remains uncertain. Nonetheless, until better diagnostic tests are available, all clues should be considered seriously.

D. K. Stevenson, MD

The Association of Third-Generation Cephalosporin Use and Invasive Candidiasis in Extremely Low Birth-Weight Infants
Cotten CM, for the National Institute for Child Health and Human Development Neonatal Research Network (Duke Univ, Durham, NC; et al)
Pediatrics 118:717-722, 2006   5–10

Objectives.—Previous studies have shown that incidence of invasive candidiasis varies substantially among centers, and previous use of broad-spectrum antibiotics is a risk factor for candidiasis in extremely low birth-weight infants. Differences in center practices, such as antibiotic strategies and the effects of these strategies on center incidence of candidiasis, are not reflected in assessments of an individual's risk of candidiasis. We evaluated the relationship between empirical antibiotic practices for extremely low birth-weight infants and center incidence of candidiasis.

Methods.—We studied a cohort of extremely low birth-weight infants who survived ≥72 hours and were admitted to 1 of 12 tertiary centers between 1998 and 2001. Multivariable logistic regression was used to validate previous broad-spectrum antibiotics use as a risk factor for subsequent candidiasis in individual infants. We calculated correlation coefficients to assess the relationship between center incidence of candidiasis with antibiotic practice patterns.

Results.—There were 3702 infants from 12 centers included, and 284 (7.7%) developed invasive candidiasis. Broad-spectrum antibiotics use was associated with candidiasis for individual infants. Center candidiasis incidence ranged from 2.4% to 20.4%. Center incidence of candidiasis was correlated with average broad-spectrum antibiotics use per infant and average use of broad-spectrum antibiotics with negative cultures per infant.

Conclusions.—Center incidences of invasive candidiasis differ substantially, and antibiotic practice differences are possible contributors to center variation in candidiasis risk.

▶ Invasive infection in preterm neonates is associated with an increased risk of morbidity and mortality.[1] Candidiasis can be particularly debilitating to this population, often resulting in death or survival with neurodevelopmental impairment.[2] In contrast to the majority of organisms responsible for nosocomial infection in preterm neonates (eg, coagulase-negative *Staphylococcus*), there is significant center-to-center variation in the prevalence of neonatal candidiasis. Differences in center practices likely contribute to the inconsistencies observed.

One possible risk factor for candidiasis in preterm neonates is the frequent, empiric use of broad-spectrum antibiotics. Approximately one third of very low birthweight (VLBW, BW <1500 g) neonates undergo at least 1 evaluation for the presence of invasive infection after the third day of life, and more than half receive at least 1 course of antibiotics in the postnatal period.[1] To date, no consensus statement or guidelines exist for the choice or duration of empiric antibiotic therapy to initiate while awaiting the results of diagnostic testing. As a result, a great deal of variability exists among centers, and individual neonatologists, as to the choice and duration of empiric antimicrobial therapy. For some, this treatment includes the use of broad-spectrum antibiotics such as the third generation cephalosporins.[3] There are data to indicate that repeated, prolonged exposure to broad-spectrum antimicrobials can result in an increase in the prevalence of virulent, antibiotic-resistant organisms in the NICU, including species of *Candida*.[4]

The report by Cotten et al correlates center incidence of candidiasis with the average use of broad-spectrum antibiotics per infant. These findings stress the need for individual institutions to conduct ongoing surveillance of healthcare-associated infections in an attempt to identify potential associated risk factors. In centers with a high incidence of candidiasis, particular attention should be paid to the identification and improvement of center practices, such as the frequent use of third generation cephalosporins, which may contribute to the problem.

M. J. Bizzarro, MD

References

1. Stoll BJ, Hansen N, Fanaroff AA, et al. Late-onset sepsis in very low birth weight neonates: the experience of the NICHD Neonatal Research Network. *Pediatrics.* 2002;110:285-291.
2. Benjamin DK Jr, Stoll BJ, Fanaroff AA, et al. Neonatal candidiasis among extremely low birth weight infants: risk factors, mortality rates, and neurodevelopmental outcomes at 18 to 22 months. *Pediatrics.* 2006;117:84-92.
3. Rubin LG, Sánchez PJ, Siegel J, Levine G, Saiman L, Jarvis WR, for the Pediatric Prevention Network. Evaluation and treatment of neonates with suspected late-onset sepsis: a survey of neonatologists' practices. *Pediatrics.* 2002;110:e42.
4. Saiman L, Ludington E, Dawson JD, et al. Risk factors for *Candida* species colonization of neonatal intensive care unit patients. *Pediatr Infect Dis J.* 2001;20: 1119-1124.

Medical and Economic Impact of a Respiratory Syncytial Virus Outbreak in a Neonatal Intensive Care Unit

Halasa NB, Williams JV, Wilson GJ, et al (Vanderbilt Univ, Nashville, Tenn)
Pediatr Infect Dis J 24:1040-1044, 2005   5–11

Background.—Respiratory syncytial virus (RSV) causes frequent nosocomial outbreaks in general pediatric wards but is less commonly reported in neonatal intensive care units (NICUs). We investigated an outbreak of RSV infection in a NICU and its impact on health care delivery, outcomes and costs.

Methods.—Retrospective chart review was performed after an RSV outbreak occurred in the NICU. A case was defined as an infant with a nasopharyngeal aspirate positive for RSV by viral culture. Nucleotide sequencing of the isolates was done to determine relatedness. Hospital bills for all RSV culture-positive infants were reviewed.

Results.—Nine infants (mean age, 34 days; mean birth weight, 1757 g; and mean estimated gestational age 31 weeks and 5 days) were infected with RSV subgroup B during this outbreak. By nucleotide sequencing, the isolates were identical. Clinical manifestations included cough, congestion, increased oxygen requirement, apnea and respiratory failure. The 5 infants requiring intubation had a significantly lower mean birth weight (1301 g versus 2328 g, $P = 0.027$), mean estimated gestational age (28 weeks and 5 days versus 35 weeks and 2 days, $P = 0.014$) and mean weight at onset of symptoms (2093 g versus 2989 g, $P = 0.049$) than the 4 nonintubated infants. More than 1.15 million dollars in hospital charges were attributable to the outbreak. All infants survived.

Conclusion.—Infants in a NICU who develop cough, congestion or apnea should be tested for RSV and other common respiratory viruses during the winter respiratory season. Even in a closed NICU, nosocomial outbreaks of these viruses can occur and have a major effect on healthcare delivery, costs and outcomes.

▶ Epidemics in the NICU represent the worst nightmares for the NICU management team. Prevention of infection is a high priority and units are judged and ranked according to their nosocomial infection rates. It is fortunate that in this study, there were no fatalities, and the cost estimates are presented in financial, not in human tragedy, terms. It has been reassuring to have the ability to ameliorate RSV infections among the population born prematurely, and the mortality toll from RSV among infants with bronchopulmonary dysplasia has virtually disappeared with RSV prophylaxis. It is a select population that is receiving prophylaxis with the RSV monoclonal antibody. On a population basis, the burden of respiratory viruses is enormous as noted in the two articles cited below.[1,2]

Ehlken et al,[1] as part of the PRIDE Study Group, evaluated the economic burden of lower respiratory viral infections in Germany. They concluded that the treatment of lower respiratory tract infections caused by RSV, parainfluenza virus, and influenza virus in the first 3 years of life was in excess of 213 million Euros (approximately $280 million) annually. These data will be helpful in determining the cost benefits of preventive strategies for these viruses.

Paramore et al documented that the treatment of RSV infection-related illness represents a significant health care burden in the United States.[2] They estimated that in 2000, there were approximately 86,000 hospitalizations, 1.7 million office visits, 402,000 emergency room visits, and 236,000 hospital outpatient visits for children less than 5 years old that were attributable to RSV infection. Total annual direct medical costs for all RSV infection for children less than 5 years old were estimated at $652 million, including hospitalization ($394 million) and other medical encounters ($258 million). Therefore, if an ounce of prevention is worth a pound of cure, we need to challenge the scientists to develop a vaccine against RSV that can be applied to a broader segment of the population.

A. A. Fanaroff, MD

References

1. Ehlken B, Ihorst G, Lippert B, for the PRIDE Study Group. Economic impact of community acquired and nosocomial lower respiratory tract infections in young children in Germany. *Eur J Pediatr*. 2005;164:607-615.
2. Paramore LC, Ciuryla V, Ciesla G, Liu L. Economic impact of respiratory syncytial virus-related illness in the US: an analysis of national databases. *Pharmacoeconomics*. 2004;22:275-284.

Response of Preterm Newborns to Immunization With a Hexavalent Diphtheria–Tetanus–Acellular Pertussis–Hepatitis B Virus–Inactivated Polio and *Haemophilus influenzae* Type b Vaccine: First Experiences and Solutions to a Serious and Sensitive Issue

Omeñaca F, Garcia-Sicilia J, García-Corbeira P, et al (La Paz Hosp, Madrid; GlaxoSmithKline, Tres Cantos, Madrid)

Pediatrics 116:1292-1298, 2005   5–12

Objective.—Preterm infants are at increased risk from infections and should be vaccinated at the usual chronological age. The aim of the study was to evaluate the immunogenicity and reactogenicity of a hexavalent diphtheria–tetanus–acellular pertussis–hepatitis B virus–inactivated polio and *Haemophilus influenzae* type b (DTPa-HBV-IPV/Hib) vaccine in preterm infants.

Methods.—In a comparative trial, 94 preterm infants between 24 and 36 weeks (mean ± SD gestational age: 31.05 ± 3.45 weeks; mean birth weight: 1420 ± 600 g) and a control group of 92 full-term infants were enrolled to receive 3 doses of a DTPa-HBV-IPV/Hib vaccine at 2, 4, and 6 months. Immunogenicity was assessed in serum samples that were taken before and 4 weeks after primary vaccination. Evaluation of reactogenicity was based on diary cards.

Results.—All preterm ($n = 93$) and full-term ($n = 89$) infants who were included in the immunogenicity analysis had seroprotective titers to diphtheria; tetanus; and polio virus types 1, 2, and 3. The immune response to the Hib and hepatitis B components was lower in preterm than in full-term infants: 92.5% versus 97.8% and 93.4% versus 95.2%, respectively. Vaccine response rates for pertussis antigens were >98.9% in both study groups. Although most geometric mean titers were lower in preterm infants, titers were similar for pertussis, a major threat for premature infants. The vaccine was well tolerated, and there were no differences in reactogenicity between groups. Some extremely immature infants experienced transient cardiorespiratory events within the 72 hours after the first vaccination with no clinical repercussion.

Conclusions.—Preterm infants who were immunized with the hexavalent DTPa-HBV-IPV/Hib vaccine at 2, 4, and 6 months displayed good immune response to all antigens. The availability of this vaccine greatly facilitates the vaccination of premature infants.

▶ As the number of routine childhood immunizations rises, decreasing the number of injections an individual child receives has become an important part of improving the acceptability of vaccine regimens. Premature infants are less likely to receive their immunizations on time than term infants, and any strategy that improves vaccine acceptability might ameliorate this disparity. Vaccines that combine a number of unrelated antigens into one preparation are a means to this end, but some combination vaccines may have decreased immunogenicity. For instance, the introduction of a DTPa-HBV-IPV/Hib combination vaccine, which may result in lower anti-Hib antibody titers, was associated with a rise in invasive Hib disease in Britain near the turn of this century.[1-3] Premature infants, especially those born below about 30 weeks' gestation, mount lower antibody titers to a number of vaccine antigens, although there has been little evidence of clinically significant differences in protection from disease. The dual factors of combination vaccines and prematurity, however, may pose a higher risk for vaccine failure.

Omeñaca et al evaluated the immunogenicity of a hexavalent vaccine, combining DTPa, Hib, inactivated polio and hepatitis B antigens, given at 2, 4, and 6 months of age in a group of premature infants born between 24 and 36 weeks' gestation, with generally reassuring results. Similar numbers of premature and term infants achieved titers consistent with seroprotection to most of the vaccine antigens. There are some notable patterns in the responses, however. The authors point out that the proportion of infants achieving seroprotective titers to Hib (anti-polyribosylribitol [PRP] antibody levels ≥ 1 μg/mL) was fully 10% lower in premature than in term infants. The magnitude of the antibody response (as measured by the geometric mean titer [GMT] of antibody) to several of the vaccine antigens, most notably Hib, diphtheria, and polio serotypes 1 and 3, was lower in premature than in term infants. This could impact seroprotection as the antibody levels decay over time.

Premature newborn infants are at risk for late vaccine administration, lower vaccine immunogenicity, and more frequent and/or severe disease from vaccine-preventable pathogens. The art of medicine consists of balancing these conflicting factors to provide the broadest and most efficacious vaccine coverage possible for these infants. In the United States, a similar, pentavalent combination vaccine (which does not include the Hib component) is currently licensed and available, and might both save needle sticks and provide adequate immunogenicity. Caution would be justified, however, in using the full hexavalent vaccine (including Hib), particularly in the smallest premature infants.

C. T. D'Angio, MD

References

1. Eskola J, Ward J, Dagan R, Goldblatt D, Zepp F, Siegrist CA. Combined vaccination of *Haemophilus influenzae* type b conjugate and diphtheria-tetanus-pertussis containing acellular pertussis. *Lancet*. 1999;354:2063-2068.
2. Daum RS, Zenko CE, Given GZ, Ballanco GA, Parikh H, Germino K. Magnitude of interference after diphtheria-tetanus toxoids-acellular pertussis/*Haemophilus influenzae* type b capsular polysaccharide-tetanus vaccination is related to the number of doses administered. *J Infect Dis*. 2001;184:1293-1299.
3. McVernon J, Andrews N, Slack MP, Ramsay ME. Risk of vaccine failure after *Haemophilus influenzae* type b (Hib) combination vaccines with acellular pertussis. *Lancet*. 2003;361:1521-1523.

Potential costs and benefits of newborn screening for severe combined immunodeficiency
McGhee SA, Stiehm ER, McCabe ERB (UCLA, Los Angeles)
J Pediatr 147:603-608, 2005   5–13

Objective.—Severe combined immunodeficiency (SCID) is a rare, treatable disorder of the immune system. The incidence is unknown but may be more common than published estimates because infants frequently die of infection before diagnosis. SCID is a candidate for universal newborn screening, so there is a need to determine under which circumstances screening would be cost-effective.

Study design.—We assumed a screening program for SCID would use T-cell lymphopenia as the screening criterion and performed a cost-utility analysis comparing universal screening with screening only those with a family history of SCID.

Results.—Assuming society is willing to pay $50,000 for every quality-adjusted life-year saved, a SCID screening test that cost less than $5 with a false-negative rate of 0.9% and a false-positive rate of 0.4% would be considered cost-effective. A nationwide screening program would cost an additional $23.9 million per year for screening costs but would result in 760 years of life saved per year of screening. The cost to detect 1 case of SCID would be $485,000.

Conclusion.—SCID screening could result in a large benefit to detected individuals, making screening relatively cost-effective in spite of the low incidence of the disease. However, an adequate test is critical to cost-effectiveness.

▶ Severe combined immune deficiency (SCID) is considered a neonatal emergency, but it is often not diagnosed during the neonatal period because there are few physical findings at birth.[1,2] Unfortunately, in most cases, the diagnosis is not made until the infant has failure to thrive or life-threatening infection. Recent studies have provided important insights into SCID, in particular, that all forms of SCID are associated with severe decreases in the number of T cells in the neonate,[3,4] that there are only 10 gene mutations that account for greater than 90% of all cases of SCID,[4] and that, if performed within the first 28 days of life, hematopoietic stem cell transplantation results in a 95% survival rate.[5] A recent review by the Centers for Disease Control and Prevention approaches the problem of primary immune deficiencies in general, and SCID in particular, from a public health perspective and provides impetus for the development of neonatal screening tests.[3] The true incidence of SCID is unknown because many affected infants die of infection before diagnosis. Estimates suggest an incidence in the range of 1 in 100,000 live births. Active research is focusing on the development of screening tests that would be based on the T-cell deficiency in SCID neonates and could be performed on the dried blood spots now collected to screen for multiple metabolic defects. A polymerase chain reaction test for the small piece of circular DNA excised when the T-cell receptor gene is rearranged is one example of such a strategy.[6] In this paper, McGhee et al use mathematical modeling to perform a cost-benefit analysis of including SCID in current screening protocols if such a test was available. The authors conclude that, despite the rarity of this condition, screening for SCID could be cost-effective if a sufficiently specific test is developed.

M. Berger, MD, PhD

References

1. Buckley RH, Schiff RI, Schiff SE, et al. Human severe combined immunodeficiency: genetic, phenotypic, and functional diversity in one hundred eight infants. *J Pediatr.* 1997;130:378-387.
2. Rosen FS. Severe combined immunodeficiency: a pediatric emergency. *J Pediatr.* 1997;130:345-346.
3. Lindegren ML, Kobrynski L, Rasmussen SA, et al. Applying public health strategies to primary immunodeficiency diseases: a potential approach to genetic disorders. *MMWR Recommen Rep.* 2004;53:1-29.
4. Buckley RH. The multiple causes of human SCID. *J Clin Invest.* 2004;114:1409-1411.
5. Myers LA, Patel DD, Puck JM, Buckley RH. Hematopoietic stem cell transplantation for severe combined immunodeficiency in the neonatal period leads to superior thymic output and improved survival. *Blood.* 2002;99:872-878.
6. Chan K, Puck JM. Development of population-based newborn screening for severe combined immunodeficiency. *J Allergy Clin Immunol.* 2005;115:391-398.

6 Cardiovascular System

Characteristics of Arterial Stiffness in Very Low Birth Weight Premature Infants
Tauzin L, Rossi P, Giusano B, et al (Université de la Méditerranée, Marseille, France)
Pediatr Res 60:592-596, 2006   6–1

Premature birth is a factor of increased blood pressure in adulthood. Little is known about the physiologic characteristics of the arterial bed in neonates. The aim of this study was to characterize *in vivo* the arterial compliance in neonates and its maturation profile in very low birth weight (VLBW) premature infants. A group of stable, VLBW premature infants was compared with a control group of near term neonates. The abdominal aortic wall distensibility coefficient (DC) and whole-body arterial compliance (WBAC) were determined using specifically designed noninvasive methods, based on ultrasonic measurements in combination with synchronous, beat-to-beat recording of aortic pulse pressure (PP). On the fifth day of life, WBAC and the CD were lower in VLBW premature infants than in controls. Furthermore, WBAC and the DC remained unchanged in VLBW premature infants 7 wk after birth. In conclusion, VLBW premature infants are characterized as early as the fifth day of life by high arterial stiffness, which persists when they reach their theoretical term. It can be speculated that early alteration of arterial elastic properties may pave the way for long-term elevation of arterial pressure in VLBW premature infants.

▶ Although the Barker hypothesis was based on the identification of a relationship between low birth weight and the increased risk of arterial hypertension, carotid arteriosclerosis, and mortality by coronary heart disease or stroke in adulthood, there is some evidence that preterm birth itself is also related to cardiovascular or metabolic disorders in adult life. In fact, an inverse relationship between adult blood pressure and gestational age has been found in both adult men and women who were born prematurely. This article is interesting because it looks directly at the physiologic characteristics of the arterial bed in neonates and suggests that high arterial stiffness in very low birth weight premature infants is seen as early as the fifth day of life and persists through term gestation. Once again, the womb sets the stage. The physical properties of the arterial bed are changed before birth. The authors present data on abdominal aortic wall DC and WBAC as surrogates for this predetermination. The fields of neonatology and maternal–fetal medicine are becoming recognized as increasingly relevant in the effort to improve the long-term outcomes in the adult human population with regard to cardiovascular disease. Perhaps more resources should be invested in the health of the fetus and newborn rather than in the aging adult, or, at least, equalize the investments.

D. K. Stevenson, MD

Nitric oxide augments fetal pulmonary artery endothelial cell angiogenesis in vitro

Balasubramaniam V, Maxey AM, Fouty BW, et al (Univ of Colorado, Denver; Univ of South Alabama, Mobile)
Am J Physiol Lung Cell Mol Physiol 290:1111-1116, 2006   6–2

Growth and development of the lung normally occur in the low oxygen environment of the fetus. The role of this low oxygen environment on fetal lung endothelial cell growth and function is unknown. We hypothesized that low oxygen tension during fetal life enhances pulmonary artery endothelial cell (PAEC) growth and function and that nitric oxide (NO) production modulates fetal PAEC responses to low oxygen tension. To test this hypothesis, we compared the effects of fetal (3%) and room air (RA) oxygen tension on fetal PAEC growth, proliferation, tube formation, and migration in the presence and absence of the NO synthase (NOS) inhibitor N^{ω}-nitro-L-arginine (LNA), and an NO donor, S-nitroso-N-acetylpenicillamine (SNAP). Compared with fetal PAEC grown in RA, 3% O_2 increased tube formation by over twofold ($P < 0.01$). LNA treatment reduced tube formation in 3% O_2 but had no affect on tube formation in RA. Treatment with SNAP increased tube formation during RA exposure to levels observed in 3% O_2. Exposure to 3% O_2 for 48 h attenuated cell number (by 56%), and treatment with LNA reduced PAEC growth by 44% in both RA and 3% O_2. We conclude that low oxygen tension enhances fetal PAEC tube formation and that NO is essential for normal PAEC growth, migration, and tube formation. Furthermore, we conclude that in fetal cells exposed to the relative hyperoxia of RA, 21% O_2, NO overcomes the inhibitory effects of the increased oxygen, allowing normal PAEC angiogenesis and branching. We speculate that NO production maintains intrauterine lung vascular growth and development during exposure to low O_2 in the normal fetus. We further speculate that NO is essential for pulmonary angiogenesis in fetal animal exposed to increased oxygen tension of RA and that impaired endothelial NO production may contribute to the abnormalities of angiogenesis seen in infants with bronchopulmonary dysplasia.

▶ This article provides *in vitro* evidence that low O_2 tension during normal fetal development facilitates the formation of blood vessels in the lung by stimulating proliferation and migration of PAECs and, in so doing, causes these cells to form tubelike structures (simulating blood vessels) when grown in culture. The study suggests that NO signaling may play an important role in regulating angiogenesis within the fetal lung. The authors speculate that NO production during intrauterine development is critical for normal lung vascular growth, and that NO, by counteracting the antiangiogenic effects of exposure to air or increased O_2 after birth, plays a pivotal role in the normal postnatal development of the pulmonary circulation.

Applying *in vitro* data taken from studies in which cultured PAECs of fetal sheep were exposed to either pharmacologic inhibition of NOS or treatment with an NO donor to model *in vivo* growth and development of lung blood vessels requires a leap of faith. Furthermore, speculating from this work that NO is essential for blood vessel formation in fetal animals exposed to air (as opposed to the low O_2 environment of the fetus) and that impaired endothelial NO production may contribute to defective angiogenesis in infants with bronchopulmonary dysplasia demands an even greater leap of faith. Nevertheless, these studies promote the notion that NO may modulate lung endothelial cell function, thereby affecting the growth and development of the pulmonary circulation in ways that have not been routinely considered. These and other recent studies clearly indicate that NO is much more than an effective vasodilator that can reverse neonatal pulmonary hypertension: it may also have an important role in the formation of lung capillaries and alveoli. Stay tuned for emerging new insights on NO in the lung during development and in newborn lung disease.

R. D. Bland, MD

Hemodynamics of the Cerebral Arteries of Infants With Periventricular Leukomalacia

Fukuda S, Kato T, Kakita H, et al (Nagoya City Univ, Japan)
Pediatrics 117:1-8, 2006   6–3

Objective.—This study investigated the developmental changes in blood flow in each cerebral artery among infants with and without periventricular leukomalacia (PVL), to elucidate the time of onset of PVL.

Methods.—Eight of 67 low birth weight infants were diagnosed through ultrasonography as having PVL with cyst formation. The mean cerebral blood flow velocities (CBFVs) in the anterior cerebral artery, middle cerebral arteries (MCAs), posterior cerebral arteries (PCAs), internal carotid arteries (ICAs), and basilar artery were measured with Doppler ultrasonography at postnatal days 0, 1, 2, 3, 4, 5, 7, 10, 14, 21, 28, 42, 56, and 70. Four of 8 infants with cyst formation and 1 of 59 infants without cyst formation developed cerebral palsy.

Results.—The mean CBFVs of infants with PVL were significantly lower in the anterior cerebral artery (days 14–70), the right MCA (days 14–70), the left MCA (days 14–70), the right PCA (days 7–70), the left PCA (days 5–70), the right ICA (days 7–70), the left ICA (days 7–70), and the basilar artery (days 14 and 28–70). The CBFVs in all arteries were also lower among those with PVL than among intact infants on day 0. The CBFVs increased postnatally in the PCAs of infants with intact brains, whereas they remained unchanged after day 14 or 21 among infants with PVL. There was a significant difference in the prevalence of cerebral palsy between the 2 groups.

Conclusions.—We suggest that the total cerebral blood supply is decreased in cases of cystic PVL and that this reduction occurs just after birth, in a defined sequence, in the cerebral arteries. We conclude that the insult resulting in PVL might occur close to the time of birth.

▶ It is not surprising that cerebral blood flow velocities in infants with PVL are lower than in those without PVL given the potential contribution of ischemia to the development of PVL and white matter changes. Decreased cerebral perfusion shortly after birth may alternatively occur to areas of preexisting injured brain, perhaps as a result of infection. The exact timing of injury may require fetal Doppler studies in addition to serial postnatal ultrasonography. This study further raises questions about the focality of PVL in association with regional perfusion deficits from specific cerebral arteries.

V. Chock, MD

A Double-Blind, Randomized, Controlled Study of a "Stress Dose" of Hydrocortisone for Rescue Treatment of Refractory Hypotension in Preterm Infants

Ng PC, Lee CH, Bnur FL, et al (Chinese Univ of Hong Kong; Prince of Wales Hosp, Hong Kong; United Christian Hosp, Hong Kong)
Pediatrics 117:367-375, 2006   6–4

Objective.—To assess the effectiveness of a "stress dose" of hydrocortisone for rescue treatment of refractory hypotension and adrenocortical insufficiency of prematurity in very low birth weight (VLBW) infants. We hypothesized that significantly more VLBW infants who were receiving dopamine ≥ 10 μg/kg per min could wean off vasopressor support 72 hours after treatment with hydrocortisone.

Methods.—A double-blind, randomized, controlled study was conducted in a university neonatal center. Forty-eight VLBW infants who had refractory hypotension and required dopamine ≥ 10 μg/kg per min were randomly assigned to receive a stress dose of hydrocortisone (1 mg/kg every 8 hours for 5 days; $n = 24$) or an equivalent volume of the placebo solution (isotonic saline; $n = 24$).

Results.—The baseline clinical characteristics were similar between the groups. Serum cortisol concentrations were very low immediately before randomization in both groups of infants. Significantly more VLBW infants who were treated with hydrocortisone weaned off vasopressor support 72 hours after starting treatment. The use of volume expander, cumulative dose of dopamine, and dobutamine were significantly less in hydrocortisone-treated infants compared with control infants. In addition, the median duration of vasopressor treatment was halved in hydrocortisone-treated patients. Two versus 11 infants in the hydrocortisone and control groups required a second vasopressor for treatment of refractory hypotension. The trend (linear and quadratic) of the mean arterial blood pressure was also significantly and consistently higher in hydrocortisone-treated infants.

Conclusions.—A stress dose of hydrocortisone was effective in treating refractory hypotension in VLBW infants. Although routine and prophylactic use of systemic corticosteroids could not be recommended because of their potential adverse effects, this relatively low dose of hydrocortisone would probably be preferable to high-dose dexamethasone for treatment of refractory hypotension in emergency and life-threatening situations.

▶ This double-blind, randomized, controlled study of 48 VLBW infants with refractory hypotension requiring 10 µg/kg dopamine or more per minute tested the hypothesis that more infants receiving a "stress dose" of hydrocortisone (1 mg/kg per dose every 8 hours for 5 days) could be weaned off vasopressor support 72 hours after steroid treatment. Thus, the study was designed with a physiologic outcome as the primary one and leaves open the question as to whether such an approach might improve long-term pulmonary or neurodevelopmental outcome. The fact that hydrocortisone can be administered safely with respect to short-term complications is not surprising or new, and it is also not surprising that blood pressure improves with its administration. What is more important to understand is what blood pressure means in terms of cardiac output and perfusion of vital organs and whether the changes that occur with the administration of hydrocortisone are, in fact, good for the infant in a more consequential way. Nonetheless, a decreased need for volume expansion, exposure to other vasoactive pharmaceuticals, and improvement in pulmonary function that lessens the need for mechanical ventilation and leads to earlier extubation are short-term potential benefits. What is also interesting about the VLBW infant is that cortisol levels may not be sufficient for understanding the capacity of the infant to respond to stress and that the relative increase in cortisol in response to stress may be insufficient to meet physiologic demands under some conditions. In fact, lower blood pressure may be a surrogate for this failure to respond adequately, but it also may not be the most sensitive surrogate. Moreover, the current study does not address the question of whether a shorter duration of treatment or even a lower dose might be possible to affect the desired change. The fact that the protocol design also included proton pump inhibitor administration leaves open the question as to whether this pharmaceutical intervention is needed in this context. Trading one set of drugs for another may or may not achieve a risk benefit ratio that is favorable in practice.

D. K. Stevenson, MD

Pilot study of milrinone for low systemic blood flow in very preterm infants

Paradisis M, Evans N, Kluckow M, et al (Univ of Sydney)
J Pediatr 148:306-313, 2006   6–5

Objectives.—To examine the hemodynamic effects of milrinone given prophylactically to very preterm infants at high risk of low superior vena cava (SVC) flow and to investigate the preliminary efficacy and safety of an optimal dose.

Study Design.—This was a prospective, open-label study in two stages. The first involved dose escalation in two cohorts. Milrinone infusions of 0.25 µg/kg per minute (n = 8) and then 0.5 µg/kg per minute (n = 11) were administered from 3 to 24 hours of age. Population pharmacokinetic modeling was used to develop an optimized dose regimen. Ten infants then were loaded with 0.75 µg/kg per minute for 3 hours, followed by 0.2 µg/kg per minute maintenance until 18 hours of age. Infants were monitored for blood pressure, serial echocardiograms, and blood milrinone levels. The primary outcome was maintenance of SVC flow greater than 45 mL/kg per minute through the first 24 hours.

Results.—Low SVC flow developed in 36% of babies at both 0.25 µg/kg per minute and 0.5 µg/kg per minute of milrinone. Blood levels on these two regimens were slow to reach the target range and accumulated above this range by 24 hours. At 0.75 to 0.2 µg/kg per minute, no infant had SVC flow below 45 mL/kg per minute, compared with 61% in historic control subjects. Four infants needed an additional inotrope to support blood pressure. Blood levels were within the target range in 9 of 10 babies.

Conclusions.—We used population pharmacokinetic modeling to develop an optimal dosing regimen for milrinone. The efficacy and safety in this novel preventative approach to circulatory support is encouraging but inconclusive. We do not recommend the use of milrinone in preterm infants outside a research setting.

▶ Low blood pressure in the preterm newborn is often treated with fluid boluses and dopamine, although there is no clear evidence for the benefit of either treatment. This study proposes a potential role for milrinone to augment systemic blood flow in these patients. Milrinone is being used in neonates after cardiac surgery to treat and prevent the low cardiac output syndrome, a state that the authors propose is similar to that of the newborn preterm infant. Although this report introduces a new, potentially useful therapy, it also serves to highlight the lack of knowledge in this field. Some questions that are raised include the following: What is the most useful measure of blood flow in the newborn preterm infant, particularly to gauge cerebral perfusion? (It is probably not the mean arterial pressure, which is likely most commonly used.) Does the low-flow state really cause intraventricular hemorrhage and poor neurodevelopmental outcome, or are they just associations? That is, is this something we really need to treat? If low flow does cause intraventricular hemorrhage, does it need to be prevented from birth, or can one treat it in a timely fashion when it happens? There is a need for more studies to answer such questions, ideally randomized, controlled trials with relevant long-term outcomes.

H. C Lee, MD

Early Low Cardiac Output Is Associated with Compromised Electroencephalographic Activity in Very Preterm Infants
West CR, Groves AM, Williams CE, et al (Univ of Auckland, New Zealand; Starship Hosp, Auckland, New Zealand)
Pediatr Res 59:610-615, 2006   6–6

Low cerebral blood flow in preterm infants has been associated with discontinuous electroencephalography (EEG) activity that in turn has been associated with poor long-term prognosis. We examined the relationships between echocardiographic measurements of blood flow, blood pressure (BP), and quantitative EEG data as surrogate markers of cerebral perfusion and function with 112 sets of paired data obtained over the first 48 h after birth in 40 preterm infants (24–30 wk of gestation, 510–1900 g at delivery). Echocardiographic measurements of right ventricular output (RVO) and superior vena caval (SVC) flow were performed serially. BP recordings were obtained from invasive monitoring or oscillometry. Modified cotside EEGs were analyzed for quantitative amplitude and continuity measurements. RVO 12 h after birth was related to both EEG amplitude at 12 and 24 h and continuity at 24 h. Mean systemic arterial pressure (MAP) at 12 and 24 h was related to continuity at 12 and 24 h after birth. Multiple regression analyses revealed that RVO at 12 h was related to median EEG amplitude at 24 h and diastolic BP at 24 h was related to simultaneous EEG continuity. In addition, at 12 h, infants in the lowest quartile for RVO measurements (<282 mL/kg/min) had lower EEG amplitude and those in the lowest quartile for MAP measurements (<31 mm Hg) had lower EEG continuity. These results suggest a relationship between indirect measurements of cerebral perfusion and cerebral function soon after birth in preterm infants.

▶ The authors explored the potential relationship between low systemic blood flow and discontinuous EEG activity by obtaining simultaneous or nearly simultaneous echocardiographic measurements, BP, and EEGs. Echocardiography for the sole purpose of measuring cardiac function in premature newborns and modified EEGs to measure cerebral function are not yet in wide use in most neonatal units, although various studies are pointing to more widespread applications.

In this analysis, BP appeared to be similar in efficacy as RVO in terms of predicting discontinuous EEG activity. Considering that finding, perhaps BP is not such a useless measurement after all. These results may support the general practice of treating low BP in newborn premature infants. Or at least, it encourages us to continue the exploration of what is considered a low BP and how to treat it.

Despite the risk adjustment, because this is an observational study, it is not certain that these are causal relationships. Perhaps a future clinical trial investigating the treatment of BP or cardiac output could incorporate EEG measurement as an outcome variable.

H. C. Lee, MD

Oxygen saturation in healthy infants immediately after birth

Kamun COF, O'Donnell CPF, Davis PG, et al (Royal Women's Hosp, Melbourne; Univ of Melbourne; Murdoch Children's Research Inst, Melbourne)
J Pediatr 148:585-589, 2006   6–7

Objective.—Because the optimal concentration of oxygen (FiO_2) required for stabilization of the newly born infant has not been established, the FiO_2 is commonly adjusted according to the infant's oxygen saturation (SpO_2). We aimed to determine the range of pre-ductal SpO_2 in the first minutes of life in healthy newborn infants.

Study Design.—We applied an oximetry sensor to the infant's right palm or wrist of term and preterm deliveries immediately after birth. Infants who received any resuscitation or supplemental oxygen were excluded. SpO_2 was recorded at 60 second intervals for at least 5 minutes and until the SpO_2 was >90%.

Results.—A total of 205 deliveries were monitored; 30 infants were excluded from the study. SpO_2 readings were obtained within 60 seconds of age

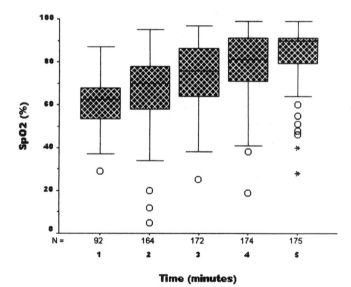

Time (minutes)

FIGURE 2.—Box plots showing the median, quartiles, range (1.5 times the quartile on that side), outliers, and extreme values for SpO_2 at each minute after birth for the first 5 minutes (N = number of patients in whom SpO_2 was obtained). A number <175 indicates that SpO_2 was not obtained in all cases. (Courtesy of Kamun COF, O'Donnell CPF, Davis PG, et al. Oxygen saturation in healthy infants immediately after birth. *J Pediatr*. 148:585-589. Copyright 2006 by Elsevier.)

from 92 of 175 infants (53%). The median (interquartile range) SpO$_2$ at 1 minute was 63% (53%-68%). There was a gradual rise in SpO$_2$ with time, with a median SpO$_2$ at 5 minutes of 90% (79%-91%) (Fig 2).

Conclusion.—Many newborns have an SpO$_2$ <90% during the first 5 minutes of life. This should be considered when choosing SpO$_2$ targets for infants treated with supplemental oxygen in the delivery room.

▶ As pulse oximeters are increasingly used in the delivery room setting, the importance of normative data cannot be underestimated. The authors clearly demonstrate the gradual rise in SpO$_2$ with time in a large population of healthy infants who did not require resuscitation, including supplemental oxygen (Fig 2). Despite the potential difficulty of securing the probe and obtaining an adequate tracing quickly enough to obtain immediate data, the total time from birth to first data was remarkably short, with a mean of 74 seconds and standard deviation of 22 seconds, allowing accurate data for more than half of the infants at 1 minute, and for the majority of infants at 2 minutes. Other investigators have also reported that healthy neonates breathing room air often require more than 5 minutes to achieve an SpO$_2$ greater than 90%.[1] Such normative data will be particularly useful in the further investigation of the use of pulse oximetry in the sick newborn, including the establishment of more precise, evidence-based guidelines for the use of oxygen in the delivery room setting.[2]

R. L. Chapman, MD

References

1. Rabi Y, Yee W, Chen SY, Singhal N. Oxygen saturation trends immediately after birth. *J Pediatr.* 2006;148:590-594.
2. Saugstad OD. Oxygen saturations immediately after birth. *J Pediatr.* 2006;148:569-570.

Prevalence of Spontaneous Closure of the Ductus Arteriosus in Neonates at a Birth Weight of 1000 Grams or Less
Koch J, Hensley G, Roy L, et al (Univ of Texas, Dallas; Children's Med Ctr, Dallas)
Pediatrics 117:1113-1121, 2006   6–8

Objective.—Ductus arteriosus (DA) closure occurs within 96 hours in >95% of neonates >1500 g in birth weight (BW). The prevalence and postnatal age of spontaneous ductal closure in neonates ≤1000 g in BW (extremely low birth weight [ELBW] neonates) remain unclear, as does the incidence of failure to close with indomethacin. Therefore, we prospectively examined the prevalence, postnatal age, and clinical variables associated with spontaneous DA closure, occurrence of persistent patent DA, and indomethacin failure in ELBW neonates.

Methods.—Neonates delivered at Parkland Memorial Hospital from February 2001 through December 2003 were studied. Those with congenital

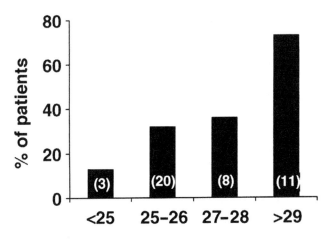

Gestational age, wk

FIGURE 3.—The relationship between EGA by obstetric dates and the occurrence of spontaneous permanent closure of the DA in ELBW neonates. Bars represent the percent of neonates in each age group that spontaneously closed the DA; values in parentheses are the number of neonates at each age. As gestational age advances, spontaneous closure of the DA increases more than fivefold ($P = .002$). (Reproduced with permission from Koch J, Hensley G, Roy L, et al. Prevalence of spontaneous closure of the ductus arteriosus in neonates at a birth weight of 1000 grams or less. *Pediatrics*. 2006;117:1113-1121.)

heart defects or death <10 days postnatally were excluded. Echocardiograms were performed 48 to 72 hours postnatal and every 48 hours until 10 days postnatally.

Results.—We studied 122 neonates with BW of 794 ± 118 (SD) g and estimated gestational age (EGA) of 26 ± 2 weeks. Spontaneous permanent DA closure occurred in 42 (34%) neonates at 4.3 ± 2 days postnatally, with 100% closure by 8 days. These neonates were more mature, less likely to have received antenatal steroids or have hyaline membrane disease (HMD; 52% vs 79%), and more likely to be growth restricted (31% vs 5%) and delivered of hypertensive women. Using regression analysis, EGA and absence of antenatal steroids and HMD predicted ductal closure. Ten (8%) neonates with early DA closure reopened and required medical/surgical closure. Eighty neonates had persistent patent DA; 7 were surgically ligated, and 5 remained asymptomatic, with 4 of 5 closing after 10 days postnatally. Sixty-eight (85%) received indomethacin at 6.2 ± 4 days postnatally; 41% failed therapy and had no distinguishing characteristics (Fig 3).

Conclusions.—Spontaneous permanent DA closure occurs in >34% of ELBW neonates and is predicted by variables related to maturation, for example, EGA and an absence of HMD, whereas indomethacin failure could not be predicated.

▶ Optimal timing of pharmacologic intervention for a patent ductus arteriosus (PDA) remains quite controversial in extremely low birthweight (ELBW) infants. Koch and associates take us one step closer to resolution of this issue by quantifying the magnitude of the problem. Of particular note was the observation that spontaneous permanent ductal closure occurred in less than 40% of patients at 28 weeks' gestation at birth, with a clearly observable increment in closure rate with advancing gestation from <25 to >29 weeks. Therefore, there is a high rate of ductal patency in this population that may well contribute to morbidity in ELBW infants.

Several opportunities for pharmacologic intervention exist. Indomethacin therapy, unfortunately, may be complicated by impaired renal function, although ibuprofen has emerged as an alternate approach without evidence of resultant oliguria.[1] Ibuprofen, in turn, does not benefit the incidence of severe intraventricular hemorrhage (IVH) as is the case for indomethacin. Surgical ligation should probably be a last resort as this therapy is associated with greater morbidity in what are admittedly nonrandomized trials.

A recent commentary by Clyman and colleagues[2] notes how practice in this area has been altered by inconsistent data regarding a possible beneficial effect of indomethacin on severe intracranial hemorrhage. They note that indomethacin use decreased after publication of the TIPP Trial,[3] which failed to show improved long-term neurodevelopmental benefit of indomethacin despite short-term benefit on severe IVH. Of particular note is their observation that the effect size proposed and not reached by the TIPP investigators was unrealistically high. It would, therefore, appear that definitive recommendations regarding prophylactic indomethacin or ibuprofen use in ELBW infants remain elusive, although postponing PDA closure until surgery becomes inevitable as a result of failed pharmacologic therapy is not a good idea.

R. J. Martin, MD

References

1. Van Overmeire B, Smets K, Lecoutere D, et al. A comparison of ibuprofen and indomethacin for closure of patent ductus arteriosus. *N Engl J Med.* 2000;343: 674-681.
2. Clyman RI, Saha S, Jobe A, Oh W. Indomethacin prophylaxis for preterm infants: the impact of 2 multicentered randomized controlled trials on clinical practice. *J Pediatr.* 2007;150:46-50.
3. Schmidt B, Davis P, Moddemann D, et al. Long-term effects of indomethacin prophylaxis in extremely-low-birth-weight infants. *N Engl J Med.* 2001;344: 1966-1972.

Combined Treatment With a Nonselective Nitric Oxide Synthase Inhibitor (L-NMMA) and Indomethacin Increases Ductus Constriction in Extremely Premature Newborns

Keller RL, Tacy TA, Fields S, et al (Univ of California, San Francisco; Wayne State Univ, Detroit)
Pediatr Res 58:1216-1221, 2005   6–9

Studies in premature animals suggest that 1) prolonged tight constriction of the ductus arteriosus is necessary for permanent anatomic closure and 2) endogenous nitric oxide (NO) and prostaglandins both play a role in ductus patency. We hypothesized that combination therapy with an NO synthase (NOS) inhibitor [N^G-monomethyl-L-arginine (L-NMMA)] and in-domethacin would produce tighter ductus constriction than indomethacin alone. Therefore, we conducted a phase I and II study of combined treatment with indomethacin and L-NMMA in newborns born at <28 weeks' gestation who had persistent ductus flow by Doppler after an initial three-dose prophylactic indomethacin course (0.2, 0.1, 0.1 mg/kg/24 h). Twelve infants were treated with the combined treatment protocol [three additional indomethacin doses (0.1 mg/kg/24 h) plus a 72-hour L-NMMA infusion]. Thirty-eight newborns received three additional indomethacin doses (without L-NMMA) and served as a comparison group. Ninety-two percent (11/12) of the combined treatment group had tight ductus constriction with elimination of Doppler flow. In contrast, only 42% (16/38) of the comparison group had a similar degree of constriction. L-NMMA infusions were limited in dose and duration by acute side effects. Doses of 10–20 mg/kg/h increased serum creatinine and systemic blood pressure. At 5 mg/kg/h, serum creatinine was stable but systemic hypertension still limited L-NMMA dose. We conclude that combined inhibition of NO and prostaglandin synthesis increased the degree of ductus constriction in newborns born at <28 weeks' gestation. However, the combined administration of L-NMMA and indomethacin was limited by acute side effects in this treatment protocol.

▶ In 2003 Keller and Clyman reported that "Newborns who are <28 weeks' gestational age and develop a recurrent, symptomatic PDA after completion of an initial indomethacin course rarely respond to multiple courses of indomethacin if there was persistent Doppler evidence of ductus flow after completion of the initial course. Additional indomethacin treatment is unlikely to produce permanent ductus closure."[1] It is, thus, logical to attempt to supplement the indomethacin with additional agents. Although adding NO synthase (NOS) inhibitor [N^G-monomethyl-L-arginine (L-NMMA)] to the second course of indomethacin constricted the ductus, the side effects were unacceptable. Surgical ligation, too, has its own set of problems, and Kabra et al,[2] in an analysis from the Trial of Indomethacin Prophylaxis in Preterm (TIPP) Trial, noted a 53% handicap amongst 95 infants who survived PDA ligation compared with 34% of 245 infants who survived after receiving only medical therapy (adjusted odds ratio 1.98; 95% confidence interval 1.18-3.30; p = .0093). This has sparked a new debate on the management of the patent ductus arteriosus in the very low birth weight infant.

A. A. Fanaroff, MD

References

1. Keller RL, Clyman RI. Persistent Doppler flow predicts lack of response to multiple courses of indomethacin in premature infants with recurrent patent ductus arteriosus. *Pediatrics*. 2003;112:583-587.

2. Kabra NS, Schmidt B, Roberts RS, Doyle LW, Papile L, Fanaroff A, for the Trial of Indomethacin Prophylaxis in Preterm (TIPP) Investigators. Neurosensory impairment after surgical closure of patent ductus arteriosus in extremely low birth weight infants: results from the Trial of Indomethacin Prophylaxis in Preterms. *J Pediatr.* 2007;150:229-234.

Oral Sildenafil in Infants With Persistent Pulmonary Hypertension of the Newborn: A Pilot Randomized Blinded Study

Baquero H, Soliz A, Neira F, et al (Universidad del Norte, Barranquilla, Colombia; Miami Children's Hosp, Fla; Emory Univ, Atlanta, Ga)
Pediatrics 117:1077-1083, 2006   6–10

Background.—Persistent pulmonary hypertension (PPHN) occurs in as many as 6.8 of 1000 live births. Mortality is ~10% to 20% with high-frequency ventilation, surfactant, inhaled nitric oxide, and extracorporeal membrane oxygenation but is much higher when these therapies are not available. Sildenafil is a phosphodiesterase inhibitor type 5 that selectively reduces pulmonary vascular resistance.

Objective.—Our goal was to evaluate the feasibility of using oral sildenafil and its effect on oxygenation in PPHN.

Design.—This study was a proof-of-concept, randomized, masked study in infants >35.5 weeks' gestation and <3 days old with severe PPHN and oxygenation index (OI) >25 admitted to the NICU (Hospital Niño Jesús, Barranquilla, Colombia). The sildenafil solution was prepared from a 50-mg tablet. The first dose (1 mg/kg) or placebo was given by orogastric tube <30 minutes after randomization and every 6 hours. Preductal saturation and blood pressure were monitored continuously. OI was calculated every 6 hours. The main outcome variable was the effect of oral sildenafil on oxygenation. Sildenafil or placebo was discontinued when OI was <20 or if there was no significant change in OI after 36 hours.

Results.—Six infants with an OI of >25 received placebo, and 7 received oral sildenafil at a median age of 25 hours. All infants were severely ill, on fraction of inspired oxygen 1.0, and with similar ventilatory parameters. Intragastric sildenafil and placebo were well tolerated. In the treatment group, OI improved in all infants within 6 to 30 hours, all showed a steady improvement in pulse oxygen saturation over time, and none had noticeable effect on blood pressure; 6 of 7 survived. In the placebo group, 1 of 6 infants survived.

Conclusions.—Oral sildenafil was administered easily and tolerated as well as placebo and improved OI in infants with severe PPHN, which suggests that oral sildenafil may be effective in the treatment of PPHN and underscores the need for a large, controlled trial.

▶ This is a provocative study, one of considerable interest to any neonatologist who manages infants with severe persistent pulmonary hypertension of the neonate (PPHN). In the United States, inhaled nitric oxide (iNO) is the primary vasodilator utilized in newborns with PPHN and severe hypoxic respiratory failure (HRF). Twelve prospective randomized trials in the United States and abroad have shown iNO to be efficacious as a selective pulmonary vasodilator in PPHN.[1] While it does not decrease mortality in affected infants, iNO does reduce their need for ECMO by 35% to 40%. Because iNO remains prohibitively expensive in many parts of the world, alternative treatments, such as sildenafil, remain attractive.

Sildenafil is a phosphodiasterase/5 (PDE5) inhibitor. It enhances pulmonary vasodilation by impeding the degradation of cyclic GMP (cGMP), the primary mediator of pulmonary vascular relaxation. At low doses it appears to have some pulmonary selectivity, such that systemic hypotension, priapism, and visual disturbances have not been commonly seen.

In this prospective, masked, pilot study ECMO-sick (OI >40) neonates were randomized to receive either 1 to 2 mg/kg/dose of sildenafil every 6 hours or sham control for up to 48 hours. All seven treated patients (mean OI 56 at study entry) showed improved oxygenation without significant hypotension or other identifiable adverse events; six of the seven (86%) survived. However, only one of six control patients (mean OI 46 at study entry) survived, as iNO or ECMO were not available as rescue therapies in this Colombian hospital. These results were more dramatic than the authors expected and resulted in closing the study far short of the planned 25-patient enrollment.

The authors review the various adverse events associated with sildenafil use in animal and human adult studies. They particularly caution against combining iNO and sildenafil until more newborns have been studied as the potentiation of pulmonary vascular relaxation may come at the expense of serious hypotension. Despite these concerns, sildenafil has proven to be efficacious in older patients with primary pulmonary hypertension.[2]

This drug should be studied in a large multicenter cohort, preferably where iNO and ECMO are available. If sildenafil works half as well as this small, but elegant, study reports, the cost savings would be enormous! My Rite Aid® pharmacist tells me that one 50-mg tablet of sildenafil costs only $14.99 and therefore would provide enough drug for a 48-hour treatment course in a 3-kg newborn. A comparable course of iNO costs $4800 or more in the United States, not to mention the additional cost if the baby subsequently requires ECMO support. If the safety and efficacy profiles hold up in larger trials, sildenafil may become the drug to replace the "ancient" tolazoline.

The number of PPHN cases requiring ECMO support over the past three years has fallen to between 720 and 740 infants per year, which is half the number of cases reported in 1992.[3] We are doing a better job of managing newborns with PPHN with more conservative ventilation practices, surfactant, iNO, and vigilant support of cardiac output. The possibility of expanding our therapeutic choices for this serious condition is a welcome prospect, indeed.

E. K. Stork, MD

References

1. Finer NN, Barrington KJ. Nitric oxide for respiratory failure in infants born at or near term. *Cochrane Database Syst Rev.* 2006;4:CD000399.

2. Sastry BK, Narasimhan C, Reddy NK, Raju BS. Clinical efficacy of sildenafil in primary pulmonary hypertension: a randomized, placebo-controlled, double-blind, crossover study. *J Am Coll Cardiol.* 2004;43:1149-1532.
3. ECMO Registry Report of the Extracorporeal Life Support Organization (ELSO). International summary. Ann Arbor, MI: January, 2007.

Prenatal diagnosis and outcome for fetuses with congenital absence of the pulmonary valve
Galindo A, Gutiérrez-Larraya F, Martínez M, et al (Hosp Universitario "12 de Octubre," Madrid; Universitat de Barcelona)
Ultrasound Obstet Gynecol 28:32-39, 2006   6–11

Objectives.—To analyze fetal echocardiographic findings of absent pulmonary valve syndrome (APVS), its association with chromosomal and extracardiac anomalies including nuchal translucency (NT) and the outcome after diagnosis.

Methods.—Data of 14 fetuses with confirmed APVS retrospectively collected in two tertiary referral centers between 1998 and 2004 were analyzed. The variables examined were: reason for referral, gestational age at diagnosis and associated abnormalities, including first trimester NT thickness. Cardiac evaluation included measurement of cardiothoracic ratio, diameter of pulmonary arteries and Doppler flow in the pulmonary trunk. Information was retrieved from clinical files, recorded videotapes and stored images. Karyotyping including examination for the 22q11 deletion was performed in all cases.

Results.—Mean gestational age at diagnosis was 28 weeks, with 5/14 (36%) diagnosed before 22 weeks. In 13/14 (93%) there was an associated ventricular septal defect (subaortic in 12 fetuses and inlet-type in one) and all 13 had tetralogy of Fallot. Enlargement of the central pulmonary arteries and cardiomegaly were present in all cases diagnosed after 22 weeks. Of the five fetuses in which APVS was detected before 22 weeks, four (80%) had a normal pulmonary trunk diameter, two (40%) had normal pulmonary branches and three (60%) had normal cardiac size. The arterial duct was absent in 11/14 (79%). A correlation between presence of the arterial duct and the size of the central pulmonary arteries or cardiomegaly could not be established. Increased NT was observed in 4/10 cases (40%) for which this information was available. 22q11 microdeletion was diagnosed in three fetuses (21%). There were five terminations of pregnancy, one intrauterine death, five neonatal deaths and one infant death. Of the six neonates with respiratory distress, only one (17%) survived and of the eight babies in whom there was an intention to treat, two survived (25%) (Fig 2).

Conclusions.—APVS can be accurately diagnosed by fetal echocardiography but screening ultrasound in the mid-second trimester is likely to have a low detection rate, probably due to the incomplete expression of the disease at this point. Many fetuses with APVS have an increased NT in the first trimester and this may help an earlier recognition of the defect. The most common associated karyotype anomaly is 22q11 microdeletion. Enlargement of

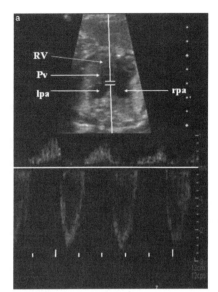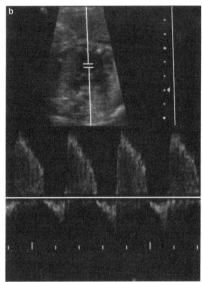

FIGURE 2.—Pulsed Doppler recording showing antegrade and retrograde flow in (a) the pulmonary trunk and (b) the right ventricle. lpa, left pulmonary artery; Pv, pulmonary valve; rpa, right pulmonary artery; RV, right ventricle. (Courtesy of Galindo A, Gutiérrez-Larraya F, Martínez M, et al. Prenatal diagnosis and outcome for fetuses with congenital absence of the pulmonary valve. *Ultrasound Obstet Gynecol.* 2006;28:32-39. Copyright International Society of Ultrasound in Obstetrics & Gynecology. Reproduced with permission. Permission is granted by John Wiley & Sons Ltd on behalf of the ISUOG.)

the central pulmonary arteries is mainly related to the gestational age at diagnosis. Our results confirm that the outlook for these patients is extremely poor.

▶ This is an interesting series from Galindo et al that confirms the associated features and poor prognosis for fetuses with absent pulmonary valves. Increased nuchal thickness must now alert the clinician to this entity as well as the usual anomalies, including trisomy 21, Turner's syndrome, etc.

Congenital absence of the pulmonary valve is a relatively rare anomaly that is usually associated with a ventricular septal defect and a restrictive pulmonary annulus with severe pulmonary regurgitation. Not infrequently, the association is with tetralogy of Fallot. The to-and-fro flow across the right ventricular outflow tract produces enormously dilated and pulsatile pulmonary arteries that cause severe respiratory distress and tracheomalacia by compression of the trachea and primary bronchi.[1] Norgaard et al[2] accumulated a series of 25 patients over 25 years with follow-up for approximately 10 years and reported 19% mortality. Zucker et al,[3] on the basis of a series of 18 patients with absence of the pulmonary valve, noted that patients with a ventricular septal defect and phenotypic features of tetralogy of Fallot have a strong family history of congenital cardiac disease, develop respiratory symptoms during infancy, and exhibit a variable prognosis, despite cardiac surgery. Patients with an intact ventricular septum are usually asymptomatic, present later in life, and show a relatively benign prognosis. On the other hand, according to Galindo et al, if they present early with respiratory distress, the prognosis is awful.

Volpe et al,[4] on the basis of a series of 21 cases, concluded that absent pulmonary valve syndrome can be reliably diagnosed and characterized prenatally. They confirmed the association with major chromosomal anomalies or 22q11 microdeletion. They attributed the relatively poor survival rate to the high rate of terminations, associated genetic anomalies, and bronchomalacia, which is a characteristic accompaniment in the overwhelming majority of cases featuring cardiomegaly and marked branch pulmonary dilatation. The condition can be recognized with certainty, but the outlook at present is grim.

A. A. Fanaroff, MD

References

1. Brown JW, Ruzmetov M, Vijay P, Rodefeld MD, Turrentine MW. Surgical treatment of absent pulmonary valve syndrome associated with bronchial obstruction. *Ann Thorac Surg.* 2006;82:2221-2226.
2. Norgaard MA, Alphonso N, Newcomb AE, Brizard CP, Cochrane AD. Absent pulmonary valve syndrome. Surgical and clinical outcome with long-term follow-up. *Eur J Cardiothorac Surg.* 2006;29:682-687.
3. Zucker N, Rozin I, Levitas A, Zalzstein E. Clinical presentation, natural history, and outcome of patients with the absent pulmonary valve syndrome. *Cardiol Young.* 2004;14:402-408.
4. Volpe P, Paladini D, Marasini M, et al. Characteristics, associations and outcome of absent pulmonary valve syndrome in the fetus. *Ultrasound Obstet Gynecol.* 2004;24:623-628.

7 Respiratory Disorders

Congenital bronchial atresia in infants and children
Morikawa N, Kuroda T, Honna T, et al (Natl Ctr for Child Health and Development, Tokyo)
J Pediatr Surg 40:1822-1826, 2005   7–1

Background/Purpose.—Congenital bronchial atresia (CBA) usually presents incidentally in asymptomatic young male adults but is rarely diagnosed in children. The aim of this study was to clarify the clinical characteristics of CBA in childhood and to describe the spectrum of this condition.

Methods.—The clinical features in 29 patients with CBA, aged from 1 day to 13 years (median, 4 years), were reviewed retrospectively. Diagnosis was confirmed by pathological findings of a blind-ending bronchus associated with distal mucous-filled bronchocele surrounded by hyperinflated lung parenchyma.

Results.—All but 1 patient were symptomatic. The most frequent symptom was productive cough and fever owing to recurrent pneumonia found in 26 children. Two infants suffered from respiratory distress. Chest x-ray showed various findings of infiltrative pneumonia, emphysema, and a large cyst. Computed tomography, bronchography, and bronchoscopy were useful modalities for demonstrating bronchocele associated with hyperinflated lung or proximal blind-ending bronchus even in infected cases. The right lower lobe was predominantly affected in 12 cases, followed by left or right upper lobe in 7 cases. Lobectomy or segmentectomy resulted in remarkable clinical improvement.

Conclusions.—Congenital bronchial atresia presents differently in children than in young adults. Modern imaging techniques and careful pathological analyses lead to an accurate diagnosis of bronchial atresia, which may be misdiagnosed as intralobar sequestration or pulmonary bronchial cysts. Bronchial atresia is a distinct pathological entity that accounts for recurrent pneumonia or respiratory distress in childhood, requiring surgical treatment.

▶ "Individually, congenital abnormalities of the lung are rare but collectively they form an important group of conditions."[1] Bronchial atresia (BA), like most lung developmental anomalies, fits that description. Although it may be suspected from a plain radiograph of the chest, it takes CT to determine all the related vascular, bronchial, osseous, and parenchymal abnormalities. MRI has a limited role. BA may be suspected antenatally from US findings[2] of a round cystic mass (caused by fluid collection in the distal lung). BA results from an antenatal vascular insult leading to atresia of a lobar, segmental, or even subsegmental bronchus. Consequently, the intervening segments of bronchus or bronchi between the atretic regions form bronchoceles progressively because of retained secretions leading to mucoid impaction. The lung distal to atresia may develop normally but shows paucity of blood vessels and is hyperinflated because of unilateral collateral air drift through pores of Kohn and canals of Lambert from the adjacent normal lung. These collateral channels act as check valves allowing air entry only. Hence, the distension and possibility of an air leak, chest radiograph may show the bronchocele, presenting as a tubular, round, ovoid or branching structure, close to the hilum, with or without a fluid level. The distal lung is always overinflated with sparse vascular shadows. BA is more common in males and the most common site for BA is the apico posterior segment of left upper lobe although Morikawa et al found the right lower lobe to be the most common site in their series. BA is usually asymptomatic, or the subjects are seen with carrying combinations of cough, wheezing, hemoptysis, shortness of breath, recurrent infection, or pneumothorax. Associated anomalies include hypoplastic ribs and pectus excavatum. Riedlinger et al,[3] in a careful study with extensive pulmonary dissection under the microscope, demonstrated that BA and congenital cyst adenomatous malformation (CCAM) of the lung nearly always coexist.[4] This was confirmed by Kunisaki et al[5] who stated, "Bronchial atresia is a common, unrecognized component of prenatally diagnosed congenital cystic adenomatoid malformations, bronchopulmonary sequestrations, congenital lobar emphysemas, and lesions of mixed pathology. Most congenital lung masses may be part of a spectrum of anomalies linked to obstruction of the developing fetal airway as an underlying component in their pathogenesis."

As noted by Morikawa, whose series presents good insight into the condition, BA should be surgically corrected if and when it is complicated by infection.

A. A. Fanaroff, MD

References

1. Wallis C. Clinical outcomes of congenital lung abnormalities. *Paediatr Respir Rev.* 2000;4:328-335.
2. Kamata S, Sawai T, Usui N, et al. Case of congenital bronchial atresia detected by fetal ultrasound. *Pediatriac Pulmonol.* 2003;35:227-229.
3. Riedlinger WF, Vargas SO, Jennings RW, et al. Bronchial atresia is common to extralobar sequestration, intralobar sequestration, congenital cystic adenomatoid malformation, and lobar emphysema. *Pediatr Dev Pathol.* 2006;9:361-373.
4. Calvert JK, Boyd PA, Chamberlain PC, Syed S, Lakhoo K. Outcome of antenatally suspected congenital cystic adenomatoid malformation of the lung: 10 years' experience 1991-2001. *Arch Dis Child Fetal Neonatal Ed.* 2006;91:F26-F28.
5. Kunisaki SM, Fauza DO, Nemes LP, et al. Bronchial atresia: the hidden pathology within a spectrum of prenatally diagnosed lung masses. *J Pediatr Surg.* 2006;41:61-65.

Sustainable use of continuous positive airway pressure in extremely preterm infants during the first week after delivery

Booth C, Premkumar MH, Yannoulis A, et al (Imperial College London; Queen Charlotte's and Chelsea Hosp, London)

Arch Dis Child Fetal Neonatal Ed 91:398-402, 2006   7–2

Background.—Early use of nasal continuous positive airway pressure (nCPAP) may reduce lung damage, but it is not clear how many extremely preterm infants can be cared for without mechanical ventilation on the first days after delivery.

Objectives.—To describe our experience of nCPAP in infants born at <27 weeks' gestation and to determine the chance of reintubation of this group of extremely preterm infants.

Methods.—A retrospective, observational study examined the period from November 2002 to October 2003, when efforts were made to extubate infants to nCPAP at the earliest opportunity. Data were collected on all infants born at <27 weeks' and gestation admitted to The Neonatal Intensive Care Unit, Queen Charlotte's and Chelsea Hospital, London, UK. The chance of an individual infant requiring reintubation within 48 h of delivery was estimated, calculating the predictive probability using a Bayesian approach, and oxygen requirements at 36 weeks' postmenstrual age were examined.

Results.—60 infants, 34 inborn and 26 ex utero transfers, were admitted; 7 infants admitted 24 h after birth were excluded and 5 died within 48 h. The mean birth weight was 788 g and the gestational age was 25.3 weeks. Extubation was attempted on day 1 in 21 of 52 infants on ventilators and was successful in 14; and on day 2 in 14 of 35 and successful in 10 of infants extubated within 48 h of delivery survived to discharge. 5 of 23 infants on mechanical ventilation at 48 h of age were on air at 36 weeks postmenstrual age, and 12 of 26 of those were on nCPAP at 48 h of age. The probability of an individual baby remaining on nCPAP was 66% (95% CI 46% to 86%) on day 1 and 80% (95% CI 60% to 99%) on day 2. The smallest infant to be successfully extubated was 660 g and the youngest gestational age was 23.8 weeks.

Conclusions.—Extremely preterm infants can be extubated to nCPAP soon after delivery, with a reasonable probability of not requiring immediate reintubation.

▶ Duration of endotracheal intubation is a known risk factor for the development of bronchopulmonary dysplasia (BPD). Therefore, it is hoped that the incidence of BPD can be reduced by respiratory support strategies that facilitate early extubation to nCPAP (or nasal intermittent positive pressure ventilation [IPPV]) or alleviate the need for endotracheal intubation. This retrospective study describes a single institution's experience in which efforts were made to extubate infants, <27 weeks' gestation, to nCPAP at the earliest opportunity. The study objective was to determine how many extremely low gestational age neonates could be successfully extubated within the first several days of life. The birth weights of the study population ranged from 420 to 1200 g and the gestational ages from 23.1 to 26.6 weeks. The early management of all 34 inborn infants was standardized and included elective intubation in the delivery room (DR) with prophylactic administration of surfactant, common conventional mechanical ventilation strategies, and extubation criteria. Although the early management of the 19 outborn infants was more variable, all received surfactant within 30 minutes of birth and were admitted to the study NICU within 24 hours of delivery. Accepting the limits of a retrospective study, it is still intriguing that although no infant weighing <660 g at birth sustained nCPAP without requiring reintubation, 25% of the infants born at 23 to 24 weeks' gestation were successfully extubated. Several large random control trials comparing initiation of nCPAP in the DR with early/prophylactic surfactant on the incidence of survival without BPD in infants <29 weeks' gestation are in progress. The results of these investigations should clarify the risks and benefits of these strategies and may shed light on how the interplay between birth weight and gestational age influences successful early treatment with nCPAP and the need for reintubation.

R. A. Ehrenkranz, MD

Low-Dose Dexamethasone Facilitates Extubation Among Chronically Ventilator-Dependent Infants: A Multicenter, International, Randomized, Controlled Trial
Doyle LW, Davis PG, Morley CJ, et al (Univ of Melbourne; Royal Women's Hosp, Melbourne; Women's and Children's Hosp, Adelaide, Australia; et al)
Pediatrics 117:75-83, 2006   7–3

Objective.—Postnatal corticosteroid therapy is controversial. The aim of this study was to determine the short-term effects of low-dose dexamethasone treatment among chronically ventilator-dependent neonates.

Methods.—Very preterm (gestational age: <28 weeks) or extremely low birth weight (birth weight: <1000 g) infants who were ventilator dependent after the first 1 week of life were eligible and were assigned randomly to receive masked dexamethasone (0.89 mg/kg over 10 days) or saline placebo. Data on ventilator and oxygen requirements and deaths were recorded.

Results.—Seventy infants were recruited from 11 centers, at a median age of 23 days. More infants were extubated successfully by 10 days of treatment in the dexamethasone group (60%, 21 of 35 patients) than in the control group (12%, 4 of 34 patients) (odds ratio [OR]: 11.2; 95% confidence interval [CI]: 3.2–39.0). Ventilator and oxygen requirements improved substantially, and the duration of intubation was shorter. There was little evidence for a reduction in either the mortality rate (dexamethasone group: 11%; control group: 20%; OR: 0.52; 95% CI: 0.14–1.95) or the rate of oxygen dependence at 36 weeks (dexamethasone group: 85%; control group: 91%; OR: 0.58; 95% CI: 0.13–2.66). There were no obvious effects of low-dose dexamethasone on blood glucose concentrations, blood pressure, or other complications. No infant experienced intestinal perforation.

Conclusions.—Low-dose dexamethasone treatment after the first 1 week of life clearly facilitates extubation and shortens the duration of intubation among ventilator-dependent, very preterm/extremely low birth weight infants, without any obvious short-term complications. Combined with recent evidence that infants at very high risk of bronchopulmonary dysplasia may benefit in the long term, our study reopens debate regarding the role of low-dose, late postnatal, corticosteroid therapy.

▶ There is nothing new under the sun. Moreover, it seems like we just cannot avoid using steroids of some sort for an indication of some sort in the neonate. Certainly, low-dose dexamethasone seems, on the face of it, better than high-dose dexamethasone, but even low-dose dexamethasone (without sulfite preservatives, no less) may not be risk free. The study is too small to be sure. On the other hand, nothing is probably risk free, certainly not being born prematurely, and some medical assistance can be at least rationalized if not proven to be helpful, although the proof is infrequently achieved based on sufficient evidence. There is no question that the short-term physiologic status of premature infants with lung disease can be altered significantly so that pulmonary function is improved and extubation is easier. The real question is whether such "therapy" has consequential long-term effects. The authors make a sophisticated argument that the infants in their study with higher rates of bronchopulmonary dysplasia might be more likely to benefit from corticosteroids with improvement in the composite outcome of death or cerebral palsy compared with ones with less BPD. However, the answer to this question is not addressed by the current report, and the authors indicate their intention to follow these infants. Unfortunately, the number of infants in the study is insufficient for addressing this important question. This is another example of how a primary physiologic outcome might drive a change in physician behavior with insufficient information about the actual impact of the intervention on long-term neurodevelopmental outcome.

D. K. Stevenson, MD

Predicting successful extubation of very low birthweight infants
Kamlin COF, Davis PG, Morley CJ (Royal Women's Hosp, Melbourne; Univ of Melbourne)
Arch Dis Child Fetal Neonatal Ed 91:F180-F183, 2006   7–4

Objective.—To determine the accuracy of three tests used to predict successful extubation of preterm infants.
Study Design.—Mechanically ventilated infants with birth weight <1250 g and considered ready for extubation were changed to endotracheal continuous positive airway pressure (ET CPAP) for three minutes. Tidal volumes, minute ventilation ($\dot{V}E$), heart rate, and oxygen saturation were recorded before and during ET CPAP. Three tests of extubation success were evaluated: (a) expired $\dot{V}E$ during ET CPAP; (b) ratio of $\dot{V}E$ during ET CPAP to $\dot{V}E$ during mechanical ventilation ($\dot{V}E$ ratio); (c) the spontaneous breath-

ing test (SBT)—the infant passed this test if there was no hypoxia or brady-cardia during ET CPAP. The clinical team were blinded to the results, and all infants were extubated. Extubation failure was defined as reintubation within 72 hours of extubation.

Results.—Fifty infants were studied and extubated. Eleven (22%) were reintubated. The SBT was the most accurate of the three tests, with a sensitivity of 97% and specificity of 73% and a positive and negative predictive value for extubation success of 93% and 89% respectively.

Conclusion.—The SBT used just before extubation of infants <1250 g may reduce the number of extubation failures. Further studies are required to establish whether the SBT can be used as the primary determinant of an infant's readiness for extubation.

▶ Duration of ET intubation is a known risk factor for the development of bron-chopulmonary dysplasia. Therefore, there has been an increased interest in limiting endotracheal intubation in very low birth weight infants, and especially extremely low birth weight infants, who require assisted ventilation. Permissive ventilation strategies that facilitate extubation have been adopted and aggressive weaning to NCPAP or nasal IPPV is common place. This report by Kamlin et al compares 3 tests evaluating readiness for extubation in 50 preterm infants less than 1250 g birth weight; the objective of this study was to determine the accuracy of these tests to predict successful extubation. Because up to 40% of extremely low birth weight infants who are extubated on the basis of such widely used criteria as clinical assessment, blood gases, and ventilator settings, a simple test that predicted successful extubation with high sensitivity and high positive predictive value should find its way into clinical practice.

The authors reported that, for infants considered ready for extubation, a 3-minute period of spontaneous breathing on ET CPAP without either brady-cardia for more than 15 seconds and/or a fall in SPO_2 below 85% (despite a 15% increase in inspired oxygen) demonstrated readiness for successful extubation. By extension, failure of the spontaneous breathing test identified most infants who would fail extubation and require reintubation. Although further studies will be necessary to demonstrate the spontaneous breathing test's potential, it is clear that reducing the morbidities associated with extubation failure by knowing who not to extubate is as important as knowing when extubation is likely to succeed.

R. A. Ehrenkranz, MD

Facilitation of neonatal endotracheal intubation with mivacurium and fentanyl in the neonatal intensive care unit
Dempsey EM, Hazzani FA, Faucher D, et al (Mcgill Univ, Montreal, Canada)
Arch Dis Child Fetal Neonatal Ed 91:279-282, 2006   7–5

Background.—Endotracheal intubation in the neonate is painful and is associated with adverse physiological effects. Some premedication regimens

TABLE 2.—Characteristics of Each Individual Intubation Attempt
Determined by Level of Experience

	Inexperience	Prior Experience	p Value
Number of intubations	26	31	
Success rate (%)	38	74	0.029
Duration of each attempt (seconds)	49 (29)	36 (23)	0.09
Number of desaturations <80%	17	12	0.04
Duration of desaturation (seconds)	21 (38)	14 (35)	0.5
Lowest saturation (%)	66 (22)	77 (20)	0.07
Number of bradycardia <100 beats/min	2	1	0.4

Values are number or mean (SD).
(Courtesy of Dempsey EM, Hazzani FA, Faucher D, et al. Facilitation of neonatal endotracheal intubation with mivacurium and fentanyl in the neonatal intensive care unit. *Arch Dis Child Fetal Neonatal Ed.* 2006;91:279-282. Reproduced with permission from the BMJ Publishing Group.)

have been shown to reduce these effects, but the optimal regimen is not yet determined.

Method.—Data on semi-elective intubations were prospectively collected in the neonatal intensive care unit over a six month period. Patients received 20 µg/kg atropine, 200 µg/kg mivacurium (a non-depolarising muscle relaxant) followed by 5 µg/kg fentanyl.

Results.—Thirty three patients were electively intubated during this time period (Table 2). The primary reason for intubation was surfactant administration (53%). Median (range) birth weight, gestational age, and age at intubation were 1360 g (675–4200), 29 weeks (25–38), and 33 hours (1–624) respectively. Twenty two of the infants were intubated on the first attempt. Median duration from initial insertion of the laryngoscope to successful intubation was 60 seconds (15 seconds to 20 minutes). In 18 cases, the first attempt was by a trainee with no previous successful intubation experience, 10 of whom intubated within two attempts. Muscle relaxation occurred at a mean (SD) of 94 (51) seconds, and mean (range) time to return of spontaneous movements was 937 seconds (480–1800). Intubation conditions were scored as excellent using a validated intubation scale.

Conclusion.—Effective analgesia can be administered and intubation performed with some brief desaturations, even when junior personnel are being taught their first intubation. In this first report of mivacurium for intubation in the newborn, effective bag and mask ventilation was easily achieved during muscle relaxation and was associated with excellent intubation conditions, permitting a high success rate for inexperienced personnel.

▶ The authors report their experience with a premedication cocktail routinely used in their NICU for elective and semielective intubations. They report results over a 6-month period on 33 neonates ranging in gestational age from 25 to 38 weeks at the time of birth. The rationale for the study was in part a neonatal quality improvement initiative and in part to evaluate the rate of successful intubations by residents having no prior experience with the procedure. Ample data exist, based on the extent of neurodevelopment of preterm and term neonates and their physiologic responses to stimuli known to be painful to older children and adults to support the premise that even premature neonates can experience pain.[1] Thus, it is incumbent on those caring for these patients to take steps to minimize pain whenever possible. Tracheal intubation falls into the category of stressful/painful procedures in which such steps are warranted, although many NICUs do not use premedication for this procedure.

The cocktail used in this study consisted of atropine, mivacurium, and fentanyl. These agents were chosen to reduce bradycardia (atropine), for short-acting muscle relaxation (mivacurium), and for short-acting analgesia (fentanyl). Furthermore, mivacurium does not have the adverse effects of succinylcholine.[2] The current study is observational. As such the only legitimate comparisons are between the experienced and inexperienced personnel performing the procedure. As expected, those with experience were able to intubate more quickly and with fewer adverse effects (eg, number of desaturations below 80% [Table 2]). However, other randomized, controlled studies have documented the benefits of premedication for intubation of neonates. This is the first reported use of mivacurium for this purpose. The lack of complications from its use is encouraging. A more recent randomized, controlled study by Roberts et al[3] supports the effectiveness of mivacurium and its lack of side effects. Long-term benefits would be much harder to demonstrate.

We must be more cognizant of the stress and pain we cause in neonates as we perform procedures whose goals are to maintain physiologic stability. This article and others indicate that, if we are experienced in managing an airway, our own stress stemming from our fear of not being able to intubate a patient after administering a muscle relaxant is unwarranted. Given the documented immediate physiologic benefits of premedication for elective and semielective intubation, premedication should be used even in the most premature patients under our care. The advantage of mivacurium is the short duration of action (about 50% shorter than that of vecuronium). Although not officially approved for use in children under 2 years of age, it has been used in younger children, including premature infants, and it is safer to use in children than succinylcholine. The cocktail suggested by Dempsey et al seems prudent pending further randomized, controlled studies designed to determine an optimal premedication cocktail with one change. Fentanyl at a dose of 5 µg/kg can cause respiratory depression. Because the purpose of the fentanyl is analgesia, there seems to be no advantage to giving more than 3 µg/kg of fentanyl.

H. C. Jacobs, MD

References

1. Shah V, Ohlsson A. The effectiveness of premedication for endotracheal intubation in mechanically ventilated neonates: A systemic review. *Clin Perinatol.* 2002;29:535-554.
2. McAllister JD, Gnauck KA. Rapid sequence intubation of the pediatric patient: fundamentals of practice. *Pediatr Clin North Am.* 1999;46:1249-1284.

3. Roberts KD, Leone TA, Edwards WH, Rich WD, Finer NN. Premedication for nonemergent neonatal intubations: a randomized, controlled trial comparing atropine and fentanyl to atropine, fentanyl, and mivacurium. *Pediatrics.* 2006;118: 1583-1591.

NF-κB in tracheal lavage fluid from intubated premature infants: association with inflammation, oxygen, and outcome

Bourbia A, Cruz MA, Rozycki HJ (Virginia Commonwealth Univ, Richmond)
Arch Dis Child Fetal Neonatal Ed 91:36-39, 2006   7–6

Objectives.—To determine if tracheal lavage concentrations of the transcription factor NF-κB, which is activated by risk factors associated with bronchopulmonary dysplasia (BPD) and induces expression of cytokines associated with BPD, is related to BPD in premature infants.

Design.—Serial tracheal lavage samples from intubated premature infants were analysed for cell count and concentrations of interleukin (IL)8 and NF-κB, corrected for dilution by secretory component concentrations.

Setting.—Level III university hospital neonatal intensive care unit.

Patients.—Thirty three intubated infants (mean (SD) birth weight 903 (258) g, median gestation 27 weeks (range 24–31)) in the first 14 days of life.

Main Outcome Measures.—Tracheal effluent NF-κB, IL8, and cell counts, corrected for dilution by secretory component measurement.

Results.—Square root transformed NF-κB concentrations were significantly related to signs of inflammation (cell count, p = 0.002; IL8, p = 0.019) and to simultaneous fraction of inspired oxygen in samples from the first 3 days of life ($r = 0.512$, p<0.003). Of the 32 subjects with samples in the first 3 days of life, the half who either died or had BPD had higher NF-κB concentrations than those without BPD (square root concentration 0.097 (0.043) v 0.062 (0.036) µg/µg protein/µg secretory component, p = 0.018).

Conclusions.—Tracheobronchial lavage NF-κB concentrations are related to lung inflammation, oxygen exposure, and pulmonary outcome in intubated preterm infants. NF-κB activation may be an early critical step leading to BPD.

▶ NF-κB is a transcription factor that is known to regulate the production of several proinflammatory cytokines and to control tissue injury and cell death. In this study, tracheal aspirate levels of NF-κB (corrected for dilution using the IgA secretory component), cell counts and IL-8 were measured in preterm infants who had BPD develop/died (n = 16) or no BPD (n = 16). Expectedly, infants with BPD or died were of significantly younger gestational age, than those who did not have BPD develop. In the samples collected in the first 3 days of life, the groups did not differ with respect to cell counts and IL-8 levels. Although NF-κB levels were significantly higher in the BPD/death group, this difference did not persist when gestational age was taken into account.

Unfortunately, attempting to identify a diagnostic marker in the tracheal aspirates of premature infants who had BPD develop has been fraught with problems. Similar to this report by Bourbia et al, the majority of studies have been conducted in a small number of infants, with the tracheal aspirate collected at a variable number of time points, and with measurements of single markers usually performed, with or without "normalization," and with variable definitions of BPD. Furthermore, many of these studies have not been replicated in different populations or with sufficient sample size; others have reported conflicting results. Not surprisingly, none of these markers for BPD are in general clinical use.

V. Bhandari, MD, DM

IL-1α Causes Lung Inflammation and Maturation by Direct Effects on Preterm Fetal Lamb Lungs
Sosenko IRS, Kallapur SG, Nitsos I, et al (Univ of Miami, Fla; Univ of Cincinnati, Ohio; Univ of Western Australia, Crawley)
Pediatr Res 60:294-298, 2006   7–7

Intra-amniotic endotoxin induces IL-1, causes chorioamnionitis, lung inflammation, lung injury and lung maturation in preterm lambs. Intra-amniotic IL-1α also causes chorioamnionitis, lung inflammation and lung maturation. We asked if IL-1α effects on the preterm lung are mediated by direct signaling to the lung rather than by indirect effects from the chorioamnionitis. To study IL-1 effects independently of chorioamnionitis, the lungs and the amniotic fluid were surgically separated in fetal sheep by diverting fetal lung fluid *via* a tracheostomy tube to a sialastic bag. A mini-osmotic pump delivered an intratracheal infusion of recombinant sheep IL-1α (10 μg) or saline (control) over 24 h. Preterm lambs were delivered 1d or 7d after the start of the infusion at 124d gestational age (Term = 150d). IL-1α recruited inflammatory cells and increased proinflammatory cytokine mRNA expression in the fetal lungs. Compared with controls, IL-1α did not alter lung antioxidant enzyme activity or alveolar numbers. IL-1α had minimal effects on the mRNA or protein expression of proteins essential for vascular development. IL-1α induced large increases in alveolar surfactant saturated phosphatidylcholine and increased lung gas volumes. Lung inflammation and maturation result from direct exposure of the fetal lung to a single cytokine - IL-1α.

▶ Over the past decade, this group of investigators has contributed greatly to our understanding of the relationship between fetal exposure to infection and subsequent changes in lung structure and function that affect the susceptibility to acute and chronic respiratory distress after premature birth. However, the precise mechanisms that link chorioamnionitis and subsequent bronchopulmonary dysplasia remain obscure. In this article, we learn that, in the absence of chorioamnionitis, direct exposure of the fetal lamb lung to a continuous, low-dose infusion of IL-1α induced lung expression of proinflammatory cytokines and an influx of leukocytes into potential airspaces. These changes were accompanied by increased saturated phosphatidylcholine levels and greater quasi-static lung compliance compared with control lungs. It is noteworthy, however, that no differences in lung epithelial surface area or alveolar number were found between IL-1α–exposed and control lungs, nor were differences in the activity of antioxidant enzymes present. These findings imply that intrapulmonary release of a specific cytokine, IL-1α, without associated chorioamnionitis, can induce lung inflammation and functional changes related to surfactant release, without evidence of reduced lung septation or a response to oxidant stress, which typify lung injury associated with endotoxin-induced chorioamnionitis in sheep. The studies reported here, however, do not rule out the possibility that a longer period of exposure to IL-1α or a longer time interval after cytokine exposure might result in structural changes consistent with impaired lung growth, as seen in bronchopulmonary dysplasia.

R. D. Bland, MD

Respiratory distress syndrome-associated inflammation is related to early but not late peri/intraventricular hemorrhage in preterm infants
Krediet TG, Kavelaars A, Vreman HJ, et al (Wilhelmina Children's Hosp, Utrecht, The Netherlands; Stanford Univ, Calif)
J Pediatr 148:740-746, 2006　　　　　　　　　　　　　　　　7–8

Objective.—To investigate whether or not peri/intraventricular hemorrhages (PIVHs) occurring in the first 12 hours of life (early PIVHs) are related to respiratory distress syndrome (RDS)-associated inflammatory factors in contrast to PIVHs developing after 12 hours of life (late PIVHs).

Study Design.—Blood samples obtained at 0 to 12 hours, 48 to 72 hours, and 168 hours of life were evaluated for determination of the proinflammatory cytokines interleukin (IL)-8 and IL-6, tumor necrosis factor (TNF)-α, and malondialdehyde (MDA) as measures of lipid peroxidation. Simultaneously, cranial ultrasonography was performed in 114 neonates under 32 weeks gestational age.

Results.—Out of the total study group of 114 neonates, 67 (59%) had RDS. Early PIVH occurred in 16 neonates, 14 of whom (88%) had RDS. Late PIVHs occurred in 12 neonates. Neonates with RDS had higher IL-8 and IL-6 levels at 0 to 12 hours ($P < .0001$; $< .0001$) and at 48 to 72 hours ($P < .001$; $< .01$) than those without RDS. Neonates with early PIVH had higher IL-8 ($P < .02$), IL-6 ($P < .02$), and MDA ($P < .01$) levels at 0 to 12 hours than those with late PIVH or no PIVH. Those with early PIVH had higher IL-8 levels at 48 to 72 hours than those without PIVH ($P < .02$). Multiple linear regression revealed an association between RDS/early PIVH and IL-8, IL-6, and MDA levels.

Conclusions.—An RDS-associated increase in proinflammatory cytokine and MDA levels was associated with early PIVHs, but not with late PIVHs, suggesting a different etiopathogenesis in early versus late PIVHs.

▶ These investigators evaluated the levels of serum proinflammatory cytokines (TNF-α, IL-6, IL-8) and a marker for oxidative stress (MDA) in a cohort of 114 premature infants. The levels were then correlated with the diagnosis of RDS and presence of PIVH. The first cranial ultrasound and serum markers were performed within the first 12 hours of life. Expectedly, infants with RDS (n = 47), were of significantly younger gestational age, than those without RDS (n = 67). And, not surprisingly, infants with RDS had more PIVH (n = 22), than those without RDS (n = 6). Infants with early PIVH (<12 hours) had a higher incidence of premature rupture of membranes with spontaneous onset of labor, histologic chorioamnionitis, were of younger gestational age, and more likely to have severe bleeds. With the use of multiple linear regression analysis, IL-6 and IL-8 had a positive relationship with RDS, and IL-8 and MDA levels were significantly associated with early PIVH.

The major limitation of this study is the use of serum markers as a surrogate for events occurring in the brain because of the difficulty in inferring a cause and effect relationship. In addition, the number of infants in this study was small. Nonetheless, these results suggest that proinflammatory cytokines and oxidative stress may play a role in the development of early PIVH in preterm neonates with RDS.

V. Bhandari, MD, DM

Non-invasive measurement of reduced ventilation:perfusion ratio and shunt in infants with bronchopulmonary dysplasia: a physiological definition of the disease
Quine D, Wong CM, Boyle EM, et al (Royal Infirmary of Edinburgh, UK; Univ of Cambridge, UK)
Arch Dis Child Fetal Neonatal Ed 91:409-414, 2006   7–9

Background.—An objective definition of bronchopulmonary dysplasia (BPD) is required to interpret trial outcomes and provide a baseline for prognostic studies. Current definitions do not quantify disease severity. The cardinal measures of impaired gas exchange are a reduced ventilation: perfusion ratio (V_A:Q) and increased right to left shunt. These can be determined non-invasively by plotting arterial oxygen saturation (SpO_2) against inspired oxygen pressure (PIO_2).

Aims.—To describe the reduced V_A):Q and shunt in infants with BPD and evaluate these as graded measures of pulmonary dysfunction.

Methods.—21 preterm infants with BPD were studied. PIO_2 was changed stepwise to vary SpO_2 between 86% and 94%. Pairs of PIO_2 and SpO_2 data points for each infant were plotted and analysed to derive reduced V_A:Q ratio and shunt.

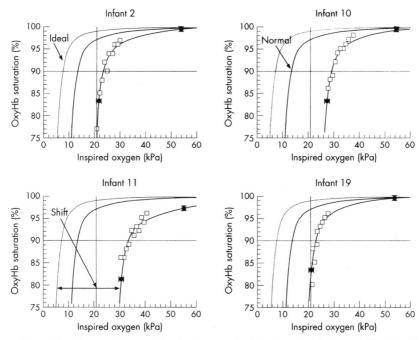

FIGURE 2.—Plots of oxyhaemoglobin (OxyHb) saturation (SpO$_2$) versus inspired oxygen (PIO$_2$, kPa) for infants 2, 10, 11 and 19. Reference grid lines are added at an SpO$_2$ of 90% and a PIO$_2$ of 21 kPa. The haemoglobin oxygen dissociation curve (ideal lung) is the reference point for derivation of shift. The normal SpO$_2$–PIO$_2$ curve is also included for comparison. (Courtesy of Quine D, Wong CM, Boyle EM, et al. Non-invasive measurement of reduced ventilation:perfusion ratio and shunt in infants with bronchopulmonary dysplasia: a physiological definition of the disease. *Arch Dis Child Fetal Neonatal Ed.* 2006;21:409-414. Reproduced with permission from the BMJ Publishing Group.)

Results.—In every infant, the SpO$_2$ versus PIO$_2$ curve was shifted to the right of the normal because of a reduced V$_A$:Q. The mean (SD) shift was 16.5 (4.7) kPa (normal 6 kPa). Varying degrees of shunt were also present, but these were less important in determining SpO$_2$ within the studied range. The degree of shift was strongly predictive of the PIO$_2$ required to achieve any SpO$_2$ within the range 86–94% (R^2>0.9), permitting shift and V$_A$:Q to be determined from a single pair of PIO$_2$ and SpO$_2$ values in this range.

Conclusions.—The predominant gas exchange impairment in BPD is a reduced V$_A$:Q, described by the right shift of the SpO$_2$ versus PIO$_2$ relationship. This provides a simpler method for defining BPD, which can grade disease severity (Fig 2, Table 3).

▶ Although defining BPD by receipt of supplemental inspired oxygen at 36 weeks' postmenstrual age (PMA) is common, wide practice variation with respect to oxygen treatment has diminished the use of that definition in clinical practice, especially in clinical investigation. The incorporation of an oxygen reduction challenge at 36 weeks' PMA to define oxygen "need" has helped to decrease the subjectivity of the definition.[1] The National Institutes of Health (NIH) consensus severity-based definition of BPD[2] recommended the use of

TABLE 3.—Right Shift (kPa) of the Arterial Oxygen Saturation (SpO$_2$) Versus Partial Pressure of Inspired Oxygen (PIO$_2$) Relationship for Different Pairs of PIO$_2$ and SpO$_2$ Values

PIO$_2$ (kPa)	SpO$_2$ (%)								
	86	87	88	89	90	91	92	93	94
21	13.1	12.8	12.5	12.2	11.8	11.4	10.9	10.3	9.5
22	14.1	13.8	13.6	13.2	12.8	12.4	11.8	11.2	10.4
23	15.2	14.9	14.6	14.2	13.8	13.3	12.8	12.1	11.2
24	16.2	15.9	15.6	15.2	14.8	14.3	13.7	13.0	12.0
25	17.2	16.9	16.6	16.2	15.8	15.3	14.6	13.8	12.8
26	18.2	17.9	17.6	17.2	16.8	16.2	15.6	14.7	13.6
27	19.3	19.0	18.6	18.2	17.8	17.2	16.5	15.6	14.5
28	20.3	20.0	19.7	19.3	18.8	18.2	17.4	16.5	15.3
29	21.3	21.0	20.7	20.3	19.8	19.1	18.3	17.4	16.1
30	22.4	22.1	21.7	21.3	20.7	20.1	19.3	18.3	16.9
31	23.4	23.1	22.7	22.3	21.7	21.1	20.2	19.2	17.7
32	24.4	24.1	23.7	23.3	22.7	22.0	21.1	20.0	18.6
33	25.5	25.2	24.7	24.3	23.7	23.0	22.1	20.9	19.4
34	26.5	26.2	25.8	25.3	24.7	24.0	23.0	21.8	20.2
35	27.5	27.2	26.8	26.3	25.7	24.9	23.9	22.7	21.0
36	28.6	28.2	27.8	27.3	26.7	25.9	24.9	23.6	21.8
37	29.6	29.3	28.8	28.3	27.7	26.9	25.8	24.5	22.7
38	30.6	30.3	29.8	29.3	28.7	27.8	26.7	25.3	23.5
39	31.7	31.3	30.8	30.3	29.7	28.8	27.7	26.2	24.3
40	32.7	32.4	31.9	31.4	30.7	29.8	28.6	27.1	25.1

(Courtesy of Quine D, Wong CM, Boyle EM, et al. Non-invasive measurement of reduced ventilation:perfusion ratio and shunt in infants with bronchopulmonary dysplasia: a physiological definition of the disease. *Arch Dis Child Fetal Neonatal Ed.* 2006;21:409-414. Reproduced with permission from the BMJ Publishing Group.)

such a physiologic assessment at 36 weeks' PMA to determine the need for oxygen therapy; the consensus was found to correlate with the spectrum of adverse pulmonary and neurodevelopmental outcomes observed in infants who had BPD develop.[3,4]

In this article, Quine et al analyzed gas exchange in 21 infants with BPD and described another physiologic assessment defining BPD. After varying the pulse oximetry measurements (SpO$_2$) between 86% and 94% by changing the inspired oxygen concentration (PIO$_2$) in a stepwise manner, SpO$_2$ was plotted against PIO$_2$ to determine the extent to which ventilation perfusion (V$_A$:Q) abnormalities or right-to-left shunting contributed to the need for supplemental inspired oxygen. The analyses demonstrated that the V$_A$:Q ratio abnormalities primarily accounted for gas exchange impairment, shifting the PIO$_2$ vs SpO$_2$ curve to the right a mean of 16.5 ± 4.7%. Fig 2 displays the plots constructed from 4 patients. Table 3 permits the V$_A$:Q ratio shift to be calculated from any pair of SpO$_2$ and PIO$_2$ values. To obtain the paired measurements employed in their analyses, the investigators used incubators with oxygen under servo control. It is unclear whether such a device is required to ensure "stable" measurements or whether the effective inspired oxygen concentration for infants receiving supplemental oxygen via a nasal cannula could be estimated by the method adapted for use in the STOP-ROP trial.[5] Future studies will hopefully demonstrate the utility of this physiologic assessment in defining the severity of BPD.

R. A. Ehrenkranz, MD

References

1. Walsh MC, Yao Q, Gettner PA, et al. Impact of a physiologic definition on bronchopulmonary dysplasia rates. *Pediatrics.* 2004;114:1305-1311.
2. Jobe AH, Bancalari E. Bronchopulmonary dysplasia. *Am J Respir Crit Care Med.* 2001;163:1723-1729.
3. Ehrenkranz RA, Walsh MC, Vohr BR, et al. Validation of the National Institutes of Health consensus definition of bronchopulmonary dysplasia. *Pediatrics.* 2005;116:1353-1360.
4. Hjalmarson O, Sandberg KL. Lung function at term reflects severity of bronchopulmonary dysplasia. *J Pediatr.* 2005;146:86-90.
5. Supplemental Therapeutic Oxygen for Prethreshold Retinopathy of Prematurity (STOP-ROP), a randomized, controlled trial. I: primary outcomes. *Pediatrics.* 2000;105:295-310.

Serum levels of seven cytokines in premature ventilated newborns: correlations with old and new forms of bronchopulmonary dysplasia
Vento G, Capoluongo E, Matassa PG, et al (Università Cattolica del Sacro Cuore, Rome; Università Cattolica, Rome; Gen Hosp S Giovanni Calibita, Rome)
Intensive Care Med 32:723-730, 2006   7–10

Objective.—In addition to the previous classification of chronic lung disease (CLD) O_2 dependency at 36 weeks of postmenstrual age, a new definition of CLD has recently been proposed: new bronchopulmonary-dysplasia (BPD). This uses total duration of O_2 supplementation and positive pressure requirements to delineate three degrees of severity (mild, moderate, and severe) according to the respiratory status at 36 weeks postmenstrual age. We analyzed the balance of serum proinflammatory and profibrotic/angiogenic cytokine concentrations in relation to CLD and the new BPD definition.

Design and Setting.—Descriptive study in a third-level neonatal ICU.

Patients.—Thirty-one preterm neonates with a gestational age of 24–29 weeks were studied to evaluate their serum cytokine concentration; they were previously enrolled in a randomized clinical trial to compare the effects of high-frequency oscillatory ventilation vs. intermittent mandatory ventilation in terms of pulmonary mechanics and lung cytokines. Serum samples were collected on days 1, 3, and 5 after birth until extubation to detect the levels of three proinflammatory cytokines plus four profibrotic/angiogenic cytokines, and correlations were examined to old CLD and new BPD. Ventilation treatments were distributed homogeneously between the groups and did not interfere with the results presented here.

Results and Conclusions.—Old CLD development, mainly corresponding to the moderate/severe forms of new BPD, was associated with increased proinflammatory and profibrotic/angiogenic cytokines, while mild forms of new BPD were characterized only by increases in profibrotic/angiogenic cytokines, suggesting a different balance of two pathogenic mechanisms in different phases of the disease.

▶ Vento et al observed that the higher serum concentrations of selected cytokines early in the postnatal period were associated with the severity of BPD in a small sample of preterm infants. Cytokines mediate acute lung injury,[1] exacerbate ventilator-induced lung injury (VILI),[2] and modulate host defense.[3] Therefore, it is indeed possible that these cytokines play a role in the pathophysiology of BPD. However, observational studies such as this study only demonstrate association and do not indicate a causal or direct role for the selected cytokines in pathophysiology, as it is possible that higher concentrations of the selected cytokines are just a marker for more severe lung injury. If these cytokines are involved in the pathophysiology of BPD, it needs to be determined whether the increase in cytokine concentrations is the result of a stronger stimulus (eg, greater ventilator induced lung injury) or whether it is due to increased cytokine production for the same stimulus. There is a substantial genetic component to the development of BPD.[4] Genetic variability in the production (or in the response to) particular cytokines, such as occurs with tumor necrosis factor-α[5] and interferon γ,[6] may lead to either higher or lower cytokine concentrations for the same stimulus. This genetic variability may augment or attenuate subsequent lung injury and BPD.

There is currently limited knowledge on: (a) which of the many known cytokines are crucial mediators of normal fetal and postnatal lung development; (b) the temporal profile of these cytokines during normal development and when the lung is injured; and (c) the effects that these cytokines modulate in the newborn lung. These important cytokines need to be identified by screening techniques such as multiplex luminex assays that can be performed on small samples, or by proteomic and/or genomic techniques. Studies should be performed on a large population of preterm infants to sort out the potential associations because of the many confounding variables. Subsequent basic research using conditional transgenic animal models and gene silencing/overexpression models will likely be required to determine the role of these cytokines in lung development and injury.

N. Ambalavanan, MD

References

1. Goodman RB, Pugin J, Lee JS, Matthay MA. Cytokine-mediated inflammation in acute lung injury. *Cytokine Growth Factor Rev.* 2003;14:523-535.
2. Belperio JA, Keane MP, Lynch JP 3rd, Strieter RM. The role of cytokines during the pathogenesis of ventilator-associated and ventilator-induced lung injury. *Semin Respir Crit Care Med.* 2006;27:350-364.
3. Strieter RM, Belperio JA, Keane MP. Cytokines in innate host defense in the lung. *J Clin Invest.* 2002;109:699-705.
4. Bhandari V, Bizzarro MJ, Shetty A, et al, for the Neonatal Genetics Study Group. Familial and genetic susceptibility to major neonatal morbidities in preterm twins. *Pediatrics.* 2006;117:1901-1906.
5. Kazzi SN, Kim UO, Quasney MW, Buhimschi I. Polymorphism of tumor necrosis factor-alpha and risk and severity of bronchopulmonary dysplasia among very low birth weight infants. *Pediatrics.* 2004;114:e243-e248.

6. Bokodi G, Derzbach L, Bányász I, Tulassay T, Vásárhelyi B. Association of interferon gamma T+874A and interleukin 12 p40 promoter CTCTAA/GC polymorphism with the need for respiratory support and perinatal complications in low birthweight neonates. *Arch Dis Child Fetal Neonatal Ed.* 2007;92:F25-F29.

The Effects of Hypercapnia on Cerebral Autoregulation in Ventilated Very Low Birth Weight Infants
Kaiser JR, Gauss CH, Williams DK (Univ of Arkansas, Little Rock)
Pediatr Res 58:931-935, 2005   7–11

Permissive hypercapnia, a strategy allowing high $PaCO_2$, is widely used by neonatologists to minimize lung damage in ventilated very low birth weight (VLBW) infants. While hypercapnia increases cerebral blood flow (CBF), its effects on cerebral autoregulation of VLBW infants are unknown. Monitoring of mean CBF velocity (mCBFv), $PaCO_2$, and mean arterial blood pressure (MABP) from 43 ventilated VLBW infants during the first week of life was performed during and after 117 tracheal suctioning procedures. Autoregulation status was determined during tracheal suctioning because it perturbs cerebral and systemic hemodynamics. The slope of the relationship between mCBFv and MABP was estimated when $PaCO_2$ was fixed at 30, 35, 40, 45, 50, 55, and 60 mm Hg. A slope near or equal to 0 suggests intact autoregulation, *i.e.* CBF is not influenced by MABP. Increasing values >0 indicate progressively impaired autoregulation. Infants weighed 905 ± 259 g and were 26.9 ± 2.3 wk gestation. The autoregulatory slope increased as $PaCO_2$ increased from 30 to 60 mm Hg. While the slopes for $PaCO_2$ values of 30 to 40 mm Hg were not statistically different from 0, slopes for $PaCO_2$ ≥45 mm Hg indicated a progressive loss of cerebral autoregulation. The autoregulatory slope increases with increasing $PaCO_2$, suggesting the cerebral circulation becomes progressively pressure passive with hypercapnia. These data raise concerns regarding the use of permissive hypercapnia in ventilated VLBW infants during the first week of life, as impaired autoregulation during this period may be associated with increased vulnerability to brain injury.

▶ The investigators observed potentially impaired cerebral autoregulation at $PaCO_2$ levels of 45 to 60 mm Hg during episodes of tracheal suctioning. The continuous measurements of CBF, MABP, and blood gas monitoring combined with signal analysis allowed for estimations of the impact of $PaCO_2$ on cerebral autoregulation. It is difficult to extrapolate the clinical implications of these findings for a few reasons. First, the measurements taken in this study were surrounding suctioning episodes. Suctioning episodes would presumably have been associated with increased carbon dioxide and blood pressure. The relationship of carbon dioxide and cerebral autoregulation may be different in cases in which there is a sudden rise in carbon dioxide compared with when there is a relatively constant carbon dioxide level. Perhaps there is an impact of change in carbon dioxide as well as actual carbon dioxide value on autoregulation. Second, the incidence of intraventricular hemorrhage and severe intraventricular hemorrhage in this observational study was low. In this cohort of

VLBW infants who were presumably sick enough to require mechanical venti-lation and who were treated practicing a strategy of permissive mild hypercap-nia, there did not appear to be an obvious negative clinical consequence to that strategy.

The authors rightly point out that it would be too early to recommend avoid-ing permissive hypercapnia after their study as they did not assess long-term neurodevelopmental outcome. Furthermore, hypocapnia has also been asso-ciated with intraventricular hemorrhage, periventricular leukomalacia, and poor neurodevelopmental outcome. Indeed, this study did not compare differ-ent strategies of carbon dioxide targets in ventilated VLBW infants. However, the investigators demonstrated that important information on CBF and auto-regulation can be obtained from noninvasive techniques such as Doppler US. Continuous measurements of CBF in relation to systemic blood pressure as obtained in this study could be applied to other areas of research in neonatol-ogy. Although neonatologists have various methods to manipulate blood pres-sure as well as blood gas measurements in VLBW infants, the effects of many of these treatments on CBF are not well known.

H. C. Lee, MD

Pulmonary Nitric Oxide Synthases and Nitrotyrosine: Findings During Lung Development and in Chronic Lung Disease of Prematurity
Sheffield M, Mabry S, Thibeault DW, et al (Univ of Missouri-Kansas City)
Pediatrics 118:1056-1064, 2006   7–12

Background.—Nitric oxide mediates and modulates pulmonary transi-tion from fetal to postnatal life. NO is synthesized by 3 nitric oxide synthase isoforms. One key pathway of nitric oxide metabolism results in nitrotyro-sine, a stable, measurable marker of nitric oxide production.

Objective.—The purpose of this study was to assess, by semiquantitative immunohistochemistry, nitric oxide synthase isoforms and nitrotyrosine at different airway and vascular tree levels in the lungs of neonates at different gestational ages and to compare results in control groups to those in infants with chronic lung disease.

Design/Methods.—Formalin-fixed, paraffin-embedded, postmortem lung blocks were prepared for immunohistochemistry using antibodies to each nitric oxide synthase isoform and to nitrotyrosine. Blinded observers evaluated the airway and vascular trees for staining intensity (0–3 scale) at 5 levels and 3 levels, respectively. The control population consisted of infants from 22 to 42 weeks' gestation who died in <48 hours. Results were com-pared with gestation-matched infants with varying severity of chronic lung disease.

Results.—In control and chronic lung disease groups, 22 to 42 weeks' ges-tation, staining for all 3 of the nitric oxide synthase isoforms was found in the airway epithelium from the bronchus to the alveolus or distal-most air-space. The abundance or distribution of nitric oxide synthase-3 staining in the airways did not show significant correlation with gestational age or severity of chronic lung disease. In the vascular tree, intense nitric oxide synthase-3 and moderate nitric oxide synthase-2 staining was found; nitric oxide synthase-1 was not consistently stained. Nitrotyrosine did stain in the pulmonary tree. Compared with controls where nitrotyrosine staining was minimal, regardless of gestation, in infants with chronic lung disease there was more than fourfold increase between severe chronic lung disease ($n = 12$) and either mild chronic lung disease or control infants ($n = 16$).

Conclusions.—All 3 of the nitric oxide synthase isoforms and nitrotyrosine are detectable by immunohistochemistry early in lung development. Nitric oxide synthase ontogeny shows no significant changes in abundance or distribution with advancing gestational age nor with chronic lung disease. Nitrotyrosine is significantly increased in severe chronic lung disease.

▶ This article describes immunohistochemical staining to detect both the presence or absence and distribution of NO synthase (NOS) isoforms and nitrotyrosine (NT), a stable metabolite of NO, in lung tissue obtained at autopsy from infants who died of neonatal chronic lung disease (CLD) compared with age-matched control infants, between 22 and 42 weeks of gestation, who died within 48 hours of birth. A clinical scoring system was used to determine the severity of CLD. Immunostaining data for control infants and infants with CLD were not significantly different, except that NOS-3 (endothelial NOS) staining at the respiratory bronchiolar level was decreased and NT staining as a percentage of tissue area was increased in the lungs of infants with severe CLD compared with gestational age–matched control infants.

Immunohistochemistry is a useful method for detecting the presence or absence and the distribution of a given protein in tissue, but it is not so useful for determining the amount of protein in tissue. This caveat aside, the article by Sheffield et al largely confirms results of previous studies performed with lung tissue from animals during development and from animal models of CLD, showing that all 3 NOS isoforms are expressed in the lungs during development, that bronchiolar expression of eNOS protein (and perhaps also pulmonary vascular expression) may be diminished in severe cases of CLD, and that the lung abundance of NT is increased in severe CLD. The finding of abundant NT in lungs of infants with severe CLD, none of whom were treated with inhaled NO, serves as a reminder that such infants already have evidence of pulmonary oxidant injury and, therefore, might be vulnerable to further damage imposed by increased exposure to NO in the presence of increased inspired O_2.

This study underscores the value of a careful and comprehensive assessment of human pathology to determine the validity of findings derived from animal models of development and/or disease. The article lends support to these models, but it also provides new information defining the pulmonary distribution of the NOS isoforms during human lung development and in CLD.

A possible shortcoming of the study was the inability to exclude, as controls, infants who may have been exposed to O_2 or mechanical ventilation for up to 48 hours after birth. For assessing the normal developmental pattern of NO isoforms and NT, it would have been useful to include immunostaining of age-matched fetal lungs, unaffected by postnatal breathing, O_2 exposure, or assisted ventilation. The absence of such a control group probably reflects the difficulty of obtaining fresh lung tissue for immunohistochemical analysis soon after fetal demise. Because data were obtained from lungs of infants that lived for up to 2 days, it is possible that some of the differences described in the lungs of these infants, compared with the lungs of normal mammalian fetuses in prior publications, could be explained by postnatal events that may have affected lung histopathology in the control infants. This article, however, is an important contribution to our knowledge of lung pathology in CLD.

R. D. Bland, MD

Early Inhaled Nitric Oxide Therapy in Premature Newborns with Respiratory Failure

Kinsella JP, Cutter GR, Walsh WF, et al (Univ of Colorado, Denver; Children's Hosp, Denver; Univ of Alabama at Birmingham; et al)
N Engl J Med 355:354-364, 2006   7–13

Background.—The safety and efficacy of early, low-dose, prolonged therapy with inhaled nitric oxide in premature newborns with respiratory failure are uncertain.

Methods.—We performed a multicenter, randomized trial involving 793 newborns who were 34 weeks of gestational age or less and had respiratory failure requiring mechanical ventilation. Newborns were randomly assigned to receive either inhaled nitric oxide (5 ppm) or placebo gas for 21 days or until extubation, with stratification according to birth weight (500

TABLE 2.—Incidence of Death or Bronchopulmonary Dysplasia at 36 Weeks of Postmenstrual Age

Variable	Inhaled Nitric Oxide (N = 398)	Placebo (N = 395)	P Value	Relative Risk (95% CI)*
	No./Total No. (%)			
All patients				
Death	78/394 (19.8)	98/392 (25.0)	0.08	0.79 (0.61-1.03)
Bronchopulmonary dysplasia	212/326 (65.0)	210/309 (68.0)	0.43	0.96 (0.86-1.09)
Death or bronchopulmonary dysplasia	282/394 (71.6)	295/392 (75.3)	0.24	0.95 (0.87-1.03)
Birth weight of 500-749 g				
Death	55/191 (28.8)	66/189 (34.9)	0.20	0.82 (0.61-1.11)
Bronchopulmonary dysplasia	113/144 (78.5)	100/132 (75.8)	0.59	1.04 (0.91-1.18)
Death or bronchopulmonary dysplasia	162/191 (84.8)	159/189 (84.1)	0.85	1.01 (0.92-1.10)
Birth weight of 750-999 g				
Death	15/138 (10.9)	24/139 (17.3)	0.13	0.63 (0.35-1.15)
Bronchopulmonary dysplasia	82/125 (65.6)	76/120 (63.3)	0.71	1.04 (0.86-1.25)
Death or bronchopulmonary dysplasia	95/138 (68.8)	95/139 (68.3)	0.93	1.01 (0.86-1.18)
Birth weight of 1000-1250 g				
Death	8/65 (12.3)	8/64 (12.5)	0.97	0.98 (0.39-2.46)
Bronchopulmonary dysplasia	17/57 (29.8)	34/57 (59.6)	0.001	0.50 (0.32-0.79)
Death or bronchopulmonary dysplasia	25/65 (38.5)	41/64 (64.1)	0.004	0.60 (0.42-0.86)

*CI denotes confidence interval.

(Reprinted by permission from Kinsella JP, Cutter GR, Walsh WF, et al. Early inhaled nitric oxide therapy in premature newborns with respiratory failure. *N Engl J Med.* 355:354-364. Copyright 2006, Massachusetts Medical Society. All rights reserved.)

to 749 g, 750 to 999 g, or 1000 to 1250 g). The primary efficacy outcome was a composite of death or bronchopulmonary dysplasia at 36 weeks of postmenstrual age. Secondary safety outcomes included severe intracranial hemorrhage, periventricular leukomalacia, and ventriculomegaly.

Results.—Overall, there was no significant difference in the incidence of death or bronchopulmonary dysplasia between patients receiving inhaled nitric oxide and those receiving placebo (71.6 percent vs. 75.3 percent, P = 0.24) (Table 2). However, for infants with a birth weight between 1000 and 1250 g, as compared with placebo, inhaled nitric oxide therapy reduced the incidence of bronchopulmonary dysplasia (29.8 percent vs. 59.6 percent); for the cohort overall, such treatment reduced the combined end point of intracranial hemorrhage, periventricular leukomalacia, or ventriculomegaly (17.5 percent vs. 23.9 percent, P = 0.03) and of periventricular leukomalacia alone (5.2 percent vs. 9.0 percent, P = 0.048). Inhaled nitric oxide therapy did not increase the incidence of pulmonary hemorrhage or other adverse events.

Conclusions.—Among premature newborns with respiratory failure, low-dose inhaled nitric oxide did not reduce the overall incidence of bronchopulmonary dysplasia, except among infants with a birth weight of at least 1000 g, but it did reduce the overall risk of brain injury.

Inhaled Nitric Oxide in Preterm Infants Undergoing Mechanical Ventilation
Ballard RA, for the NO CLD Study Group (Children's Hosp of Philadelphia; et al)
N Engl J Med 355:343-353, 2006   7–14

Background.—Bronchopulmonary dysplasia in premature infants is associated with prolonged hospitalization, as well as abnormal pulmonary and neurodevelopmental outcome. In animal models, inhaled nitric oxide improves both gas exchange and lung structural development, but the use of this therapy in infants at risk for bronchopulmonary dysplasia is controversial.

Methods.—We conducted a randomized, stratified, double-blind, placebo-controlled trial of inhaled nitric oxide at 21 centers involving infants with a birth weight of 1250 g or less who required ventilatory support between 7 and 21 days of age. Treated infants received decreasing concentrations of nitric oxide, beginning at 20 ppm, for a minimum of 24 days. The primary outcome was survival without bronchopulmonary dysplasia at 36 weeks of postmenstrual age.

Results.—Among 294 infants receiving nitric oxide and 288 receiving placebo birth weight (766 g and 759 g, respectively), gestational age (26 weeks in both groups), and other characteristics were similar. The rate of survival without bronchopulmonary dysplasia at 36 weeks of postmenstrual age was 43.9 percent in the group receiving nitric oxide and 36.8 percent in the placebo group (P = 0.042). The infants who received inhaled nitric oxide were discharged sooner (P = 0.04) and received supplemental

TABLE 2.—Incidence of the Primary Outcome

Outcome	Inhaled Nitric Oxide	Placebo	P Value	Relative Benefit (95% CI)*
	No./Total No. (%)			
Overall population				
Survival without chronic lung disease	129/294 (43.9)	106/288 (36.8)	0.04	1.23 (1.01-1.51)
Death or survival with chronic lung disease	165/294 (56.1)	182/288 (63.2)		
Chronic lung disease	149/294 (50.7)	164/288 (56.9)		
Death	16/294 (5.4)	18/288 (6.3)		
Birth weight of 500-799 g				
Survival without chronic lung disease	85/197 (43.1)	74/197 (37.6)	0.14	1.20 (0.94-1.54)
Death or survival with chronic lung disease	112/197 (56.9)	123/197 (62.4)		
Chronic lung disease	99/197 (50.3)	108/197 (54.8)		1.01 (0.96-1.07)
Death	13/197 (6.6)	15/197 (7.6)		1.30 (0.91-1.87)
Birth weight of 800-1250 g				
Survival without chronic lung disease	44/97 (45.4)	32/91 (35.2)	0.14	1.00 (0.95-1.06)
Death or survival with chronic lung disease	53/97 (54.6)	59/91 (64.8)		
Chronic lung disease	50/97 (51.5)	56/91 (61.5)		
Death	3/97 (3.1)	3/91 (3.3)		

*CI denotes confidence interval.

oxygen therapy for a shorter time (P = 0.006). There were no short-term safety concerns (Table 2).

Conclusions.—Inhaled nitric oxide therapy improves the pulmonary outcome for premature infants who are at risk for bronchopulmonary dysplasia when it is started between 7 and 21 days of age and has no apparent short-term adverse effects.

▶ Initial clinical studies in preterm infants with severe respiratory failure[1] and with developing or established bronchopulmonary dysplasia[2,3] found that inhaled nitric oxide improved oxygenation, similar to its dramatic effect in term infants with hypoxic respiratory failure. In subsequent animal studies, inhaled nitric oxide was shown to improve surfactant function,[4] attenuate hyperoxic lung injury,[5] reduce lung inflammation,[6] and promote lung growth.[7,8] These findings suggested that administration of inhaled nitric oxide to preterm infants might prevent lung injury through mechanisms in addition to improved gas exchange by selective pulmonary vasodilatation, and stimulated additional studies in this population.

The trials of inhaled nitric oxide in infants with a birth weight of 500 to 1250 g reported by Kinsella et al (Abstract 7–13) and Ballard et al (Abstact 7–14) are the largest to date. The average gestational age of enrolled subjects in the two trials was 25 to 26 weeks, a group at high risk of lung and brain injury. In the trial of Kinsella et al, mechanically ventilated infants who were less than 48 hours of age were randomly assigned to receive inhaled nitric oxide at a dose of 5 ppm, or nitrogen placebo for 21 days, or until they no longer needed mechanical ventilation. The incidence of death or bronchopulmonary dysplasia, the primary outcome, was not different between groups. In prespecified subgroup analyses stratified by birth weight, the combined primary outcome and bronchopulmonary dysplasia alone were reduced in treated infants with birth weight 1000 to 1250 g, a group that accounted for only 16% of the subjects and would be expected to be at much lower risk for these outcomes than the other two weight groups. Treatment with inhaled nitric oxide also reduced overall ultrasonographic evidence of brain injury (severe intracranial hemorrhage, periventricular leukomalacia, or ventriculomegaly), a secondary outcome.

In the trial of Ballard et al, infants who continued to require mechanical ventilation at 7 to 21 days of age or, if they were in the lowest birth weight group, remained on continuous positive airway pressure, were randomly assigned to a 24-day course of nitrogen placebo or inhaled nitric oxide at an initial dose of 20 ppm for 48 to 96 hours, then weaned at weekly intervals to 10, 5, and 2 ppm. Survival at 36 weeks postmenstrual age without bronchopulmonary dysplasia, the primary outcome, was improved in the treated group and the duration of oxygen therapy and hospitalization was reduced. In a post hoc analysis, the benefit was limited to the approximately 40% of infants who were 7 to 14 days old at randomization. Complications of prematurity, including evolution of cranial ultrasonographic findings, did not differ between groups.

Although inhaled nitric oxide does not appear to improve outcome in the most critically ill extremely low birth weight infants,[9] these two studies suggest a possible role in the treatment of preterm infants with respiratory failure who are less critically ill. However, questions remain regarding the selection of infants most likely to benefit and the most effective time of initiation, as well as the optimal dose and duration of treatment. Although cranial US abnormalities appeared to be less in the treatment group in the study of Kinsella et al and the evolution of US findings was not different between groups in the study of Ballard et al, long-term follow-up is essential to document improvement or no difference in neurodevelopmental outcome. Furthermore, the high cost of inhaled nitric oxide treatment makes it more difficult to justify its use until benefit is proven. For these reasons, use in preterm infants should be limited to clinical trials until more data are available, especially longer term follow-up of the children in these two trials.

A. Stark, MD

References

1. Kinsella JP, Walsh WF, Bose CL, et al. Inhaled nitric oxide in premature neonates with severe hypoxaemic respiratory failure: a randomized controlled trial. *Lancet.* 1999;354:1061-1065.
2. Banks BA, Seri I, Ischiropoulos H, Merrill J, Rychik J, Ballard RA. Changes in oxygenation with inhaled nitric oxide in severe bronchopulmonary dysplasia. *Pediatrics.* 1999;103:610-618.
3. Clark PL, Ekekezie II, Kaftan HA, Castor CA, Truog WE. Safety and efficacy of nitric oxide in chronic lung disease. *Arch Dis Child Fetal Neonatal Ed.* 2002;86:F41-F45.
4. Ballard PL, Gonzales LW, Godinez RI, et al. Surfactant composition and function in a primate model of infant chronic lung disease: effects of inhaled nitric oxide. *Pediatr Res.* 2006;59:157-162.
5. Cotton RB, Sundell HW, Zeldin DC, et al. Inhaled nitric oxide attenuates hyperoxic lung injury in lambs. *Pediatr Res.* 2006;59:142-146.
6. Kang JL, Park W, Pack IS, et al. Inhaled nitric oxide attenuates acute lung injury via inhibition of nuclear factor-kappa B and inflammation. *J Appl Physiol.* 2002;92:795-801.
7. McCurnin DC, Pierce RA, Chang LY, et al. Inhaled NO improves early pulmonary function and modifies lung growth and elastin deposition in a baboon model of neonatal chronic lung disease. *Am J Physiol Lung Cell Mol Physiol.* 2005;288: L450-L459.
8. Tang JR, Markham NE, Lin YJ, et al. Inhaled nitric oxide attenuates pulmonary hypertension and improves lung growth in infant rats after neonatal treatment with a VEGF receptor inhibitor. *Am J Physiol Lung Cell Mol Physiol.* 2004;287:L344-L351.
9. Van Meurs KP, Wright LL, Ehrenkranz RA, et al. Inhaled nitric oxide for premature infants with severe respiratory failure. *N Engl J Med.* 2005;353:13-22.

Inhaled nitric oxide in very preterm infants with severe respiratory distress syndrome

Dani C, Bertini G, Pezzati M, et al (Careggi Univ, Florence, Italy)
Acta Paediatr 95:1116-1123, 2006   7–15

Aim.—To test the hypothesis that inhaled nitric oxide therapy can decrease the incidence of bronchopulmonary dysplasia and death in preterm infants with severe respiratory distress syndrome; to evaluate the possible predictive factors for the response to inhaled nitric oxide therapy.

Methods.—Preterm infants (less than 30 weeks' gestation) were randomized to receive during the first week of life inhaled nitric oxide, or nothing, if they presented severe respiratory distress syndrome. Then, the treated infants were classified as non responders and responders.

Results.—Twenty infants were enrolled in the inhaled nitric oxide therapy group and 20 in the control group. Bronchopulmonary dysplasia and death were less frequent in the inhaled nitric oxide group than in the control group (50 vs. 90%, p = 0.016). Moreover, nitric oxide treatment was found to decrease as independent factor the combined incidence of death and BPD (OR = 0.111; 95% C.I. 0.02–0.610). A birth weight lower than 750 grams had a significant predictive value for the failure of responding to inhaled nitric oxide therapy (OR 12; 95% C.I. 1.3–13.3).

Conclusion.—Inhaled nitric oxide decreases the incidence of bronchopulmonary dysplasia and death in preterm infants with severe respiratory distress syndrome. Birth weight may influence the effectiveness of inhaled nitric oxide therapy in promoting oxygenation improvement in preterm infants.

▶ The conclusions of the recently reported random control trials[1-4] evaluating treatment of preterm infants with respiratory distress syndrome (RDS) with inhaled nitric oxide (iNO) are not straightforward. Differences in study design, and especially of patient eligibility, have led to conclusions that iNO either reduced the incidence of BPD or death,[1] or did not alter the incidence of BPD or death.[2-4] Furthermore, subgroup analyses have suggested that infants >1000 g birth weight may be more likely to respond to iNO, resulting in a decreased incidence of BPD or death in the subset of treated infants.[2,4]

The results described by Dani et al in this report are consistent with these observations. On the basis of OIs at enrollment, 16.4 ± 5.1 in the iNO group and 15.1 ± 4.9 in the control group, the severity of illness experienced by the infants recruited into the trial by Dani et al falls between the OIs at enrollment in the Kinsella et al and the Van Meurs et al trials. Interestingly, non-iNO responders in the Dani et al trial tended to have lower birth weights and higher OIs; a birth weight <750 g was predictive of a non-iNO responder. Unfortunately, the impact of the data is limited by the small sample size. However, inclusion of the data into a meta-analysis, or into the planned individual patient meta-analysis, should enhance the value of the respective analyses.

R. A. Ehrenkranz, MD

References

1. Schreiber MD, Gin-Mestan K, Marks JD, Huo D, Lee G, Srisuparp P. Inhaled nitric oxide in premature infants with the respiratory distress syndrome. *N Engl J Med.* 2003;349:2099-2107.
2. Van Meurs KP, Wright LL, Ehrenkranz RA, et al. Inhaled nitric oxide for premature infants with severe respiratory failure. *N Engl J Med.* 2005;353:13-22.

3. Field D, Elbourne D, Truesdale A, et al, for the INNOVO Trial Collaborating Group. Neonatal ventilation with inhaled nitric oxide versus ventilatory support without inhaled nitric oxide for preterm infants with severe respiratory failure: the INNOVO multicenter randomised controlled trial. *Pediatrics.* 2005;115:926-936.
4. Kinsella JP, Cutter GR, Walsh WF, et al. Early inhaled nitric oxide therapy in premature newborns with respiratory failure. *N Engl J Med.* 2006;355:354-364.

Substrate utilization and kinetics of surfactant metabolism in evolving bronchopulmonary dysplasia
Spence KL, Zozobrado JC, Patterson BW, et al (Washington Univ, St Louis)
J Pediatr 147:480-485, 2005   7–16

Objectives.—To use stable isotopically labeled precursors of pulmonary surfactant phospholipids to measure precursor utilization and surfactant turnover in premature infants who required mechanical ventilation at birth, 2 weeks, and >4 weeks of age.

Study Design.—Infants of ≤28 weeks' gestation received simultaneous 24-hour intravenous infusions of $[1,2,3,4-^{13}C_4]$ palmitate and $[1-^{13}C_1]$ acetate at birth, 2 weeks, and ≥4 weeks of life. Disaturated phospholipids were extracted from sequential tracheal aspirate samples obtained over a period of 2 weeks. Fractional catabolic rate (a measure of total turnover) and the fractional synthetic rates from plasma palmitate and de novo synthesis (acetate) were measured.

Results.—The fractional catabolic rate increased from 25.3% ± 7.0% per day at birth to 53.8% ± 14.4% per day at 4 weeks ($P = .001$). The combined contribution from plasma palmitate and de novo synthesis to total synthesis increased from 44.2% ± 19.8% at birth to 85.2% ± 32.8% at 4 weeks ($P = .03$).

Conclusions.—Total surfactant turnover increased in premature infants with evolving bronchopulmonary dysplasia. The increasing contributions from acetate and plasma palmitate suggest a decrease in surfactant phospholipid recycling.

▶ Chronically ventilated preterm infants with bronchopulmonary dysplasia (BPD) have been shown to have transient episodes of abnormal surfactant function characterized by decreased surface tension, lowering ability and deficiency of surfactant proteins B and C but not surfactant phospholipids. These episodes appeared to be temporally associated with episodes of infection and respiratory deterioration.[1]

Spence et al have examined surfactant kinetics in infants with BPD. This complex study concludes that surfactant turnover is increased in premature infants who are ventilated in the first month after birth and that this phenomenon is largely due to new surfactant synthesis rather than recycling of secreted surfactant. The findings are limited by methodological problems; for example, interpretation of the data was dependent on assumptions relating to surfactant pool size. Nonetheless, because administration of exogenous surfactant is being considered as a treatment for infants with evolving BPD,[1,2] these observations may be useful.

I. Gross, MD

References

1. Merrill JD, Ballard RA, Cnaan A, et al. Dysfunction of pulmonary surfactant in chronically ventilated premature infants. *Pediatr Res.* 2004;56:918-926.
2. Pandit PB, Dunn MS, Kelly EN, Perlman M. Surfactant replacement in neonates with early chronic lung disease. *Pediatrics.* 1995;95:851-854.

Tracheotomy in Very Low Birth Weight Neonates: Indications and Outcomes
Sisk EA, Kim TB, Schumacher R, et al (Univ of Michigan, Ann Arbor)
Laryngoscope 116:928-933, 2006   7–17

Objective/Hypothesis.—To review incidence of, indications for, and outcomes of tracheotomy in very low birth weight (VLBW) infants.

Study Design.—Retrospective review in tertiary care hospital.

Methods.—Eighteen VLBW (<1,500 g) infants with bronchopulmonary dysplasia undergoing tracheotomy in the neonatal intensive care unit between October 1997 and June 2002 were studied. Controls consisted of 36 VLBW infants undergoing intubation without tracheotomy, two per study infant, matched by gestational age and weight. Outcome measures included duration and number of intubation events, time to decannulation, complications, comorbidities, length of stay, and speech, language, and swallowing measures.

Results.—Infants undergoing tracheotomy had an average duration of intubation of 128.8 days with a median number of 11.5 intubation events, both significantly greater than those of controls. Percentage of those with laryngotracheal stenosis was 44% of study infants had laryngotracheal stenosis compared to 1.6% in all intubated VLBW infants. The tracheotomy group had a significantly higher incidence of gastroesophageal reflux, pulmonary hypertension, and gastrostomy tube placement. The overall tracheotomy-related complication rate was 38.9%. Three were lost to follow-up, and five deaths occurred, two possibly tracheotomy-related. Six of ten were decannulated by an average time of 3.8 years, two of six after laryngotracheal reconstruction. Four of ten remained cannulated for a variety of reasons. Disorders of speech, language, and swallowing were common.

Conclusions.—When considering tracheotomy in VLBW infants, the total number of intubation events should be monitored as well as the total duration of intubation. The relatively high incidence of laryngotracheal stenosis argues for earlier endoscopy and possibly earlier tracheotomy in infants with developing stenoses.

▶ A retrospective chart review was performed on 636 VLBW infants (361-1500 g) admitted to the neonatal intensive care unit (NICU) from October 1997 through June 2002. Of these infants, 508 (80%) required intubation and ventilation, and of these 508, 18 tracheostomies were performed (3.5% of intubated patients). The 18 patients requiring tracheostomy were compared to 36 intubated control infants, who were matched for gestational age and weight. The average duration of intubation was 128.8 days for those patients eventually receiving a tracheostomy compared with that of 44.5 days for the control patients. Though the median number of intubation events and the average length of stay were significantly greater in the tracheostomy patients compared with that of the control patients, there was no difference between the groups when the increased average duration of intubation in the tracheostomy patients was taken into account. Multiple comorbidities were found in both the study and the control groups. Only gastroesophageal reflux disease, pulmonary hypertension, and the need for a gastrostomy tube were significantly more likely to occur in the study group. At the time of tracheotomy, the infants were an average of 44.5 weeks' gestation, and all underwent a direct laryngoscopy and bronchoscopy. Abnormalities of the upper airway were noted in 17 of 18 patients, and these included glottic or subglottic edema in 7 patients, laryngeal granulation tissue in 4, tracheomalacia in 4, bronchomalacia in 4, laryngomalacia in 1, and a persistent tracheoesophageal fistula in 1.

Laryngotracheal stenosis was eventually diagnosed in 8 of 18 tracheostomy patients, and no mention is made of that diagnosis in the other intubated, VLBW infants. All tracheostomies were performed in a controlled elective setting in the operating room under general anesthesia and no perioperative complications were reported. Of the 8 patients who were eventually determined to have laryngotracheal stenosis, there was no increase in their oxygen requirement after the tracheostomy compared with that of the control patients, implying that upper-airway issues were the major determinant in the need for a tracheostomy and not bronchopulmonary dysplasia (BPD). No separate analysis is reported in these 8 patients in endoscopic findings, intubation time or events, or comorbidities. Of the 18 patients receiving a tracheostomy, 1 died at home at 18 months of age with a displaced tracheostomy tube, and 1 died at home in the postoperative period after a laryngotracheal reconstruction and stent placement. Of the remaining patients with a tracheotomy and laryngotracheal stenosis, one remained with a tracheostomy after 2 unsuccessful laryngotracheal reconstructions. This patient has had significant neuromuscular and behavioral problems. One patient was decannulated at 6.7 years of age after 3 laryngotracheal reconstructions. One patient had a successful laryngotracheal reconstruction, but remained cannulated because of neuromuscular issues. Two patients were decannulated at 3 and 4 years of age without a laryngotracheal reconstruction, the latter having had a tonsil and adenoidectomy and a Nissen fundoplication. Of the tracheostomy patients without laryngotracheal stenosis, 3 remained ventilator dependent until their deaths from cor pulmonale and respiratory failure. Three were weaned after prolonged ventilation, and 2 eventually decannulated. One remained cannulated with breath-holding spells. One patient was decannulated but required replacement of the tracheotomy within 90 days because of possible true vocal cord dysfunction. Three patients were lost to follow-up.

J. E. Arnold, MD

Surfactant Protein D Levels in Umbilical Cord Blood and Capillary Blood of Premature Infants. The Influence of Perinatal Factors
Dahl M, Holmskov U, Husby S, et al (Odense Univ, Denmark; Univ of Southern Denmark, Odense C)
Pediatr Res 59:806-810, 2006   7–18

Surfactant protein D (SP-D) is a collectin that plays an important role in the innate immune system and takes part in the surfactant homeostasis by regulating the surfactant pool size. The aims of this study were to investigate the values of SP-D in umbilical cord blood and capillary blood of premature infants and to relate the levels to perinatal conditions. A total of 254 premature infants were enrolled in the present study. Umbilical cord blood was drawn at the time of birth and capillary blood at regular intervals throughout the admission. The concentration of SP-D in umbilical cord blood and capillary blood was measured using ELISA technique. The median concentration of SP-D in umbilical cord blood was twice as high as in mature infants, 769 ng/mL (range 140–2,551), with lowest values in infants with intrauterine growth retardation (IUGR) and rupture of membranes (ROM). The median concentration of SP-D in capillary blood day 1 was 1,466 ng/mL (range 410–5,051 ng/mL), with lowest values in infants born with ROM and delivered vaginally. High SP-D levels in umbilical cord blood and capillary blood on day 1 were found to be more likely in infants in need for respiratory support or surfactant treatment and susceptibility to infections. We conclude that SP-D concentrations in umbilical cord blood and capillary blood in premature infants are twice as high as in mature infants and depend on several perinatal conditions. High SP-D levels in umbilical cord blood and capillary blood on day 1 were found to be related to increased risk of RDS and infections.

▶ Surfactant proteins A (SP-A) and D (SP-D) play roles in both surfactant homeostasis and pulmonary innate immunity. They are collagen-containing C-type (calcium dependent) lectins, called collectins, and are structurally similar to mannose-binding protein of the lectin pathway of the complement system.[1] They recognize a broad spectrum of pathogens and allergens and trigger immune responses offering protection against infection and allergenic challenge. Indeed, SP-A and SP-D have been shown to be involved in viral neutralization, clearance of bacteria, fungi, and apoptotic and necrotic cells, downregulation of allergic reaction, and resolution of inflammation. Unlike SP-A, it does not contribute to lowering surface tension. SP-D-deficient mice have no respiratory abnormalities at birth, but the deficiency causes development of emphysema and a predisposition to specific infections. No human infant or child with respiratory distress and mutation in the SP-D gene has been identified. Hilgendorff et al[2] found that serum SP-D and mannose-binding lectin serum concentrations were significantly lower in preterms less than 32 weeks' gestational age (GA), compared with those at term. In infants with respiratory distress syndrome (RDS), SP-D concentrations from tracheal aspirates were increased in preterm infants between 28 and 32 weeks, but not those less than 28 weeks' GA suffering from RDS. The data pool is further expanded by Dahl et al where elevated cord and capillary levels were present in preterm infants with RDS and infections. This is an expansion of their report[3] on 458 mature infants where they concluded that SP-D concentrations in umbilical cord blood and capillary blood are highly variable and depend on several perinatal conditions, including maternal tobacco ingestion, intrauterine growth, presence of labor and cesarean section (after which levels were elevated). The role of SP-D in the metabolism of surfactant is, as yet, quite unclear but no doubt, as soon as it is elucidated, more surfactant proteins will be identified, and the research will need to continue. Murine models suggest the possibility that the recombinant forms of SP-A and SP-D may have potential in controlling pulmonary infection, inflammation, and allergies in humans[4] and could potentially be useful therapeutically in attenuating inflammatory processes in neonatal chronic lung disease, cystic fibrosis, and emphysema. We await further developments.

A. A. Fanaroff, MD

References

1. Kishore U, Bernal AL, Kamran MF, et al. Surfactant proteins SP-A and SP-D in human health and disease. *Arch Immunol Ther Exp (Warsz)*. 2005;53:399-417.
2. Hilgendorff A, Schmidt R, Bohnert A, Merz C, Bein G, Gortner L. Host defence lectins in preterm neonates. *Acta Paediatr*. 2005;94:794-799.
3. Dahl M, Juvonen PO, Holmskov U, Husby S. Surfactant protein D in newborn infants: factors influencing surfactant protein D levels in umbilical cord blood and capillary blood. *Pediatr Res*. 2005;58:908-912.
4. Clark H, Reid K. The potential of recombinant surfactant protein D therapy to reduce inflammation in neonatal chronic lung disease, cystic fibrosis, and emphysema. *Arch Dis Child*. 2003;88:981-984.

Intratracheal Recombinant Surfactant Protein D Prevents Endotoxin Shock in the Newborn Preterm Lamb

Ikegami M, Carter K, Bishop K, et al (Univ of Cincinnati, Ohio; Genzyme Corp, Framingham, Mass)

Am J Respir Crit Care Med 173:1342-1347, 2006   7–19

Rationale.—The susceptibility of neonates to pulmonary and systemic infection has been associated with the immaturity of both lung structure and the immune system. Surfactant protein (SP) D is a member of the collectin family of innate immune molecules that plays an important role in innate host defense of the lung.

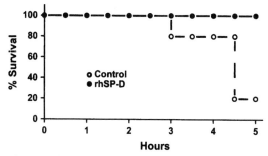

FIGURE 1.—Kaplan-Meier plot of recombinant human surfactant protein D (rhSP-D) treated group and control group. In the control group, only 20% of the lambs survived until the end of the 5-h study period. In contrast, all lambs tested with rhSP-D survived. p < 0.05 by log-rank test. (Courtesy of Ikegami M, Carter K, Bishop K, et al. Intratracheal recombinant surfactant protein D prevents endotoxin shock in the newborn preterm lamb. *Am J Respir Crit Care Med.* 2006;173:1342-1347. Official Journal of the American Thoracic Society. Copyright American Thoracic Society.)

Objectives.—We tested whether treatment with recombinant human SP-D influenced the response of the lung and systemic circulation to intratracheally administered *Escherichia* coli lipopolysaccharides.

Methods.—After intratracheal lipopolysaccharide instillation, preterm newborn lambs were treated with surfactant and ventilated for 5 h.

Measurement.—Survival rate, physiologic lung function, lung and systemic inflammation, and endotoxin level in plasma were evaluated.

Main Results.—In control lambs, intratracheal lipopolysaccharides caused septic shock and death associated with increased endotoxin in plasma. In contrast, all lambs treated with recombinant human SP-D were physiologically stable and survived (Fig 1). Leakage of lipopolysaccharides from the lungs to the systemic circulation was prevented by intratracheal recombinant human SP-D. Recombinant human SP-D prevented systemic inflammation and decreased the expression of IL-1β, IL-8, and IL-6 in the spleen and liver. Likewise, recombinant human SP-D decreased IL-1β and IL-6 in the lung and IL-8 in the plasma. Recombinant human SP-D did not alter pulmonary mechanics following endotoxin exposure. Recombinant human SP-D was readily detected in the lung 5 h after intratracheal instillation.

Conclusions.—Intratracheal recombinant human SP-D prevented shock caused by endotoxin released from the lung during ventilation in the premature newborn.

▶ The importance of this work, although done in sheep, is that it makes clear that SP-D, an innate immune protein, may be important in the defense against pneumonia and related septicemia and shock in low birth weight infants (less than 1500 g) who have been exposed to chorioamnionitis in utero. Not only does the work inform us about the pathogenesis of systemic endotoxin shock, it also suggests that intratracheal rhSP-D treatment might be useful in preventing this syndrome caused by endotoxin released from the lung during ventilation in the premature newborn. Although pulmonary inflammation was not blocked, the systemic effects of lipopolysaccharides were ameliorated in the sheep model. The authors thus conclude that rhSP-D may represent a potential therapeutic strategy for prevention of systemic inflammatory response in association with lung infection. Lambs are not people, but the reasonableness of this approach seems compelling.

D. K. Stevenson, MD

Long-term outcomes after infant lung transplantation for surfactant protein B deficiency related to other causes of respiratory failure
Palomar LM, Nogee LM, Sweet SC, et al (Washington Univ, St Louis; Johns Hopkins Univ, Baltimore, Md)
J Pediatr 149:548-553, 2006   7–20

Objective.—To determine if the outcomes of lung transplantation for infants with surfactant protein-B (SP-B) deficiency are unique.

Study Design.—From a prospective analysis to identify infants with genetic causes of surfactant deficiency, we identified 33 SP-B–deficient infants from 1993 to 2005, and, among those undergoing lung transplantation (n = 13), compared their survival, pulmonary function, and developmental progress with infants who underwent transplantation at <1 year of age for parenchymal lung disease (n = 13) or pulmonary vascular disease (n = 11).

Results.—Five-year survival rates (~50%, *P* = .3) and causes of death were similar for all three groups once the infants underwent transplantation. However, significant pretransplantation mortality decreased 5-year survival from listing to approximately 30% (*P* = .17). Pulmonary function, development of bronchiolitis obliterans, and school readiness were similar among the three groups. We detected anti SP-B antibody in serum of 3 of 7 SP-B–

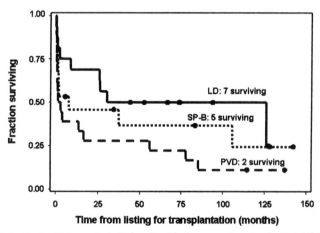

FIGURE 1.—Kaplan-Meier survival of infants listed for lung transplantation for SP-B deficiency (*SPB*), parenchymal lung disease (*LD*), and pulmonary vascular disease (*PVD*). The 5-year survival rates were 31%, 43%, and 22%, respectively. There was no statistical difference in the overall rate of survival among the three groups (*P* = .12). (Courtesy of Palomar LM, Nogee LM, Sweet SC, et al. Long-term outcomes after infant lung transplantation for surfactant protein B deficiency related to other causes of respiratory failure. *J Pediatr.* 149:548-553. Copyright 2006 by Elsevier.)

TABLE 1.—Characteristics of SP-B–Deficient Infants (n = 33)

Birth Weight (kg)		3.3 ± 0.8
Gestational age (wk)		39 ± 1
Sex		18 F:15 M
Race		C 26; AA 1; H 4; other 2
Age at diagnosis		19 (4-247) days*
Genotype	121 ins2/121 ins2	16
	121 ins2/other	10
	Homozygous other	4
	Heterozygous other	3
Listed: decline		17:15

*Excludes one infant diagnosed after lung transplantation.
Abbreviation: SP-B, Surfactant protein-B.
(Courtesy of Palomar LM, Nogee LM, Sweet SC, et al. Long-term outcomes after infant lung transplantation for surfactant protein B deficiency related to other causes of respiratory failure. *J Pediatr.* 149:548-553. Copyright 2006 by Elsevier.)

deficient infants and none of 7 SP-B–sufficient infants but could not identify any associated adverse outcomes.

Conclusions.—Long-term outcomes after infant lung transplantation for SP-B–deficient infants are similar to those of infants transplanted for other indications. These outcomes are important considerations in deciding to pursue lung transplantation for infants with disorders of alveolar homeostasis (Fig 1 and Tables 1, 2, and 3).

▶ This brief article describes outcomes of 13 infants who underwent lung transplantation between 1993 and 2005 because of respiratory failure from SP-B deficiency. It compares the outcomes of these infants to the outcomes of infants who underwent lung transplantation at younger than 1 year because of respiratory failure from parenchymal lung disease (excluding bronchopulmonary dysplasia) or pulmonary vascular disease. The numbers of infants in each group are small (12, 13, and 11), as are the number of survivors through 2005 (5, 7, and 2, respectively), which limits the value of comparing data among the groups. Thus, the conclusion remains tenuous that the long-term outcomes of infants with SP-B deficiency who undergo lung transplant surgery are similar to the outcomes of infants who receive transplanted lungs in the first year of life for conditions other than SP-B deficiency. Nearly one third of those listed for lung transplantation in this study died while awaiting surgery. The limited data on pulmonary function and neurodevelopment of infants who survived the surgery suggest that SP-B deficiency did not worsen functional outcomes when compared with the outcomes of infants who received transplanted lungs for conditions other than SP-B deficiency. However, the report that 2 of the 3 infants with SP-B–deficiency who survived more than 5 years had bronchiolitis obliterans, a life-threatening condition that was also common in the other groups, underscores the relatively bleak prognosis that confronts all infants who undergo lung transplantation in the first year of life. Missing from this article is an account of what must be the enormous economic and emo-

TABLE 2.—Transplantation Outcomes

	Surfactant Protein-B	Parenchymal Lung Disease	Pulmonary Vascular Disease	P Value
Transplanted/number listed (%)	12/17 (71)*	13/16 (81)	11/21 (52)	.18
Age at listing (days)§	28 (9-286)*†	70 (15-318)	127 (17-221)	.003
Age at transplant (days)§	76 (50-136)*‡	130 (61-374)	136 (83-278)	.03
ECMO pretransplant/total transplanted	4/13	2/13	3/11	
Survival to discharge, n (% of transplanted)	8 (67)	12 (92)	8 (73)	.17
LOS post transplant (days)§	32 (18-118)	38 (12-132)	37 (21-82)	.97
Survivors as of end 2005, n (% of transplanted)	5 (42)	7 (54)	2 (18)	.2
Cause of death				
Bronchiolitis obliterans	1		3	
Infection	3	3		
Malignancy		1	1	
Graft failure	3	1	2	
Gastroenteritis/dehydration	1		1	
Other		1	2	

*Excludes infant diagnosed after lung transplantation.
†Data available for n = 12.
‡Data available for n = 10.
§Median (range).
Abbreviations: ECMO, Extracorporeal membrane oxygenation; *LOS,* length of hospital stay.
(Courtesy of Palomar LM, Nogee LM, Sweet SC, et al. Long-term outcomes after infant lung transplantation for surfactant protein B deficiency related to other causes of respiratory failure. *J Pediatr.* 149:548-553. Copyright 2006 by Elsevier.)

TABLE 3.—Growth, Development, and Pulmonary Function of Survivors

	Surfactant Protein-B (n = 5)	Parenchymal Lung Disease (n = 12)	Pulmonary Vascular Disease (n = 8)	P Value
Interval between transplant and measurement (months, med-range)	36 (5–137)	33 (8–117)	46 (7–132)	.9
Weight Z-score, med (range)	−1.0 (−2.7–1.0)	−0.9 (−2.6–1.6)	−1.9 (−2.7–0.7)	.4
Length Z-score, med (range)	−1.3 (−3.8–1.2)	−1.9 (−3.2–0.1)	−1.4 (−3.0–0.3)	.8
FRC (mL/kg, mean ± SD)	30 ± 4	26 ± 6	25 ± 8	.7
Flow (FRC/s, mean ± SD)	1.5 ± 0.2	0.8 ± 0.6	0.8 ± 0.5	.1
Bronchiolitis obliterans (n, at any age)	3	4	4	.7
Development*				
≥ 5 y/o: No age appropriate for grade	3/3	4/6	4/4	1.0
< 5 y/o: Performance age/ chronological age†	0.8 ± 0.2	0.7 ± 0.2	1.0 ± 0.3	.3
Not available	0	3	2	

Note: Infants were given transplantation at St Louis Children's Hospital only.
*As of 12/31/2004 or at death.
†Development age (mo) determined by testing (Bayley or Vineland)/chronological age at test.
Abbreviation: FRC, Functional residual capacity.
(Courtesy of Palomar LM, Nogee LM, Sweet SC, et al. Long-term outcomes after infant lung transplantation for surfactant protein B deficiency related to other causes of respiratory failure. *J Pediatr*. 149:548-553. Copyright 2006 by Elsevier.)

tional cost that families encounter in pursuing heroic survival measures for very young infants with lethal respiratory diseases.

R. D. Bland, MD

Caffeine Therapy for Apnea of Prematurity
Schmidt B, for the Caffeine for Apnea of Prematurity Trial Group (McMaster Univ, Hamilton, Ont, Canada; et al)
N Engl J Med 354:2112-2221, 2006   7–21

Background.—Methylxanthines reduce the frequency of apnea of prematurity and the need for mechanical ventilation during the first seven days of therapy. It is uncertain whether methylxanthines have other short- and long-term benefits or risks in infants with very low birth weight.

Methods.—We randomly assigned 2006 infants with birth weights of 500 to 1250 g during the first 10 days of life to receive either caffeine or placebo, until drug therapy for apnea of prematurity was no longer needed. We evaluated the short-term outcomes before the first discharge home.

Results.—Of 963 infants who were assigned to caffeine and who remained alive at a postmenstrual age of 36 weeks, 350 (36 percent) received supplemental oxygen, as did 447 of the 954 infants (47 percent) assigned to placebo (adjusted odds ratio, 0.63; 95 percent confidence interval, 0.52 to 0.76; P<0.001) (Table 3). Positive airway pressure was discontinued one week earlier in the infants assigned to caffeine (median postmenstrual age, 31.0 weeks; interquartile range, 29.4 to 33.0) than in the infants in the placebo group (median postmenstrual age, 32.0 weeks; interquartile range, 30.3 to 34.0; P<0.001). Caffeine reduced weight gain temporarily (Fig 2). The mean difference in weight gain between the group receiving caffeine and the group receiving placebo was greatest after two weeks (mean difference, −23 g; 95 percent confidence interval, −32 to −13; P<0.001). The rates of death, ultrasonographic signs of brain injury, and necrotizing enterocolitis did not differ significantly between the two groups.

Conclusions.—Caffeine therapy for apnea of prematurity reduces the rate of bronchopulmonary dysplasia in infants with very low birth weight.

▶ Apnea of prematurity is one of the most common problems experienced by preterm infants born less than or equal to 34 weeks' gestation. Since observational treatment studies[1-3] in the 1970s reported that treatment with the methylxanthine aminophylline (or theophylline) significantly reduced the incidence and severity of apnea, methylxanthines (aminophylline/theophylline and caffeine) have been a widely used in NICUs. It has been common for preterm infants to be treated with methylxanthines until about 34 weeks' postmenstrual age (PMA), the age at which the respiratory center should have matured sufficiently to permit discontinuance of methylxanthine therapy. However, despite its long use, few clinical studies[4-6] have been performed to evaluate long-term effects, and although limited by small numbers, they have not demonstrated significant differences in neurodevelopmental or growth outcomes. There-

TABLE 3.—Outcome before the First Discharge Home*

Outcome	Caffeine Group (N = 1006)	Placebo Group (N = 1000)	Unadjusted Odds Ratio	Odds Ratio Adjusted for Center (95% CI)	P Value	Odds Ratio Adjusted for Center and Patient Characteristics (95% CI)†
Death — no. (%)	52 (5.2)	55 (5.5)	0.94	0.93 (0.63-1.38)	0.73	0.96 (0.64-1.44)
Bronchopulmonary dysplasia — no. (%)‡	350 (36.3)	447 (46.9)	0.65	0.63 (0.52-0.76)	<0.001	0.64 (0.52-0.78)
Retinopathy of prematurity — no. (%)§	322 (39.2)	362 (43.2)	0.84	0.84 (0.68-1.03)	0.09	0.88 (0.70-1.10)
Brain injury — no. (%)¶	126 (13.0)	138 (14.3)	0.90	0.90 (0.69-1.18)	0.44	0.97 (0.74-1.28)
Necrotizing enterocolitis — no. (%)	63 (6.3)	67 (6.7)	0.93	0.93 (0.65-1.33)	0.63	0.94 (0.65-1.34)
Drug therapy only for closure of patent ductus arteriosus — no. (%)‖**	293 (29.3)	381 (38.1)	0.67	0.67 (0.55-0.81)	<0.001	0.67 (0.54-0.82)
Surgical closure of patent ductus arteriosus — no. (%)**	45 (4.5)	126 (12.6)	0.33	0.32 (0.22-0.45)	<0.001	0.29 (0.20-0.43)

*CI denotes confidence interval.

†The odds ratio has been adjusted for the gestational age and sex of the infant, as well as for the presence or absence of antenatal administration of corticosteroids, a multiple birth, and an endotracheal tube at randomization.

‡This outcome is for infants who were alive at a postmenstrual age of 36 weeks (963 in the caffeine group and 954 in the placebo group).

§This outcome is for infants who were examined for retinopathy in the 35 study centers where the infants were enrolled (822 in the caffeine group and 838 in the placebo group). A total of 531 infants (53 percent) in the caffeine group and 490 infants (49 percent) in the placebo group were transferred to another hospital before their first discharge home. Data on retinal examinations performed after those transfers will be collected at the 18-month follow-up.

¶This outcome is for infants who underwent cranial ultrasonography at least once after randomization (967 in the caffeine group and 966 in the placebo group). In the caffeine group, 33 infants had intraparenchymal echodense lesions, 24 had cystic periventricular leukomalacia, 6 had a porencephalic cyst, and 93 had ventriculomegaly (with or without intraventricular hemorrhage); in the placebo group, 41 infants had intraparenchymal echodense lesions, 37 had cystic periventricular leukomalacia, 16 had porencephalic cysts, and 99 had ventriculomegaly (with or without intraventricular hemorrhage).

‖Fourteen infants in each group received ibuprofen, and 282 in the caffeine group and 372 in the placebo group received indomethacin.

**This outcome excludes infants who underwent surgical closure of a patent ductus arteriosus before randomization (five in the caffeine group and one in the placebo group).

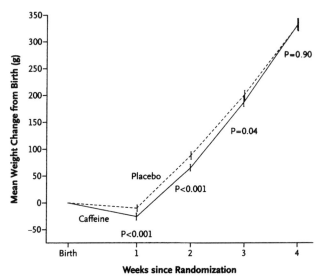

FIGURE 2.—Mean change in body weight during the first four weeks after random assignment to caffeine or placebo. The mean difference in weight gain was −16 g after one week (95 percent confidence interval, −25 to −7), −23 g after two weeks (95 percent confidence interval, −32 to −13), and −13 g after three weeks (95 percent confidence interval, −25 to −0.4). (Reprinted by permission from Schmidt B, for the Caffeine for Apnea of Prematurity Trial Group. Caffeine therapy for apnea of prematurity. *N Engl J Med.* 354:2112-2221. Copyright 2006, Massachusetts Medical Society. All rights reserved.)

fore, the goal of this multicenter, placebo-controlled RCT, to study the short- and long-term efficacy and safety of methylxanthines in ELBW infants in an adequately powered trial, is long overdue.

This report describes the short-term outcomes. As shown in Table 3, caffeine significantly reduced the frequency of BPD (defined as the need for supplemental oxygen at 36 weeks' PMA) and was associated with greater weight loss during the first 3 weeks of life (Fig 2). In addition, a post-hoc analysis demonstrated that infants who received caffeine treatment were also significantly less likely to undergo therapy, pharmacologic or surgical, to close a PDA. Although these data are certainly encouraging, conclusions about the long-term safety must wait until follow-up at corrected ages of 18 to 21 months and 5 years are completed. But, unless truly significant adverse neurodevelopmental outcomes are identified, one wonders how much the widespread use of caffeine to lessen the incidence and severity of apnea and to facilitate extubation will change. Because the 18 to 21-month corrected age follow-up of this study cohort was expected to be completed in December 2006, we may not have to wait too long.

R. A. Ehrenkranz, MD

References

1. Kuzemko JA, Paala J. Apnoeic attacks in the newborn treated with aminophylline. *Arch Dis Child.* 1973;48:404-406.

2. Shannon DC, Gotay F, Stein IM, Rogers MC, Todres ID, Moylan FM. Prevention of apnea and bradycardia in low-birthweight infants. *Pediatrics.* 1975;55:589-594.
3. Uauy R, Shapiro DL, Smith B, Warshaw JB. Treatment of severe apnea in prematures with orally administered theophylline. *Pediatrics.* 1975;55:595-598.
4. Gunn TR, Metrakos K, Riley P, Willis D, Aranda JV. Sequelae of caffeine treatment in preterm infants. *J Pediatr.* 1979;94:106-109.
5. Nelson RM, Resnick MB, Holstrum WJ, Eitzman DV. Developmental outcome of premature infants treated with theophylline. *Dev Pharmacol Ther.* 1980;1: 274-280.
6. Henderson-Smart DJ, Steer P. Methylxanthine treatment for apnea in preterm infants. *Cochrane Database Syst Rev.* 2001;3:CD000140.

Apnea Is Not Prolonged by Acid Gastroesophageal Reflux in Preterm Infants

Di Fiore JM, Arko M, Whitehouse M, et al (Case Western Reserve Univ, Cleveland, Ohio; Shaker Heights, Ohio; Salt Lake City, Utah; et al)

Pediatrics 116:1059-1063, 2005   7–22

Objective.—To examine the temporal relationship between apnea and gastroesophageal reflux (GER) and to assess the effect of GER on apnea duration.

Methods.—A total of 119 preterm infants underwent 12-hour cardiorespiratory monitoring studies using respiratory inductance plethysmography, heart rate, oxygen saturation (SaO_2), and esophageal pH. The studies were scored for GER (pH <4 for ≥5 seconds) and apnea ≥15 seconds or ≥10 seconds that occurred within 30 seconds of GER. Apnea ≥10 seconds was used to assess whether GER would prolong apnea duration.

Results.—There were 6255 episodes of GER. Only 1% of GER episodes were associated with apnea ≥15 seconds, and there was no difference in apnea rate before, during, or after GER. There was also no difference in rate of apnea ≥10 seconds before versus during GER; however, there was a decrease in apnea rate immediately after GER. The presence of GER during apnea did not prolong apnea duration, and GER had no effect on the lowest SaO_2 or heart rate during apnea.

Conclusion.—There is no evidence of a temporal relationship between acid-based GER and apnea in preterm infants. In addition, GER does not prolong apnea duration and does not exacerbate the resultant decrease in heart rate and SaO_2.

▶ Despite a paucity of data linking GER and apnea in preterm infants, or evidence that treatment of GER will alter the frequency of apnea, antireflux medications are widely prescribed for many of these preterm infants.[1] Di Fiore et al, in an elegant study of more than 6000 episodes of GER, show that only 1% of the GER episodes were associated with apnea. In addition, there was no difference in the rate or duration of the apneic episode before or during the GER. On the contrary, there appeared to be a decrease in apnea after GER, perhaps because of behavioral arousal caused by the reflux.[2] As noted by Bancalari, "GER is a normal physiologic event occurring at all ages and in the majority of preterm infants and, in most instances, is related to transient esophageal sphincter relaxation. This relaxation may be increased during episodes of apnea or by the use of drugs such as caffeine and aminophylline," which are used to treat the apnea. As the treatment of GER is neither necessarily safe nor effective, it is perhaps judicious to abandon the shotgun approach to the treatment of GER in preterm infants with apneic episodes. To quote Eduardo Bancalari, "Let's be reminded that there are maturational processes for which time is the best and safest therapy." Sounds like good advice to me.

A. A. Fanaroff, MD

References

1. Poets CF. Gastroesophageal reflux: a critical review of its role in preterm infants. *Pediatrics.* 2004;113:e128-e132.
2. Bancalari E. Apnea is not prolonged by acid gastroesophageal reflux in preterm infants. *Pediatrics.* 2005;116:1217-1218.

8 Central Nervous System and Special Senses

Intracranial Epidural Hematoma in Newborn Infants: Clinical Study of 15 Cases
Heyman R, Heckly A, Magagi J, et al (CHRU Pontchaillou, Rennes, France)
Neurosurgery 57:924-929, 2005   8–1

Objective.—Epidural hematoma (EDH) in newborn infants is rare. We have described the history of 15 newborns with EDH to provide a better understanding of this pathology.

Methods.—This is a descriptive case series study using a retrospective review of the medical records of newborns who were admitted to the Pediatric Intensive Care Unit and Neurosurgery Department with the diagnosis of birth EDH over a 24-year period (1979–2002).

Results.—There was no sex predominance, and most of the mothers were young, nulliparous women. The time latency from birth to the first signs varied from 0 to 24 hours. Clinical presentation was nonspecific: seizures and hypotonia were the main symptoms. The parietal area was the most frequent location. Surgical drainage was required in nine patients, and no deaths were reported.

Conclusion.—This report highlights the clinicoradiological characteristics of newborn EDH, which occurs more frequently in newborns that experienced difficult delivery from a nulliparous mother. Surgery is not a rule; some patients can be managed with conservative treatment. The outcome is generally good.

▶ Cleavage of the dura mater from bone, together with laceration or tearing of the major veins, venous sinuses, or branches of the middle meningeal artery, results in an epidural hematoma. Despite the torque, natural and mechanical forces applied to the fetal skull, including forceps and vacuum extractors, an epidural hematoma is, fortunately, a rare occurrence. The rarity of this condition often has been ascribed to the fact that in infants the dura mostly is contiguous with the inner periosteum and cannot be detached easily from the

165

overlying skull, together with the fact that the middle meningeal artery has not developed fully.

In over 50% of cases an epidural hematoma is accompanied by a fractured skull and cephalohematoma. It took 24 years for Heyman et al to accumulate a series of 15 patients, including one dropped on the delivery room floor, verifying how uncommon the entity is. It is often unclear whether the injury was directly caused by the forceps or had already been inflicted by uterine dystonia, or a combination of both. But excessive molding often accompanies an epidural hematoma, and trauma is the major precipitating event.[1] The clinical features, usually on the day of birth, include hypotonia often accompanied by seizures and progressive scalp swelling, together with features of raised intracranial pressure (a bulging anterior fontanel and hypotonia progressing to stupor and coma). The diagnosis is confirmed by CT or MRI as ultrasound is not reliable in diagnosing extradural hematomas in neonates. I was somewhat surprised that not all cases required surgical intervention and the prognosis, according to Heyman et al, is variable. Of the 12 patients who were available for testing, 8 children had normal neurologic and psychomotor examination at follow-up (range, 6 months to 6 years). Three children had moderate neurologic deficits or psychomotor delay and a single child had severe neurologic disability that included cerebral palsy. We must remain grateful that this is such an uncommon entity.

A. A. Fanaroff, MD

Reference

1. Hamlat A, Heckly A, Adn M, Poulain P. Pathophysiology of intracranial epidural haematoma following birth. *Med Hypotheses.* 2006;66:371-374.

Postasphyxial Hypoxic-Ischemic Encephalopathy in Neonates: Outcome Prediction Rule Within 4 Hours of Birth
Shah PS, Beyene J, To T, et al (Univ of Toronto; Hosp for Sick Children, Toronto)
Arch Pediatr Adolesc Med 160:729-736, 2006   8–2

Objectives.—To construct and validate a model and derive a simple rule that is usable in any birth location for the prediction of outcome of term infants with severe asphyxia.

Design.—Retrospective cohort study.

Setting.—Regional outborn neonatal intensive care unit.

Participants.—Infants with postintrapartum asphyxial hypoxic-ischemic encephalopathy (n = 375).

Main Exposures.—Clinical and laboratory predictors available at age 4 hours.

Main Outcome Measures.—A logistic regression model was developed and internally validated (with random sampling and based on the year of birth) for severe adverse outcome, which was defined as death or severe disability (severe cerebral palsy, severe developmental delay, sensorineural deafness, or cortical blindness singly or in combination). A simple prediction rule was derived from 3 variables.

Results.—Complete data were available for 302 (92%) of the 345 infants with known outcomes (204 infants with severe adverse outcome). Six independent predictors of outcomes were identified. Using the 3 most significant predictors (chest compressions, age at onset of respiration, and base deficit), severe adverse outcome rates were 46% (95% confidence interval, 33%-58%) with none of the 3 predictors, 64% (95% confidence interval, 54%-73%) with any 1 predictor, 76% (95% confidence interval, 66%-85%) with any 2 predictors, and 93% (95% confidence interval, 81%-99%) with all of the 3 predictors present. The internal validations revealed a robust model.

Conclusions.—This predictive model for neonatal hypoxic-ischemic encephalopathy provides a sliding scale of probabilities that could be used for prognostication and to design eligibility criteria for decision making including neuroprotective therapy.

▶ This is an excellent study evaluating a model for the prediction of outcome of term infants with severe asphyxia. This predictive model, using the 3 most significant predictors, chest compression in the delivery room, age of onset of spontaneous respiration, and base deficit on either the cord or the first postnatal blood gas, provides a sliding scale of probability that may prove useful for risk stratification of infants with hypoxic ischemic encephalopathy for clinical trials. The findings are closely matched by the NICHD Neonatal Research Network Study evaluating predictor variables and the development of scoring systems and classification trees to predict death/moderate severe disability or death in infants with hypoxic ischemic encephalopathy. In that report, Ambalavanan et al[1] used logistic regression analysis of clinical and laboratory variables available within 6 hours of birth with death or moderate/severe disability at 18 to 22 months. This secondary analysis of the Network's randomized whole body cooling trial data[2] evaluated the classification rates for the scoring systems, classification and regression tree model, and early neurologic examination. Correct classification rates were 78% for death/disability and 71% for death with the scoring systems, 80% and 77%, respectively, with the classification and regression tree models, and 67% and 73% with severe encephalopathy in the early neurological examination. Correct classification rates were similar in the hypothermia and in the control groups.

While concerns that outcome data were collected from various sources rather than from evaluations performed by certified examiners have been addressed by the authors in the discussion section, it is not always possible to exclude neonates with congenital malformations or intrauterine infections within 4 hours of birth. In addition, meconium aspiration syndrome, which is often associated with hypoxic ischemic encephalopathy, may evolve clinically and radiographically beyond 4 hours of age. Furthermore, hemorrhagic shock, which was also excluded from this analysis, may be associated with acute asphyxial injury that may or may not be reversible.

Nonetheless, the predictive model presented by Shah et al will be useful in evaluating high-risk infants for future neuroprotective trials. Cerebral function monitoring as a tool to further stratify the highest risk infants will be also available once the ongoing TOBY trial (using this modality with sample size large enough to evaluate both moderate and severe changes on the amplitude integrated EEG and 18- to 22-month outcome) is completed.[3]

S. Shankaran, MD

Reference

1. Ambalavanan N, Carlo WA, Shankaran S, et al, for the National Institute of Child Health and Human Development Neonatal Research Network. Predicting outcomes of neonates diagnosed with hypoxemic-ischemic encephalopathy. *Pediatrics.* 2006;118:2084-2093.
2. Shankaran S, Laptook AR, Ehrenkranz RA, et al. Whole-body hypothermia for neonates with hypoxic-ischemic encephalopathy. *N Engl J Med.* 2005;353:1574-1584.
3. National Perinatal Epidemiology Unit Web site. Whole body hypothermia for the treatment of perinatal asphyxial encephalopathy: the TOBY study. Available at: http://www.npeu.ox.ac.uk/Toby. Accessed May 15, 2007.

Neonatal loss of γ–aminobutyric acid pathway expression after human perinatal brain injury
Robinson S, Li Q, DeChant A, et al (Case Western Reserve Univ, Cleveland, Ohio)
J Neurosurg 104:396-408, 2006   8–3

Object.—Perinatal brain injury leads to chronic neurological deficits in children. Damage to the premature brain produces white matter lesions (WMLs), but the impact on cortical development is less well defined. Gamma–aminobutyric acid(GABA)ergic neurons destined for the cerebral cortex migrate through the developing white matter and form the subplate during late gestation. The authors hypothesized that GABAergic neurons are vulnerable to perinatal systemic insults in premature infants, and that damage to these neurons contributes to impaired cortical development.

Methods.—An immunohistochemical analysis involving markers for oligodendrocytes, GABAergic neurons, axons, and apoptosis was performed on a consecutive series of 15 human neonatal telencephalon samples obtained postmortem from infants born at 25 to 32 weeks of gestation. The tissue samples were divided into two groups based on the presence or absence of WMLs by performing routine histological analyses. The expression of GABAergic neurons was compared between the two groups by using age-matched samples. Two-tailed t-tests were used for statistical analyses. Ten infants had WMLs and five did not. Significant losses of oligodendrocytes and axons and markedly increased apoptosis were appreciated in tissue samples from the infants with WMLs. Samples from infants with WMLs also showed significant losses of glutamic acid decarboxylase–67-positive cells and calretinin-positive cells, shorter neuropeptide Y–positive neurite lengths, and losses of cells expressing $GABA_A\alpha1$, $GABA_BR1$, and N-acetylaspartate diethylamide NR1 receptors when these factors were compared with those in samples from infants without WMLs (all $p < 0.02$).

Conclusions.—In addition to oligodendrocyte loss, axonal disruption, and excess apoptosis, a significant loss of telencephalon GABAergic neuron expression was found in neonatal brains with WMLs, compared with neonates' brains without WMLs. The loss of GABAergic subplate neurons in infants with WMLs may contribute to the pathogenesis of neurological deficits in children.

▶ In the preterm neonate, hypoxic/ischemic insults result in selective white matter injury, termed periventricular leukomalacia (PVL), with little or no cortical pathology. Its pathogenesis is complex and likely involves ischemia/reperfusion in the critically ill premature infant, with impaired regulation of cerebral blood flow, as well as inflammatory mechanisms associated with maternal and/or fetal infection.[1] PVL in preterm infants is the major antecedent of cerebral palsy. However, in term babies, hypoxic encephalopathy is the most common cause of seizures and can result in cortical infarction.

Bassan et al[2] reviewed the data on some 5774 infants with a birth weight of < 2500 g and confirmed the diagnosis of periventricular hemorrhagic infarction, diagnosed by ultrasound in a total of 58 infants with 0.1% weighing between 1500 and 2500 g, 2.2% (750-1500 g), and 10% (<750 g). Gestational age–matched control infants were identified with normal cranial ultrasound. Infants with periventricular hemorrhagic infarction compared with control infants had significantly greater association with assisted conception, intrapartum factors (emergency cesarean section, low Apgar scores), early neonatal complications (patent ductus arteriosus, pneumothorax, pulmonary hemorrhage), blood gas disturbances, low blood pressure with need for pressor agents, volume infusion, and respiratory support. Neonatal mortality of this group was 40% (n = 23).

Robinson et al, as summarized above, report that in neonatal brains with white matter loss that, in addition to the loss of oligodendrocytes, there is axonal disruption, and excess apoptosis, as well as a significant loss of telencephalon GABAergic neuron expression. Glutamate receptors are developmentally regulated in both neuronal and glial cells within the brain. Extracellular glutamate accumulates in the setting of hypoxia/ischemia, and excess activation of glutamate receptors has been implicated in hypoxic/ischemic cellular death. Glutamate receptor–mediated excitotoxicity is a predominant mechanism of hypoxic ischemic injury to developing cerebral white matter, which may be ameliorated by topirimate.[3] Talos et al[4] report that for mid-gestational cases aged 20 to 24 postconceptional weeks (PCW) and for premature infants (25-37 PCW), they found that radial glia, premyelinating oligodendrocytes, and subplate neurons transiently expressed GluR2 lacking (alpha-amino-3-hydroxy-5-methyl-4-isoxazole propionic acid receptor = AMPARs). Notably, prematurity represents a developmental window of selective vulnerability for white matter injury, such as periventricular leukomalacia (PVL). During term (38-42 PCW) and post-term neonatal (43-46 PCW) periods, age windows characterized by increased susceptibility to cortical injury and seizures, GluR2 expression was low in the neocortex, specifically on cortical pyramidal and nonpyramidal neurons. Their study indicates that Ca^{++} permeable AMPAR blockade may represent an age-specific therapeutic strategy for potential use in humans. As the underlying mechanisms of injury and repair are understood, therapeutic strategies for different gestational ages and windows of opportunity can be developed. The dawning of brain intensive care is finally emerging.

A. A. Fanaroff, MD

References

1. Haynes RL, Baud O, Li J, Kinney HC, Volpe JJ, Folkerth DR. Oxidative and nitrative injury in periventricular leukomalacia: a review. *Brain Pathol.* 2005;15:225-233.
2. Bassan H, Feldman HA, Limperopoulos C, et al. Periventricular hemorrhagic infarction: risk factors and neonatal outcome. *Pediatr Neurol.* 2006;35:85-92.
3. Follett PL, Deng W, Dai W, et al. Glutamate receptor-mediated oligodendrocyte toxicity in periventricular leukomalacia: a protective role for topiramate. *J Neurosci.* 2004;24:4412-4420.
4. Talos DM, Follett PL, Folkerth RD, et al. Developmental regulation of alpha-amino-3-hydroxy-5-methyl-4-isoxazole-propionic acid receptor subunit expression in forebrain and relationship to regional susceptibility to hypoxic/ischemic injury. II. Human cerebral white matter and cortex. *J Comp Neurol.* 2006;497: 61-77.

Neuroprotective effects of topiramate after hypoxia–ischemia in newborn piglets
Schubert S, Brandl U, Brodhun M, et al (Friedrich Schiller Univ, Jena, Germany)
Brain Res 1058:129-136, 2005   8–4

Background.—Perinatal hypoxia-ischemia (HI) is associated with delayed cerebral damage, which involves receptor-mediated excitotoxicity. Until now, successful interventions to reduce excitotoxicity early after HI in experimental settings failed to transform into clinical applications owing to negative side effects. A promising new approach using the anticonvulsant Topiramate (TPM) has shown to be effective to reduce brain damage after early HI in a rodent model of combined TPM-hypothermia. Here, we used TPM solely administered 1 h after HI in a neonatal piglet model in order to verify possible neuroprotection.

Methods.—Newborn piglets were subjected to HI by transient occlusion of carotid arteries and hypotension (62–65% of baseline). Fifteen minutes later, an additional reduction of the inspired oxygen fraction to 0.06 was performed for 13 min. One cohort (VEHICLE, $n = 8$) received saline solution i.v. 1 h after HI and then twice a day. Two further cohorts were treated at same times with TPM (HI-TPM10, $n = 8$, loading dose 20 mg/kg; maintenance dose 10 mg/kg/day; HI-TPM20, $n = 8$, loading dose 50 mg/kg; maintenance dose 20 mg/kg/day). Untreated animals (CONTROL, $n = 8$) received all experimental procedures except HI. Animals were monitored 3 days after HI concerning occurrence of seizures as well as neurological and behavioral functions. After 72 h, the brains were perfused and processed to assess neuronal loss and DNA-fragments (TUNEL staining).

Results.—There was a significant reduction of neuronal cell loss in HI-TPM20 animals. However, apoptosis was increased in the frontal white matter of HI-TPM20 animals.

Conclusions.—Exclusive TPM treatment shows neuroprotection in newborn piglets after HI.

▶ Recent clinical trials support a neuroprotective role of brain hypothermia either by using a combination of head and body cooling[1] or body cooling alone[2] and suggest that management of infants with HI is changing from provision of supportive intensive care to implementation of brain-oriented specific therapies. This report examines the neuroprotective effects of TPM administered 1 hour after a defined interval of HI in newborn piglets. TPM is potentially an attractive neuroprotective drug because it targets the role of excitatory neurotransmitters during and after HI in the pathogenesis of brain injury. Although developed as an anticonvulsant, TPM provides neuroprotection *in vivo* by using adult rodent models of middle cerebral artery embolization.[3] In 10-day rat pups, TPM suppressed acute seizures induced by hypoxia and attenuated the long-term increases in susceptibility to kainite-induced seizures and seizure associated neuronal injury.[4] The extent of neuroprotection in neonatal animals remains unclear; TPM (30 mg/kg) was not effective when used 15 minutes after focal ischemia in rodents.[5] In the current study, a high dose of TPM (50 mg/kg load, 20 mg/kg/d maintenance) was associated with less damaged cells (semiquantitative assessment) and a trend toward reduced abnormalities of neurobehavior. These neuroprotective effects were accompanied by greater evidence of apoptosis compared with lower doses of TPM or vehicle infusion.

Many neuroprotection studies are performed with rodents. Performance of this study in newborn swine provides the ability to monitor systemic hemodynamics, acid-base status, respiratory gas exchange, and biochemical parameters. Furthermore, neurobehavioral assessments are more easily scored compared with newborn rodents. In this study TPM was administered by IV means, and there were no alterations in systemic variables attributable to TPM. This is attractive because neuroprotective treatments need to be initiated rapidly and result in therapeutic concentrations in brain tissue. TPM readily crosses the blood-brain barrier and results in CSF concentrations that are approximately 80% of plasma concentrations. Furthermore, TPM pharmacokinetics in newborn piglets with or without HI indicates that the half-life is long and facilitates maintenance of brain tissue concentrations.[6] However, at present TPM is not available in an IV preparation and absorption via enteral use is unpredictable in critically ill infants. The results of the current study of TPM administered after HI are encouraging but much more investigation is needed to balance the extent of neuroprotection and apoptosis.

A. Laptook, MD

References

1. Gluckman PD, Wyatt JS, Azzopardi D, et al. Selective head cooling with mild systemic hypothermia after neonatal encephalopathy: Multicentre randomized trial. *Lancet.* 2005;365:663-670.

2. Shankaran S, Laptook AR, Ehrenkranz RA, et al, for the National Institute of Child Health and Human Development Neonatal Research Network. Whole body hypothermia for neonates with hypoxic-ischemic encephalopathy. *N Engl J Med.* 2005;353:1574-1584.
3. Yang Y, Shuaib A, Li Q, Siddiqui MM. Neuroprotection by delayed administration of topiramate in a rat model of middle cerebral artery embolization. *Brain Res.* 1998;804:169-176.
4. Koh S, Jensen FE. Topiramate blocks perinatal hypoxia-induced seizures in rat pups. *Ann Neurol.* 2001;50:366-372.
5. Liu Y, Barks JD, Xu G, Silvestein FS. Topiramate extends the therapeutic window for hypothermia-mediated neuroprotection after stroke in neonatal rats. *Stroke.* 2004;35:1460-1465.
6. Galinkin JL, Kurth CD, Shi H, Priestley MA, Loepke AW, Adamson PC. The plasma pharmacokinetics and cerebral spinal fluid penetration of intravenous topiramate in newborn pigs. *Biopharm Drug Disp.* 2004;25:265-271.

The Current Etiologic Profile and Neurodevelopmental Outcome of Seizures in Term Newborn Infants

Tekgul H, Gauvreau K, Soul J, et al (Harvard Med School; Ege Univ, Izmir, Turkey)
Pediatrics 117:1270-1280, 2006   8–5

Objectives.—The objectives of this study were to delineate the etiologic profile and neurodevelopmental outcome of neonatal seizures in the current era of neonatal intensive care and to identify predictors of neurodevelopmental outcome in survivors.

Methods.—Eighty-nine term infants with clinical neonatal seizures underwent neurologic examination, electroencephalography (EEG), neuroimaging, and extensive diagnostic tests in the newborn period. After discharge, all infants underwent regular neurologic evaluations and, at 12 to 18 months, formal neurodevelopmental testing. We tested the prognostic value of seizure etiology, neurologic examination, EEG, and neuroimaging.

Results.—Etiology was found in 77 infants. Global cerebral hypoxia-ischemia, focal cerebral hypoxia-ischemia, and intracranial hemorrhage were most common. Neonatal mortality was 7%; 28% of the survivors had poor long-term outcome. Association between seizure etiology and outcome was strong, with cerebral dysgenesis and global hypoxia-ischemia associated with poor outcome. Normal neonatal period/early infancy neurologic examination was associated with uniformly favorable outcome at 12 to 18 months; abnormal examination lacked specificity. Normal/mildly abnormal neonatal EEG had favorable outcome, particularly if neonatal neuroimaging was normal. Moderate/severely abnormal EEG, and multifocal/diffuse cortical or primarily deep gray matter lesions, had a worse outcome.

Conclusions.—Mortality associated with neonatal seizures has declined although long-term neurodevelopmental morbidity remains unchanged. Seizure etiology and background EEG patterns remain powerful prognostic factors. Diagnostic advances have changed the etiologic distribution for neonatal seizures and improved accuracy of outcome prediction. Global cerebral hypoxia-ischemia, the most common etiology, is responsible for the large majority of infants with poor long-term outcome.

▶ "The more things change, the more they stay the same." In some respects, that statement fits this report describing the current etiologic profile and neurodevelopmental outcome of seizures in term newborn infants managed during a recent 38-month period. Because there have been multiple diagnostic and therapeutic advances during the past 15-20 years, Tekgul et al chose to evaluate the impact of these advances on the etiology and outcomes of neonatal seizures in term infants. Although they found that mortality of infants with seizures was substantially lower, the prevalence of adverse long-term outcomes and of later seizure recurrence in survivors was essentially unchanged from previous reports. As shown in Tables 3 and 4 of the original article, the strongest prediction of long-term outcome continues to be the underlying seizure etiology and EEG background patterns.

R. A. Ehrenkranz, MD

MRS of normal and impaired fetal brain development
Girard N, Fogliarini C, Viola A, et al (Université de la Méiterranée, Marseille, France)
Eur J Radiol 57:217-225, 2006   8–6

Cerebral maturation in the human fetal brain was investigated by in utero localized proton magnetic resonance spectroscopy (MRS). Spectra were acquired on a clinical MR system operating at 1.5 T. Body phased array coils (four coils) were used in combination with spinal coils (two coils). The size of the nominal volume of interest (VOI) was 4.5 cm^3 (20 mm $\times$ 15 mm $\times$ 15 mm). The MRS acquisitions were performed using a spin echo sequence at short and long echo times (TE = 30 ms and 135 ms) with a VOI located within the cerebral hemisphere at the level of the centrum semiovale. A significant reduction in *myo*-inositol and choline and an increase in N-acetylaspartate were observed with progressive age. The normal MR spectroscopy data reported here will help to determine whether brain metabolism is altered, especially when subtle anatomic changes are observed on conventional images. Some examples of impaired fetal brain development studied by MRS are illustrated (Fig 1).

▶ This article assesses cerebral maturation in the human fetal brain by use of proton magnetic resonance spectroscopy (MRS). The authors use 4 body phased-array coils and 2 spinal coils with a large voxel of interest (20 mm $\times$ 15 mm $\times$ 15 mm) over the mother's abdomen and spine to assess the fetal brain on a 1.5T MR scanner at 2 echo times of 30 ms and 135 ms. The authors show a reduction in *myo*-inositol and choline and an increase in N-acetyl aspartate with maturation. They conclude that these data will assist in determining whether brain metabolism is abnormal.

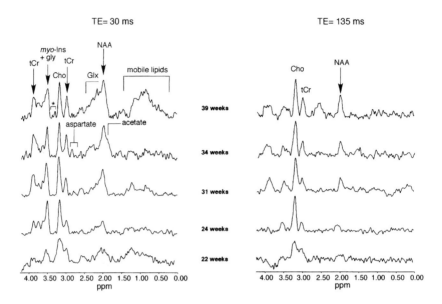

TE= 30 ms   TE= 135 ms

•: taurine + *scyllo*-Inositol

FIGURE 1.—Typical brain fetal spectra obtained with the PRESS sequence at short (left panel) and log echo times (right panel) from 22 to 39 weeks GA. (Courtesy of Girard N, Fogliarini C, Viola A, et al. MRS of normal and impaired fetal brain development. *Eur J Radiol.* 57:217-225. Copyright 2006 by Elsevier.)

This study pushes the boundaries of current MR technologies to apply MRS in the developing brain and will continue to inspire new investigators to expand on this foundation. However, there are several concerns that must be balanced in this study. (1) The sequence length of 6 minutes is clearly of limited feasibility in a healthy fetus who is active and moving. With improved acquisition speed and higher field MR (3T), then this may be reduced, making this more feasible. (2) Acquisition of MRS is clearly improved at higher field strengths and if 3T is deemed safe for the fetus then the applicability of MRS for the fetus will be greatly enhanced. (3) Voxel of interest in this study is very large and fixed in size despite marked increases in total brain size over maturation. The tissues that are being sampled—whether white matter, gray matter, deep nuclear gray matter—are unknown because no figure with the voxel placement is illustrated in the article. It is also plausible that the voxel is shifting in its location and that this may result in differing brain metabolic profiles. Improvements in acquisition speed and resolution would allow a more specific location in the brain to be analyzed across differing gestations. (4) Postacquisition quantification remains problematic in MRS with differing views of the standards for such measurements. Standard measurements and analysis tools should be agreed on to allow comparative data across MR scanners and methods.

Despite these limitations, this article applies MRS in the fetal brain to provide some very preliminary feasibility data. It has laid down the gauntlet to other investigators to consider this technique in their evaluation of the developing brain and establish the relationship of these measures to pathology and later neurodevelopmental outcomes to confirm its utility.

T. E. Inder, MD

Detection of Impaired Growth of the Corpus Callosum in Premature Infants
Anderson NG, Laurent I, Woodward LJ, et al (Christchurch Hosp, New Zealand; Hôpital Bon-Secours, Metz, France; Univ of Canterbury, Christchurch, New Zealand; et al)
Pediatrics 118:951-960, 2006   8–7

Objective.—There is an urgent need for a bedside method to assess the effectiveness of neonatal therapies designed to improve cerebral development in very low birth-weight infants. The aim of this study was to assess the impact of preterm birth on the serial growth of the corpus callosum and how soon it could be detected after birth with cranial ultrasound.

Methods.—We recruited 61 very low birth-weight infants admitted to a single regional level III NICU from 1998 to 2000. Study infants had 2 cranial sonograms ≥7 days apart in the first 2 weeks of life and further sonograms at 6 weeks and at term equivalent. At each time point, the length of the corpus callosum and cerebellar vermis was measured on midline sagittal images, with growth rates calculated in millimeters per day. We compared growth of corpus callosum and cerebellar vermis in individuals, between birth age groups, and with corrected gestational age. We used antenatal growth rate of the corpus callosum of 0.2 to 0.27 mm/day as a reference. Relationships between corpus callosum growth rates and neurodevelopmental outcome at 2 years of age (corrected) were also examined.

Results.—Growth of the corpus callosum was normal in most infants during the first 2 weeks of life but slowed after this (0.21 mm/day from 0–2 weeks vs 0.11 mm/day for weeks 2–6). Slowing of corpus callosum growth below expected reference range was consistently detectable by age 6 weeks for 96% of infants born between 23 and 33 weeks' gestation. Although some improvement in growth rate was observed for 15% of infants after 6 weeks, this was confined to infants born after 28 weeks. Vermis length correlated strongly with corpus callosum length. By 2 years of age, serious motor delay and cerebral palsy were associated with poorer growth of the length of the corpus callosum between 2 and 6 weeks after birth.

Conclusions.—The effect of preterm birth on growth of the corpus callosum is detectable by 6 weeks after delivery in preterm infants born at gestations of 23 to 33 weeks. Reduced growth of the corpus callosum in weeks 2 to 6 places these infants at elevated risks of later psychomotor delay and cerebral palsy.

▶ Impaired neurologic development of preterm infants is of the utmost concern for both neonatologists and parents. A limiting factor in developing new neuroprotective strategies is the lack of simple bedside indicators of cortical development that can be used in the first few weeks of life following preterm delivery. This study reports a simple technique for measuring the growth rate of the corpus callosum and cerebellar vermis from sequential, standard head ultrasonograms that appears to correlate with impaired motor system development. In previous work,[1] these authors found that preterm infants had corpus callosal growth rates that were reduced by about half compared with antenatal rates when calculated from birth and term equivalent measurements, which potentially reflected impaired cortical growth and connectivity. Here, the authors investigate the detailed pattern of this impaired growth in a prospective, observational study and link this pattern to impaired neurologic outcomes. Corpus callosal and cerebellar vermis growth rates were measured for 61 very low birth weight infants born between 23 and 33 weeks' gestation who had head US at less than 2 weeks (2 scans more than 7 days apart), at 6 weeks, and at term equivalent. Head MRI at term equivalence and neurodevelopmental testing at 2 years' corrected age were also performed. Compared with in utero growth rates, corpus callosal growth in most preterm infants was normal for the first 2 postnatal weeks but had slowed significantly in almost all preterm infants by 6 weeks of age, regardless of whether they had developed periventricular leukomalacia or intraventricular hemorrhage. Growth rates were reduced in the first 2 weeks only in small-for-gestational age infants. Only a few infants showed improved growth rates after 6 weeks, and this improvement was limited to those born at more than 28 weeks' gestation. Cerebellar vermis growth correlated strongly with corpus colossal length, which reinforces previous observations linking cortical and cerebellar growth and connectivity. The growth of both structures reflects both axon number and the extent of myelination. The most commonly observed growth pattern—normal initial growth followed by a dramatic delay, independent of gestational age at birth or postnatal complications—has important implications for understanding the underlying biology. This pattern implies that very low birth weight infants have decreasing axonal numbers and/or decreased myelination that develops relatively rapidly after delivery, regardless of their clinical status. Removal from the in utero environment at any time before 33 weeks' gestation results in at least several weeks of abnormal brain growth. The specific factors responsible for this decline are unknown but appear to be involved consistently across a range of preterm gestations. Furthermore, impaired callosal growth may be correlated with poor neurologic outcomes. In this study, motor but not cognitive impairment was associated with severe decreases of growth during the 2- to 6-week window, but this finding requires an increased sample size to draw a definitive conclusion. If corpus callosal growth rate monitoring becomes a standard part of neurologic follow-up, as the authors suggest, data should soon be sufficient to more fully assess the associations both with postnatal events and with long-term outcomes. The authors have provided us with an important new tool for evaluating the impact of early neuroprotective interventions and rightly emphasize the need to intervene as soon as possible postnatally to prevent ongoing changes in brain growth and connectivity.

A. Penn, MD, PhD

Reference

1. Anderson NG, Laurent I, Cook N, Woodward L, Inder TE. Growth rate of corpus callosum in very premature infants. *AJNR Am J Neuroradiol.* 2005;26:2685-2690.

Circulating Interferon-gamma and White Matter Brain Damage in Preterm Infants

Hansen-Pupp I, Harling S, Berg A-C, et al (Lund Univ, Sweden; Malmö Univ, Sweden)

Pediatr Res 58:946-952, 2005   8–8

The fetal inflammatory response has been suggested as causal in neonatal morbidity. Serial levels of circulating cytokines were evaluated in 74 infants with a mean gestational age (GA) of 27.1 wk. Pro-inflammatory [tumor necrosis factor-α (TNF-α), interferon-γ (IFN-γ), IL-1 beta, IL-2, IL-6, IL-8, IL-12] [corrected] and modulatory (IL-4, IL-10) cytokines were analyzed from cord blood, and at 6, 24 [corrected] and 72 h postnatal age. Measure of cytokine burden over time was assessed by calculating the area under curve (AUC) for analyzed levels (0–72 h). Premature rupture of membranes (PROM) was associated with higher levels of IL-2 at birth and at 6 h, of IFN-γ at 6 and 24 h postnatal age and of TNF-α at 6 and 24 h. Levels of IFN-γ at 6, 24, and 72 h were increased in infants developing white matter brain damage (WMD) compared with those without WMD. Infants with arterial hypotension requiring dopamine treatment had an increase in IL-6 with a peak at 6 h of age. Severe intraventricular hemorrhage (IVH) was associated with increase in AUC [(IL-6) and (IL-8), odds ratio (OR) 2.8 and 13.2 respectively], whereas white matter brain damage (WMD) [corrected] was associated with increase in AUC (IFN-γ; OR, 26.0) [corrected] A fetal immune response with increased postnatal levels of IFN-gamma was associated with development of WMD. PROM was associated with a T-helper 1 cytokine response with increased levels of IFN-γ. Type of inflammatory response appears of importance for subsequent morbidity.

▶ The major contribution of this study is that it confirms previous observations and experimental evidence supporting a role for circulating inflammatory molecules in the cause of WMD in the preterm newborn.[1] The major limitations of the study are its rather small sample size and that too many relationships are being evaluated. Potentially interesting information might have been lost in the publication process. For example, a more detailed description of cutoffs used for some AUC comparisons in risk analyses might have been helpful, not only for the uninitiated. Slightly more detail regarding cytokines other than interferon would have been desirable.

Nonetheless, this interesting article definitely deserves attention. Not only will it help generate important new research hypotheses, to be tested in larger studies, it might also be helpful in putting traditional etiologic paradigms in perspective. Let me suggest that those interested in blood pressure treatment–

cytokine relationships might want to take a closer look at this publication, because no support is offered for the hypothesis that arterial hypotension (or its treatment) is associated with brain damage in preterm newborn infants.

O. Dammann, Dr med, SM

Reference

1. Dammann O, Leviton A. Inflammatory brain damage in preterm newborns—dry numbers, wet lab, and causal inference. *Early Hum Dev.* 2004;79:1-15.

Noninvasive Measurements of Regional Cerebral Perfusion in Preterm and Term Neonates by Magnetic Resonance Arterial Spin Labeling
Miranda MJ, Olofsson K, Sidaros K (Copenhagen Univ, Hvidovre, Denmark)
Pediatr Res 60:359-363, 2006   8–9

Magnetic resonance arterial spin labeling (ASL) at 3 Tesla has been investigated as a quantitative technique for measuring regional cerebral perfusion (RCP) in newborn infants. RCP values were measured in 49 healthy neonates: 32 preterm infants born before 34 wk of gestation and 17 term-born neonates. Examinations were performed on unsedated infants at postmenstrual age of 39–40 wk in both groups. Due to motion, reliable data were obtained from 23 preterm and 6 term infants. Perfusion in the basal ganglia (39 and 30 mL/100 g/min for preterm and term neonates, respectively) was significantly higher ($p < 0.0001$) than in cortical gray matter (19 and 16 mL/100 g/min) and white matter (15 and 10 mL/100 g/min), both in preterm neonates at term-equivalent age and in term neonates. Perfusion was significantly higher ($p = 0.01$) in the preterm group than in the term infants, indicating that RCP may be influenced by developmental and postnatal ages. This study demonstrates, for the first time, that noninvasive ASL at 3T may be used to measure RCP in healthy unsedated preterm and term neonates. ASL is, therefore, a viable tool that will allow serial studies of RCP in high-risk neonates.

▶ The intriguing technique of MR arterial spin labeling (ASL) adds to the growing arsenal of newer neurodiagnostic technologies for evaluation of cerebral perfusion. The authors acknowledge that motion artifact is a major limitation of this technique, resulting in a 40% exclusion rate for potential study subjects. In addition, comparisons between preterm and term groups need to be interpreted with caution given the small numbers, unclear preceding clinical course of the preterm infants, and limitation of a single scan done at one moment in time. Despite these concerns, this study provides initial normative data for a new technique. Given the difficulties inherent in obtaining serial MRI scans, it will be interesting to compare MR ASL with bedside measures of cerebral blood flow such as NIRS and Doppler ultrasonography.

V. Chock, MD

Axial and Radial Diffusivity in Preterm Infants Who Have Diffuse
White Matter Changes on Magnetic Resonance Imaging at Term-
Equivalent Age
Counsell SJ, Shen Y, Boardman JP, et al (MRC Clinical Sciences Centre, London; Imperial College London; Hammersmith Hosp, London)
Pediatrics 117:376-386, 2006   8–10

Objective.—Diffuse excessive high signal intensity (DEHSI) is observed in the majority of preterm infants at term-equivalent age on conventional MRI, and diffusion-weighted imaging has shown that apparent diffusion coefficient values are elevated in the white matter (WM) in DEHSI. Our aim was to obtain diffusion tensor imaging on preterm infants at term-equivalent age and term control infants to test the hypothesis that radial diffusivity was significantly different in the WM in preterm infants with DEHSI compared with both preterm infants with normal-appearing WM on conventional MRI and term control infants.

Methods.—Diffusion tensor imaging was obtained on 38 preterm infants at term-equivalent age and 8 term control infants. Values for axial (λ_1) and radial [$(\lambda_2 + \lambda_3)/2$] diffusivity were calculated in regions of interest positioned in the central WM at the level of the centrum semiovale, frontal WM, posterior periventricular WM, occipital WM, anterior and posterior portions of the posterior limb of the internal capsule, and the genu and splenium of the corpus callosum.

Results.—Radial diffusivity was elevated significantly in the posterior portion of the posterior limb of the internal capsule and the splenium of the corpus callosum, and both axial and radial diffusivity were elevated significantly in the WM at the level of the centrum semiovale, the frontal WM, the periventricular WM, and the occipital WM in preterm infants with DEHSI compared with preterm infants with normal-appearing WM and term control infants. There was no significant difference between term control infants and preterm infants with normal-appearing WM in any region studied.

Conclusions.—These findings suggest that DEHSI represents an oligodendrocyte and/or axonal abnormality that is widespread throughout the cerebral WM.

▶ Severe neuroimaging abnormalities identifiable by cranial US, such as parenchymal hemorrhage and cystic periventricular leukomalacia, are known to be associated with adverse neurodevelopmental outcomes among preterm infants. However, a substantial proportion of impaired former preterm infants do not have a history of such significant brain injury. Much more subtle patterns of WM injury can be identified by MRI and quantified by methods such as diffusion tensor imaging (DTI). Several investigator groups are now studying whether findings by such technologies can predict neuromotor outcomes better than current, more routine methods. Counsell et al have previously reported that DEHSI is seen in most preterm infants at term-equivalent age on T2-weighted brain MRI. Using DTI, the authors now convincingly demonstrate that DEHSI is linked with abnormal WM development by showing that axial and radial diffusivity measures in preterm infants with DEHSI are significantly different from those without DEHSI or from term infants. Patient numbers were small; thus, conclusions cannot be reliably drawn with respect to clinical antecedents of DEHSI, but this question was not the main aim of the current study. Further quantitative DTI research will be needed to validate and expand on these findings. Of course, meticulous neurodevelopmental follow-up will be the most crucial component to investigating the capacity of any advanced neuroimaging marker to better predict outcomes of these extraordinarily vulnerable infants.

S. R. Hintz, MD, MS

Neonatal Intensive Care Unit Characteristics Affect the Incidence of Severe Intraventricular Hemorrhage
Synnes AR, and the Canadian Neonatal Network (Univ of British Columbia, Canada; Univ of Northern British Columbia, Canada; Univ of Toronto; et al)
Med Care 44:754-759, 2006   8–11

Objectives.—The incidence of intraventricular hemorrhage (IVH), adjusted for known risk factors, varies across neonatal intensive care units (NICU)s. The effect of NICU characteristics on this variation is unknown. The objective was to assess IVH attributable risks at both patient and NICU levels.

Study Design.—Subjects were <33 weeks' gestation, <4 days old on admission in the Canadian Neonatal Network database (all infants admitted in 1996–97 to 17 NICUs). The variation in severe IVH rates was analyzed using Bayesian hierarchical modeling for patient level and NICU level factors.

Results.—Of 3772 eligible subjects, the overall crude incidence rates of grade 3–4 IVH was 8.3% (NICU range 2.0–20.5%). Male gender, extreme preterm birth, low Apgar score, vaginal birth, outborn birth, and high admission severity of illness accounted for 30% of the severe IVH rate variation; admission day therapy-related variables (treatment of acidosis and hypotension) accounted for an additional 14%. NICU characteristics, independent of patient level risk factors, accounted for 31% of the variation. NICUs with high patient volume and high neonatologist/staff ratio had lower rates of severe IVH.

Conclusions.—The incidence of severe IVH is affected by NICU characteristics, suggesting important new strategies to reduce this important adverse outcome.

▶ This Canadian population of premature infants has been studied previously in regard to risk factors relating to the rate of grades 3 or 4 IVH and variation by individual NICU.[1] In the current study, the authors investigate what factors of NICUs may contribute to this variation.

As in the previous study of this population, treatment for acidosis and vasopressor use in the first day was associated with a higher risk of severe IVH. However, even after risk adjustment for the severity of illness, it is not possible to tease out whether it was the underlying condition requiring such treatment or the treatment itself that may have contributed more to this phenomenon.

That a larger patient volume was protective is not surprising; this has also previously been shown to be associated with decreased mortality.[2] It is interesting that a higher neonatologist–housestaff ratio also correlated with a decreased rate of severe IVH. It was not stated directly whether a full-time neonatologist equivalent meant a full-time clinical appointment or whether it might allow for a full-time neonatologist to have a decreased clinical requirement for the purposes of research or teaching. If the latter is possible, perhaps the effect of an academic setting with more full-time neonatologists per housestaff could also have been a protective factor. Although we are often tempted to invoke causality in such studies, we are only identifying associations with variables that could reflect other unidentified aspects of care. Is it possible that those hospitals with a large neonatologist–housestaff ratio have a host of unmeasured structural differences that could be the actual drivers of the reduced IVH rates?

A limitation of the study is that the models used by the authors presume that the outcome of severe IVH is largely due to neonatal factors. However, IVH may also be influenced by perinatal factors such as the use of antenatal steroids and the quality of obstetric care. The only antenatal treatment factor considered in the analysis was mode of delivery, and cesarean section conferred an advantage. Obstetric service staffing may similarly affect the development of IVH, although one would guess that the level of high-risk obstetric care would correlate with that of neonatal services, as studied by the authors.

Identifying the factors that may contribute to severe IVH and the risk of a poor neurologic outcome in this vulnerable population remains a high priority. Some factors such as birth weight are out of our control; however, this study clearly suggests that there are also factors that may be modifiable by our practice patterns, and this warrants further study.

H. C. Lee, MD

References

1. Synnes AR, Chien LY, Peliowski A, Baboolal R, Lee SK, for the Canadian NICU Network. Variations in intraventricular hemorrhage incidence rates among Canadian neonatal intensive care units. *J Pediatr.* 2001;138:525-531.
2. Phibbs CS, Bronstein JM, Buxton E, Phibbs, RH. The effects of patient volume and level of care at the hospital of birth on neonatal mortality. *JAMA.* 1996;276:1054-1059.

Prolonged Indomethacin Exposure Is Associated With Decreased White Matter Injury Detected With Magnetic Resonance Imaging in Premature Newborns at 24 to 28 Weeks' Gestation at Birth

Miller SP, Mayer EE, Clyman RI, et al (Univ of California, San Francisco; Univ of British Columbia, Vancouver, Canada)
Pediatrics 117:1626-1631, 2006   8–12

Objectives.—Newborns delivered before 28 weeks' gestation commonly have white matter lesions on MRI that are associated with adverse neurodevelopmental outcomes. Our objective was to determine the risk factors for MRI-detectable white matter injury in infants delivered before 28 weeks' gestation who were treated with prophylactic indomethacin.

Methods.—This was a prospective cohort study conducted at the intensive care nursery at University of California San Francisco Children's Hospital. Patients included 57 premature newborns between 24 and 27 (+6 days) weeks' gestation at birth (October 1998 to October 2004). We identified perinatal and neonatal risk factors associated with moderate-severe "white matter injuries" (T1 signal abnormalities >2 mm or >3 areas of T1 abnormality) and moderate-severe "brain abnormality" (moderate-severe white matter injuries, any degree of ventriculomegaly, or severe intraventricular hemorrhage) on MRI. Infants were studied with MRI at 31.1 weeks' postmenstrual age (median).

Results.—Moderate-severe white matter injuries were detected in 12 (21%) of 53 preterm newborns, and 20 (35%) of 57 had moderate-severe brain abnormality. Prolonged indomethacin exposure was the only risk factor independently associated with a lower risk of white matter injury or brain abnormality, even when adjusting for the presence of a hemodynamically significant PDA, gestational age at birth, prenatal betamethasone, systemic infection, and days of mechanical ventilation.

Conclusions.—In this observational study, a longer duration of indomethacin exposure was associated with less white matter injury in infants delivered before 28 weeks' gestation. A randomized trial of prolonged indomethacin treatment is needed to determine whether indomethacin can decrease white matter injury and neurodevelopmental abnormalities.

▶ This article studies the perinatal risk factors that are associated with white matter lesions on MR imaging in preterm infants born less than 28 weeks' gestation. The authors appear to have a priori hypothesis that prophylactic indomethacin may be associated with an alteration in the presence of white matter abnormalities on MR imaging. Of the 216 preterm infants admitted over a 6-year period, 57 were recruited with no major differences in their perinatal characteristics (although the data for this are not presented). In a similar fashion to their previous paper relating MR abnormalities to outcome, 35% of the infants had moderate to severe abnormalities with 21% having moderate to severe T1-weighted white matter (WM) abnormalities. On statistical analysis, only prolonged indomethacin use for an additional 3 to 6 doses after the initial prophylactic dose was associated with a significant reduction in the severity of

WM abnormality, even after adjustment for the presence of a hemodynami-cally significant PDA, gestational age at birth, prenatal steroids, systemic in-fection, and days of mechanical ventilation. The authors conclude that pro-longed indomethacin for 6 doses may reduce WM injury in preterm infants <28 weeks' gestation.

This study raises some provocative thoughts about the use of more pro-longed indomethacin as a neuroprotective agent for the cerebral WM. There are, however, some concerns in the study: (1) Infants with moderate to severe WM abnormalities had several characteristics that differ greatly from previous reports, including more prenatal steroid use (75% vs 51%), no chorioamnioni-tis (0% vs 27%), and no necrotizing enterocolitis, which is the most potent fac-tor in our own studies (0% vs 20%) and (2) Ventriculomegaly, which should be associated with white matter atrophy, was more common in the absent WM abnormalities group (17% vs 8%). Although neither these clinical nor radio-logic criteria were said to reach statistical significance, they do raise concerns about the nature of the population who had WM abnormalities and the etiology of their injuries. Interestingly, 75% of the infants with moderate to severe WM abnormalities had evidence of systemic infection. There is no detail about the timing of this infection in relation to the timing of the abnormalities on the early MR imaging. It is plausible, although not discussed at length by the authors, that indomethacin may be reducing the inflammatory response in the cerebral WM, particularly in response to systemic infection. It would seem worthy of further interrogation as to when the infection occurred in relation to the MR imaging. Finally, these authors have often repeated MR imaging close to term along with neuromotor examinations. Neither later MR imaging, which is re-ported in their neurodevelopmental outcome article, nor neuromotor out-comes are reported in this study. It would be of great interest to see these re-sults as well as neurodevelopmental outcomes at 2 years in this cohort. The answer as to whether additional doses of indomethacin may reduce cerebral white matter injury remains unknown, but this article certainly provokes fur-ther investigation.

T. E. Inder, MD

Plurality-dependent risk of severe intraventricular hemorrhage among very low birth weight infants and antepartum corticosteroid treatment

Blickstein I, for the Israel Neonatal Network (Kaplan Med Ctr, Rehovot, Israel; et al)

Am J Obstet Gynecol 194:1329-1333, 2006   8–13

Objective.—This study was undertaken to compare the effect of antenatal corticosteroid therapy on the risk for severe intraventricular hemorrhage (IVH grade III-IV) in preterm singleton and multiple very low birth weight (VLBW) infants.

Study Design.—The occurrence of severe IVH was recorded in 5022 singleton, 2032 twin, and 582 triplet infants, delivered at 24 to 32 weeks'

TABLE 1.—Frequency of IVH Among VLBW Infants, by Plurality (Singleton, Twins, and Triplets) and Antenatal Corticosteroid Therapy (Complete, Partial, and No Treatment)

Frequency of IVH Grade III-IV Antenatal Corticosteroid Therapy	Singletons (N = 5022)	Twins (N = 2032)	Triplets (n = 582)	Total (n = 7636)
Complete course	157/2297[a,b] (6.8)	98/1052[d,e] (9.3)	36/431[g,h] (8.3)	291/3780[i,k] (7.7)
Partial course	111/881[a,c] (12.6)	64/408[d,f] 15.7)	11/69[g,j] (15.9)	186/1358[j,l] (13.7)
None	355/1844[b,c] (19.2)	107/572[e,f] (18.7)	24/82[h,i] (29.3)	486/2498[k,l] (19.4)
Total	623/5022 (12.4)	269/2032 (13.2)	71/582 (12.2)	963/7636 (12.6)

Data presented as n/N (%). Statistics are shown as OR (95% CI). a = 0.6 (0.4-0.7); b = 0.3 (0.3-0.4); c = 0.6 (0.5-0.8); d = 0.5 (0.4-0.8); e = 0.4 (0.3-0.6); f = 0.8 (0.6-1.1); g = 0.4 (0.2-0.9); h = 0.2 (0.1-0.4); i = 0.4 (0.2-1.1); j = 0.5 (0.4-0.6); k = 0.3 (0.3-0.4); l = 0.7 (0.5-0.8).

(Courtesy of Blickstein I, for the Israel Neonatal Network. Plurality-dependent risk of severe intraventricular hemorrhage among very low birth weight infants and antepartum corticosteroid treatment. *Am J Obstet Gynecol.* 194:1329-1333. Copyright 2006 by Elseiver.)

TABLE 2.—Odds Ratio (95% CI) for IVH by Plurality and Antenatal Corticosteroids Adjusted for Covariables

Antenatal Corticosteroid Therapy	Singletons	Twins	Triplets
Complete course	Reference	1.3 (1.0-1.7)	1.5 (0.9-2.3)
Partial course	1.6 (1.2-2.1)	1.9 (1.3-2.7)	2.3 (1.0-5.2)
None	2.7 (2.1-3.3)	2.4 (1.8-3.3)	3.9 (1.9-8.2)

(Courtesy of Blickstein I, for the Israel Neonatal Network. Plurality-dependent risk of severe intraventricular hemorrhage among very low birth weight infants and antepartum corticosteroid treatment. *Am J Obstet Gynecol.* 194:1329-1333. Copyright 2006 by Elseiver.)

gestation, registered in the Israeli National VLBW infant database. Antenatal corticosteroid therapy was defined as complete, partial, or none.

Results.—The incidence of IVH grade III-IV ranged from 6.8% among singletons receiving complete course to 29.3% in triplets without antenatal corticosteroid treatment. Complete treatment significantly reduced the incidence of IVH in all plurality groups (Table 1). The adjusted risk for IVH among multiple infants who received a complete course compared with singletons was not significantly different, odds ratio (OR) 1.3, 95% CI 1.0-1.7 for twins and OR 1.5, 95% CI 0.9-2.3 for triplets (Table 2).

Conclusion.—Complete course of antenatal corticosteroid therapy was independently associated with decreased risk for severe IVH in singleton and in multiple preterm VLBW infants.

▶ Since the 1994 National Institutes of Health consensus panel on the effect of antenatal corticosteroid therapy for fetal maturation, a single course of betamethasone (12 mg intramuscular every 24 hours for 2 doses) to women at risk for preterm delivery between 24 and 34 weeks has been standard of care.[1] However, the benefits of corticosteroids in multiple pregnancies have been questioned. The latest meta-analysis of a total of 12 studies recruited 504 infants from multiple gestations[2]; it concluded that there was not enough evidence of effectiveness to support the use of antenatal corticosteroids in multiple pregnancies. It is unclear whether the questionable effects are related to inadequate dosing because of an expanded plasma volume and a higher fetal mass, more rapid clearance, or that many women are not treated or are treated only hours before delivery.

Ballabh et al,[3] in a study of the pharmacokinetics of betamethasone in 30 singleton and 21 twin pregnancies at a mean gestational age of 29 weeks, found that the volume of distribution was similar but the half-life of betamethasone was significantly shorter in twin than in singleton pregnancies. Clearance of betamethasone was greater in the twin pregnancies but did not reach statistical significance. The authors speculated that the decreased efficacy of betamethasone in twin pregnancies might be due to suboptimal dosing. The Ballabh et al results are consistent with the retrospective study by Murphy et al,[4] which compared the outcomes of prophylactic versus rescue antenatal corticosteroid treatment strategies in twin pregnancies. Seventy percent of rescue twins received no steroids. Among newborns younger than 34 weeks who had received a complete course of corticosteroids, the risk of respiratory distress syndrome (RDS) was not significantly reduced (adjusted OR, 0.59; 95% CI, 0.29-1.18), suggesting reduced bioavailability of corticosteroids in twin pregnancies. In contrast, Jobe and Soll[5] pointed out that there is no experimental evidence to support higher doses and proposed that the current dose may be too high and the schedule not optimal because the slow adsorption and long half-life (36 to 72 hours) of betamethasone phosphate (half the dose) may be of no benefit to the fetus. Jobe[6] further suggested that multiple pregnancies were less responsive because the underlying cause of preterm labor in twins and triplets might not "stress" these fetuses sufficiently for them to respond to antenatal corticosteroids.

The population-based observational cohort studies from the Israel National VLBW Infant Database between 1995 and 2001 of 24- to 32-week-old singletons, twins, and triplets have added interesting nuances to the question of the appropriate dose for corticosteroids for preterm multiple pregnancies. In the first study of 8206 VLBW infants (4,754 singletons, 2460 twins, and 906 triplets),[7] the incidence of RDS ranged from 58.2% in singleton infants who received a complete course of therapy to 81.5% in triplets who received no treatment. After adjustment for confounders, the effect of antenatal corticosteroids on RDS (not graded for severity) decreased with increasing plurality. Twins had a 1.4-fold excess risk and triplets had a 1.8-fold risk of RDS. Complete corticosteroid treatment in all plurality groups significantly reduced the risk of RDS. Partial treatment had the same effect as no treatment.

L. Wright, MD

References

1. Effect of corticosteroids for fetal maturation on perinatal outcomes. NIH Consensus Development Panel on the Effect of Corticosteroids for Fetal Maturation on Perinatal Outcomes. *JAMA*. 1995;273:413-418.
2. Roberts D, Dalziel S. Antenatal corticosteroids for accelerating fetal lung maturation for women at risk of preterm birth. *Cochrane Database Syst Rev*. 2006; 3:CD00454.
3. Ballabh P, Lo ES, Kumari J, et al. Pharmacokinetics of betamethasone in twin and singleton pregnancy. *Clin Pharmacol Ther*. 2002;71:39-45.
4. Murphy DJ, Caukwell S, Joels LA, Wardle P. Cohort study of the neonatal outcome of twin pregnancies that were treated with prophylactic or rescue antenatal corticosteroids. *Am J Obstet Gynecol*. 2002;187:483-488.
5. Jobe AH, Soll RF. Choice and dose of corticosteroid for antenatal treatments. *Am J Obstet Gynecol*. 2004;190:878-881.
6. Jobe AH. Antenatal steroids in twins [Letter]. *Am J Obstet Gynecol*. 2003; 188:856.
7. Blickstein I, Shinwell ES, Lusky A, Reichman B, for the Israel Neonatal Network. Plurality-dependent risk of respiratory distress syndrome among very-low-birth-weight infants and antepartum corticosteroid treatment. *Am J Obstet Gynecol*. 2005;192:360-364.

Early Brain Injury in Premature Newborns Detected With Magnetic Resonance Imaging Is Associated With Adverse Early Neurodevelopmental Outcome
Miller SP, Ferriero DM, Leonard C, et al (Univ of California San Francisco)
J Pediatr 147:609-616, 2005   8–14

Objective.—To determine the neurodevelopmental outcome of prematurely born newborns with magnetic resonance imaging (MRI) abnormalities.

Study Design.—A total of 89 prematurely born newborns (median age 28 weeks postgestation) were studied with MRI when stable for transport to MRI (median age, 32 weeks postgestation); 50 newborns were studied again near term age (median age, 37 weeks). Neurodevelopmental outcome was determined at 18 months adjusted age (median) using the Mental Development Index (Bayley Scales Infant Development II) and a standardized neurologic exam.

Results.—Of 86 neonatal survivors, outcome was normal in 51 (59%), borderline in 22 (26%), and abnormal in 13 (15%). Moderate/severe MRI abnormalities were common on the first (37%) and second (32%) scans. Abnormal outcome was associated with increasing severity of white matter injury, ventriculomegaly, and intraventricular hemorrhage on MRI, as well as moderate/severe abnormalities on the first (relative risk [RR] = 5.6; P = .002) and second MRI studies (RR = 5.3; P = .03). Neuromotor abnormalities on neurologic examination near term age (RR = 6.5; P = .04) and postnatal infection (RR = 4.0; P = .01) also increased the risk for abnormal neurodevelopmental outcome.

Conclusions.—In premature newborns, brain abnormalities are common on MRI early in life and are associated with adverse neurodevelopmental outcome.

▶ This article studies the neurodevelopmental outcomes of preterm infants with magnetic resonance (MR) imaging abnormalities in the cerebral white matter. The MR imaging was attempted to be undertaken in 89 preterm infants on 2 occasions, one at around 4 weeks of age (32 weeks postmenstrual age) and for half of the cohort at term equivalent. The authors find that abnormalities were common on the first MR image, including white matter injury in 50%, ventriculomegaly in 30%, IVH in 35%, and cerebellar hemorrhage in 10%. Although the absolute numbers of infants at term is half that of the earlier scan, the relative distribution of these MR abnormalities did not change. Overall, moderate severe abnormalities were found in 37% of infants on the first scan and 32% of infants on the second scan. For white matter injury the scoring remained fairly constant across the studies with 87% of infants being categorized in the same manner on each scan. Neurodevelopmental outcome was classified on the basis of a neuromotor examination scale and the Bayley Scales of Infant Development II at 12-24 months of age. Borderline was defined as MDI/PDI 70-84 or any abnormality in tone or reflexes, whereas abnormal outcome was MDI/PDI >70 or functional motor deficits. The analysis focused on the relationship of MR abnormalities to the 13 infants with abnormal outcomes—6 isolated cognitive, 1 pure motor and 6 mixed motor and cognitive. They found that abnormal outcome was associated with increasing severity of MR abnormalities on both scans. The authors concluded that brain abnormalities are common on MRI and are associated with later adverse neurodevelopmental outcome.

This study is important in providing the following evidence: (1) MR imaging is feasible in the premature infant population as early as 30 weeks' gestation without concern. It was a little disappointing to see that this study had to use sedation in 30% to 40% of their scans. MR imaging can be undertaken without sedation with feeding, bundling, and careful handling and continuous saturation monitoring; (2) MR abnormalities are very common in the preterm infant with diffuse white matter abnormalities occurring in up to 50% of infants; (3) MR abnormalities are seen as early as 4 weeks of age and may be more challenging to visualize over time. This is certainly noted for the T1 signal abnormalities, although by term there is also a better chance to visualize brain (gyral) development and white matter volumes as additional markers of abnormality; and (4) MR abnormalities are the best predictors of outcome that we currently possess and may provide the insight into the pathway to neurodevelopmental disability. These abnormalities related to both motor and cognitive outcomes. Reducing the frequency and severity of these MR abnormalities should be associated with improved neurodevelopmental outcomes.

The final challenges have been noted by the authors and should be considered as MR imaging studies move forward including (1) a truly representative population of preterm infants, (2) optimal image acquisition with fine-slice imaging at no greater than 1.5 mm slice thickness for visualization of abnormalities, (3) minimizing sedation and any risk associated with MR imaging, and (4) standardizing scoring systems for the entire MR scan including white matter evaluation for both T1 and T2 (often reported by the Hammersmith group) signal characteristics. In addition, diffusion imaging with quantifiable values for the apparent diffusion coefficient may add further information; and (5) earlier imaging in the first few weeks of life may provide critical insight into the timing of this injury so that we can determine when to offer neuroprotective interventions.

T. E. Inder, MD

Neural progenitors populate the cerebrospinal fluid of preterm patients with hydrocephalus

Krueger RC Jr, Wu H, Zandian M, et al (University of California, Los Angeles; Cedars-Sinai Med Ctr, Los Angeles)
J Pediatr 148:337-340, 2006   8–15

Objectives.—To evaluate cerebrospinal fluid (CSF) of preterm patients with hydrocephalus for neural progenitors.

Study Design.—This report describes a prospective study of CSF obtained from preterm infants, either with progressive posthemorrhagic hydrocephalus (PPHH) or without known intercranial pathology. Cells recovered by centrifugation were analyzed by reverse transcriptase-polymerase chain reaction or by immunocytometry. Alternatively, cells were cultured by using methods permissive to neural progenitor growth and analyzed by immunocytochemistry and Western blotting.

Results.—Human CSF cells were obtained from 20 preterm infants at ~27 weeks estimated gestational age (15 infants with PPHH, 5 control infants). The number of these cells removed over time from patients with PPHH were substantial, based on our calculations. Cells recovered from patients with PPHH transcribe markers for neural progenitors, all the mature cells types of the central nervous system, and a large battery of chondroitin sulfate proteoglycan genes, including the entire aggrecan/lectican family. These cells proliferated in culture, and precursor markers were detected by Western blotting, immunocytochemistry, and cytometry. Cells could not be cultured from control patients.

Conclusions.—Neural progenitor accumulation in CSF could confound the clinical interpretation of CSF cell counts in hydrocephalus and may play as yet undetermined roles in the biology of injury after hydrocephalus. These findings suggest the potential for neural stem cell propagation from CSF.

▶ The effects of hydrocephalus on ventricular neural stem cells is largely unknown. It seems likely that changes in CSF pressure or disruption of the ependymal layer might change the normal development of neural progenitors and could involve release of such progenitors into the CSF. In this study, the cellular contents of CSF from infants with PPHH was studied and compared with that from healthy infants of similar gestational ages (25 to 34 weeks' gestation). Not surprisingly, the nucleated cell content of the CSF from infants with PPHH was strikingly elevated. The cells from the PPHH patients were analyzed by fluorescence-activated cell sorting, reverse transcription polymerase chain reaction analysis, and culturing. Overall, isolated cells could express both Nestin and glial fibrillary acidic protein and proliferate in culture. Unfortunately, these assays cannot clearly distinguish neural progenitors from many other cells that would be expected in PPHH CSF, such as activated microglia or macrophages that can also express these markers. A major limitation of this study is that neither differentiation assays nor transplant assays were used to demonstrate neural progenitor capacity for the CSF cells. The study goes on to compare acutely isolated CSF cells to fetal neural stem cells in terms of RNA expression. Although the gene expression patterns are similar, the acutely isolated cells are highly likely to be a mixed cell population, so it is unclear which CSF cells are expressing individual RNA and how this corresponds to the cells that can proliferate in culture. Furthermore, cells present in normal CSF were too few to undergo any of these analyses, so it is uncertain whether these proliferative properties are induced by the PPHH environment or if the concentration of proliferative cells released into the CSF is simply increased by PPHH. It remains unclear whether the large quantities of CSF removed from preterm infants with PPHH is worth saving, as the authors are doing. This study holds out the intriguing possibility that there is a population of neural progenitors that can be released into the CSF, but the identity, capacity, and utility of the cells isolated in this study need further confirmation.

A. Penn, MD, PhD

Reoxygenation with 100% Oxygen Versus Room Air: Late Neuroanatomical and Neurofunctional Outcome in Neonatal Mice with Hypoxic-Ischemic Brain Injury
Presti AL, Kishkurno SV, Slinko SK, et al (Columbia Univ, New York; Weill-Cornell Univ, New York)
Pediatr Res 60:55-59, 2006   8–16

Study investigated neuroutcome in mice subjected at 7–8 d of life to hypoxic-ischemic brain injury (HI) followed by 30 min of reoxygenation with 100% O_2 (Re-O_2) or room air (Re-Air). At 24 h of recovery, mouse reflexes were tested. At 7 wks after HI spatial orientation and memory were assessed in the same mice. Mortality rate was recorded at 24 h and at 7 wks of recovery. In separate cohort of mice, changes in cerebral blood flow (CBF) during HI-insult and reoxygenation were recorded. Re-O_2 *versus* Re-Air mice exhibited significantly delayed geotaxis reflex. Adult Re-O_2 *versus* Re-Air mice exhibited significantly better spatial learning and orientation with strong tendency toward better preserved memory. Histopathology revealed significantly less hippocampal atrophy in Re-O_2 *versus* Re-Air mice. Following a hypoxia-induced hypoperfusion, Re-O_2 re-established CBF in the ipsilateral side to the prehypoxic level significantly faster than Re-Air. The mortality was higher among Re-O2 versus Re-Air mice, although, it did not reach statistical significance. Re-O_2 *versus* Re-Air restores CBF significantly faster and results in better late neuroutcome. However, greater early motor deficit and higher mortality rate among Re-O_2 *versus* Re-Air mice suggest that Re-O_2 may be deleterious at the early stage of recovery.

▶ The results of this investigation were mixed in regard to testing oxygen versus room air. The short-term outcome of geotaxis was better in the room air group, whereas long-term navigational learning and spatial orientation skills were better preserved with 100% oxygen. On the other hand, mortality was somewhat increased in the 100% oxygen group as well (47% vs 29%). If we are trying to best simulate natural physiology, then it does seem that excess oxygen disrupts this natural process more, as seen by the increased cerebral blood flow in the 100% oxygen group during reoxygenation. Perfusion increased to levels beyond those seen before injury. But it is difficult to know what may be optimal treatment after injury because natural processes are not always beneficial. There is also the uncertainty in many of our patients of the timing and duration of injury, which may affect the consequences of various treatments; in this experiment, the model used for brain injury was subjecting mice to 8% oxygen for 20 minutes at day 7-8 of age after right common carotid artery ligation. This model of brain injury may have more than 1 mechanism and the best strategy for oxygen use in this setting may be difficult to determine. Likewise, in a clinical setting, it may not be possible to achieve a simple overarching strategy for oxygen (or no oxygen) use.

H. C. Lee, MD

Prenatal alcohol exposure alters GABA$_A\alpha_5$ expression: A mechanism of alcohol-induced learning dysfunction
Toso L, Roberson R, Woodard J, et al (NIH, Bethesda, Md)
Am J Obstet Gynecol 195:522-527, 2006   8–17

Objective.—In a model for fetal alcohol syndrome (FAS), we have previously found an alteration in NMDA receptors suggesting mediation, at least in part, of alcohol-related learning deficit. NMDA and GABA receptors interact in a multisynaptic circuit for the regulation of the inhibitory tone through the CNS. The GABA receptor subunit GABA$_A\alpha_5$ is involved in learning and is developmentally regulated, as it is excitatory in the perinatal brain and inhibitory in the adult. We were interested to evaluate alcohol's effect on GABA$_A\alpha_5$ expression to further understand alcohol-induced learning dysfunction.

Study Design.—Timed, pregnant C57B16/J mice were treated on gestational day 8 with alcohol (25% alcohol, 0.03 mL/kg i.p.) or control (saline). Embryos and brains were harvested 10 days after treatment, and brains from adult offspring were collected after evaluation in the Morris Water Maze, a well-established test for spatial learning. Gene expression included samples from at least 3 litters per timepoint, and calibrator-normalized relative real-time polymerase chain reaction (PCR) was performed to quantify GABA$_A\alpha_5$ with GAPDH standardization. Statistical analysis included analysis of variance (ANOVA).

Results.—Prenatal alcohol exposure significantly decreased GABA$_A\alpha_5$ expression in the embryo ($P < .02$) and fetal brains ($P < .01$) 10 days after therapy. However, in adult brains GABA$_A\alpha_5$ expression was increased versus controls ($P < .01$). As previously demonstrated, prenatal alcohol exposure resulted in deficits in adults learning the Morris Water Maze with controls learning faster ($P < .05$).

Conclusion.—Prenatal alcohol exposure alters developmental GABA$_A\alpha_5$ expression. This may further explain the long-lasting damage of alcohol on learning skills. Both the alcohol-induced reduction in the GABA$_A\alpha_5$ subunit during development and up-regulation in adult brain may be related to learning deficits resulting in decreased learning potential caused by the developmental defect and an increased inhibition of learning resulting from increased expression as an adult. In combination with our previous findings, these suggest that alcohol-induced learning impairment is likely the result of alterations of both NMDA and GABA expression and function.

▶ FAS disorder is a major public health problem, and 1% of liveborns are affected. The mechanism of ethanol developmental toxicity remains unclear. In this article, another effect of ethanol is shown, a reduction in GABA$_A\alpha_5$ expression, which might help explain the learning deficits associated with FAS disorder. However, much is still to be learned. The reduction in $GABA_A\alpha_5$ was found 10 days after the exposure. If we wish to develop interventions at this point, they would need to be directed toward each deficit described. What we really need to know is the target for ethanol and how the interaction with the target leads to deficits such as reduced $GABA_A\alpha_5$ expression 10 days later. In some respects, this finding is like the Barker hypothesis. An event (eg, poor nutrition or ethanol exposure) causes a change (epigenetic) leading to an outcome (eg, high blood pressure or a learning deficit). Understanding the steps between exposure and epigenetic changes will lead to more efficacious interventions for changing a number of outcomes.

C. F. Bearer, MD, PhD

9 Behavior and Pain

Behavioral Responses to Pain Are Heightened After Clustered Care in Preterm Infants Born Between 30 and 32 Weeks Gestational Age
Holsti L, Grunau RE, Whifield MF, et al (Univ of British Columbia, Canada; Children's and Women's Health Centre of British Columbia, Vancouver, Canada; Umeå Univ, Sweden)
Clin J Pain 22:757-764, 2006   9–1

Objective.—To compare biobehavioral pain responses of preterm infants born at differing gestational ages (GAs) when pain was preceded by a rest period or by a series of routine nursing interventions.

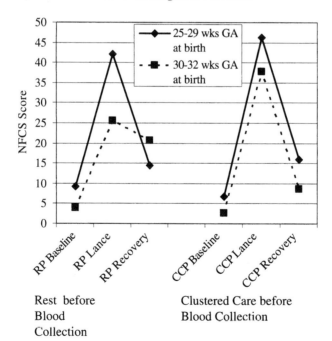

FIGURE 1.—Facial responses during phases of blood collection (Baseline, Heel Lance, and Recovery) during the 2 procedures [rest before blood collection (RP) or clustered care before blood collection (CCP)] comparing infants 25 to 29 weeks and 30 to 32 weeks gestational age at birth. (Courtesy of Holsti L, Grunau RE, Whifield MF, et al. Behavioral responses to pain are heightened after clustered care in preterm infants born between 30 and 32 weeks gestational age. *Clin J Pain.* 2006;22:757-764. Reprinted with permission from Lippincott William & Wilkins at http://lww.com.)

Methods.—In a randomized, within subjects, cross-over design, facial (Neonatal Facial Coding System), sleep/wake state and heart rate (HR) responses of 43 preterm infants [mean birth weight: 1303 g (range 590 g to 2345 g); mean GA at birth: 30 weeks (range 25 to 32)] were examined across 3 phases of blood collection (Baseline, Lance, and Recovery) under 2 conditions: pain after a 30-minute rest period versus pain after a series of routine nursing interventions (clustered care). Infant behavioral responses were coded from continuous bedside videotapes. HR was analyzed using custom physiologic signal processing software.

Results.—Infants born at earlier GA (< 30 wk) had equally intense facial responses during the Lance phase regardless of condition. However, later born infants (≥ 30 wk GA) showed heightened facial responses indicative of sensitized responses during blood collection when it was preceded by clustered care ($P = 0.05$) (Fig 1). Moreover, later born infants had significantly lower facial ($P = 0.05$) and HR ($P = 0.04$) reactivity during Recovery when blood collection followed clustered care.

Discussion.—Earlier born preterm infants showed heightened states of arousal and poor ability to modulate HR during Recovery when an invasive procedure was preceded by routine tactile nursing procedures. Alternatively, later born infants exhibited sensitized responses when clustered care preceded blood collection. Our findings support the importance of cue based individualized approaches to care (Fig 1).

▶ During the past several years pain assessment scales, such as the Neonatal Facial Coding System (NFCS), have been used to measure or score pain responses in neonates, and developmental care models, such as clustered care or the Newborn Individualized Developmental Care and Assessment Program (NIDCAP), have been widely implemented to reduce stress and behavioral responses to pain. In addition, because JACHO (Joint Commission on Accreditation for Healthcare Organizations) has referred to pain as the fifth vital sign, pain scores are commonly recorded with measurements of temperature, heart rate, respirations, and blood pressure.

The aims of this cross-over design trial were (1) to compare preterm infant responses to procedural pain (eg, heel lance) after a rest period with their responses to procedural pain after a series of routine interventions (referred to as clustered care) and (2) to examine gestational age and sex differences in infant response patterns. Fig 1 displays the NFCS score during phases of blood collection (baseline, lance, and recovery). Infants showed greater facial responses to blood collection after they had experienced clustered care. In addition, infants 25 to 29 weeks had similar patterns of NFCS responses to blood collection after a rest period or clustered care. However, the response by infants 30 to 32 weeks' gestation was different; whereas a heightened response to the lance followed clustered care, those infants also displayed a more rapid recovery. Although the goal of clustered care is to allow infants to rest for longer periods between care interventions, these findings emphasize the need to base the timing of those interventions on an infant's individualized cues rather than simply follow a developmental care strategy.

R. A. Ehrenkranz, MD

Persistence of fetal memory into neonatal life

Gonzalez-Gonzalez NL, Suarez MN, Perez-Piñero B, et al (Univ Hosp of the Canary Islands, Tenerife; Univ Hosp "Puerta del Mar," Cádiz, Spain)
Acta Obstet Gynecol Scand 85:1160-1164, 2006   9–2

Objectives.—To test the hypothesis that fetal memory persists into the neonatal period.

Study Design.—Forty-one newborns that had been repeatedly stimulated by using fetal vibroacoustic stimulation were compared with 31 controls. The same vibroacoustic stimulator was used for both fetal and neonatal stimulation tests. For the neonatal test the stimulus was applied against the mastoid of the newborn with the interposition of a specifically designed solid–liquid interface to simulate intrauterine conditions. Student's *t*-test was used.

Results.—Neonatal habituation rate (the number of consecutive stimuli applied before a baby stopped responding) was significantly higher in those newborns who had not participated in the fetal habituation study (7.0 ± 5.4 stimuli) than in those who had (4.1 ± 4.1 stimuli), $p = 0.01$.

Conclusions.—Newborns who were stimulated in utero habituated earlier than those who had not previously experienced the stimulation. These results suggest that fetal memory persists into neonatal life.

▶ This clever study demonstrates that experiences in utero can influence the behavior of newborn infants. The method relies on the phenomenon of habituation. Habituation is a decline in responsiveness to stimuli that are presented repeatedly or for long periods of time. Habituation can be conceptualized as a form of nonassociative learning.

Healthy women between 38 and 40 weeks' gestation (N = 41) were recruited for the study. With the use of US visualization, a vibroacoustic stimulus was repeatedly applied to the maternal abdomen above the fetal head at a rate of 1 s every minute until no fetal response was observed on 4 consecutive trials or until a maximum of 24 stimuli were delivered. The procedure was repeated every 48 to 72 hours until delivery: 18 fetuses experienced 3 tests, 14 had 2 tests, and 9 had 1 test. Control infants were the consecutive healthy newborns who had not experienced the vibroacoustic stimulus. One to 2 days after delivery, the same stimulus was applied to the infant's mastoid through a solid–liquid interface to mimic intrauterine conditions. The main measure was the number of presentations to habituation.

The authors documented that 95.1% of the fetuses habituated on the first test, 93.7% habituated on the second test, and 100% habituated on the third test. The mean fetal habituation rate was 7.0 ± 4.6 stimuli. The postnatal habituation rate for control babies was very similar to that of the fetuses and significantly higher than that of the babies who had participated in the fetal habituation experience (7.0 ± 5.4 stimuli for the control subjects compared with 4.1 ± 4.1 for the participants). The more rapid rate of habituation demonstrated that the exposed neonates treated the stimulus as familiar, whereas the control infants experienced the stimulus as new.

This is not the first study to demonstrate that newborns recognize stimuli they experienced as fetuses. For example, previous research has documented that newborns recognize their mothers' voices and musical sounds that they heard in utero. This study is distinctive because it used a discrete and novel stimulus for both the fetal and newborn testing. Although the authors conclude that the fetus is able to learn and memorize, a more appropriate interpretation is that a distinctive, repeated vibroacoustic stimulus in late fetal life can, indeed, influence behavior in the neonatal period. At a very general level, behavioral change as a function of experience can be classified as learning or memory. However, it is unclear what the fetuses learned. For example, would they have shown a more rapid rate of habituation if the neonatal test had used a different vibroacoustic stimulus? If a more complex stimulus had been used, could they anticipate changes in 1 of several elements? More research on the fetus's and newborn's capacity to learn is needed.

H. M. Feldman, MD, PhD

Infants in a neonatal intensive care unit: parental response
Carter JD, Mulder RT, Bartram AF, et al (Christchurch School of Medicine and Health Sciences, New Zealand)
Arch Dis Child Fetal Neonatal Ed 90:F109-F113, 2005   9–3

Objective.—To compare the psychosocial functioning of the parents (mother and father) of infants admitted to a neonatal intensive care unit (NICU) with the parents of infants born at term and not admitted to the NICU.

Design.—Random sample of NICU parents and term non-NICU parents were assessed across a variety of psychiatric and psychosocial measures shortly after the birth of their infant.

Setting.—Christchurch Women's Hospital, New Zealand. Labour ward and level III NICU.

Participants.—A total of 447 parents (242 mothers; 205 fathers) with an infant admitted to a regional NICU during a 12 month period; 189 parents (100 mothers; 89 fathers) with infants born at term and not requiring NICU admission.

Main Outcome Measures.—Depression and anxiety symptoms, psychosocial functioning.

Results.—Overall, levels of anxiety and depression were low in both parent groups. Compared with control parents, a higher percentage of NICU parents had clinically relevant anxiety and were more likely to have had a previous NICU admission and be in a lower family income bracket. Infant prematurity was associated with higher levels of symptomatology in both NICU mothers and fathers.

Conclusions.—Specific interventions are not needed for most parents who have an infant admitted to the NICU as they appear to adapt relatively successfully. Infant prematurity impacts negatively on the father as well as the mother. Consequently these parents may benefit from increased clinical attention.

▶ This report adds to the literature investigating parental response to the NICU experience. The inclusion of a control group, as well as information from fathers and parents of moderately preterm infants, add additional information regarding the adjustment of these parents. The main finding of no significant difference in depressive symptoms, but increased anxiety symptoms in the NICU parents, is in contrast to much of the previous literature, which has demonstrated significant rates of anxiety and depression among NICU parents. The difference in these results is likely explained by the inclusion of moderately preterm and term infants in the NICU group (the majority of the NICU group), because a subgroup analysis demonstrated the highest anxiety and depression scores in the subgroup of parents who had infants younger than 33 weeks' gestational age. These findings suggest that additional psychological support may be most important to those NICU parents with significantly premature infants, a finding that may be beneficial when considering staffing and resources for the provision of this type of support.

R. L. Chapman, MD

Pediatric Resident Education in Palliative Care: A Needs Assessment
Kolarik RC, Walker G, Arnold RM (Univ of Pittsburgh, Pa; Med Univ of South Carolina, Charleston)
Pediatrics 117:1949-1954, 2006   9–4

Objective.—The goal was to characterize pediatric residents' perceived educational needs for pediatric palliative care. The data generated from this study will facilitate the planning of specific educational interventions.

Methods.—All residents in the Children's Hospital of Pittsburgh pediatrics residency program were asked to complete a survey in September 2003. Participation in the study was voluntary. Residents rated their previous training, personal experience, knowledge, competence, and emotional comfort with 10 specific aspects of pediatric palliative care. This rating was followed by 13 questions related to attitudes about palliative care practices and training. The last section asked the respondents to rank 11 palliative care educational topics in order of importance.

Results.—Forty-nine of 75 eligible residents participated. Although residents thought that pediatricians should have an important role in providing palliative care, residents reported minimal training, experience, knowledge, competence, and comfort in virtually all areas of palliative care for children. We found no significant improvement in any of these areas from the pediatric level-1 year to the pediatric level-3 year. Residents wanted more training regarding pain management. After pain control, the next 4 educational needs were communication skills, namely, discussing prognosis, bad news, and code status and talking with children about end-of-life care.

Conclusions.—There is a clear need for increased efforts in pediatric palliative care education during residency training. Pediatric residents do not think that they are trained adequately in palliative care, and this perception does not improve with time. Pediatric residents view palliative care as important for primary care physicians and desire more education.

▶ This is a timely reminder that we need to enhance resident education in palliative care. The residents in this 3-year program reported they cared for an average of 19 patients with terminal illnesses during this time. However, they felt that they had minimal training in palliative care and expressed a clear need to enhance their competence, particularly with respect to pain management and communication in discussing prognoses, bad news, code status, and talking with children about end-of-life care. They also did not feel their training, experience, knowledge, competence, and comfort improved over the 3 years and felt that providing this care should not be left to oncologists and critical care or palliative care specialists alone.

The authors speculate as to why residents did not feel confident in these skills: no formal palliative care service existed at the time of the survey (2003), they received no specific mentorship or teaching of these skills in the clinical rotations, and attending staff also lacked training. The authors appropriately suggest it is unrealistic to expect substantial improvements in the absence of focused clinical experience, role modeling, and feedback.

The implications of this survey are very important: palliative care is becoming increasingly incorporated into the neonatal ICU, and residents want and perceive they need more education in this aspect of care. While educational interventions are planned and may improve matters in the authors' and others' settings, it is worth re-emphasizing the study of Sahler et al in 2000[1]: it is a shift in attitude and bias, not a shift in resources, that is most needed to implement a successful end-of-life curriculum. Role modeling, role playing, and communication skills may be more important than knowledge-based educational interventions. It may take faculty development initiatives to improve role modeling, as any planned resident-directed educational initiative highlights the need for attending staff to embrace the concept of palliative care in the ICU, neonatal ICU, and oncology units. Without changes in the "culture" of a unit or the "hidden curriculum",[2] educational interventions alone are insufficient: for when residents do not see practiced what they have learned, it can be counterproductive and may blunt any well-intentioned educational intervention.

J. Hellmann, MB, BCh, FCP(SA), FRCPC

References

1. Sahler OJ, Frager G, Levetown M, Cohn FG, Lipson MA. Medical education about end-of-life care in the pediatric setting: principles, challenges, and opportunities. *Pediatrics*. 2000;105:575-584.
2. Hafferty FW. Beyond curriculum reform: confronting medicine's hidden curriculum. *Acad Med*. 1998;73:403-407.

10 Gastrointestinal Health and Nutrition

Vacuum-assisted closure: a new method for treating patients with giant omphalocele
Kilbride KE, Cooney DR, Custer MD (Texas A and M Health Science Ctr, Temple)
J Pediatr Surg 41:212-215, 2006   10–1

Introduction.—Closure of giant omphalocele can present a surgical challenge. Neither silo, skin flap, nor primary closure has been successful in treating all patients. We present a novel application of the vacuum-assisted closure (VAC) device, which allows for improved results in these difficult cases.

Methods.—The VAC device (KCI, San Antonio, Tex) consisted of a sponge applied directly to the bowel and liver, covered with impermeable transparent dressing, and attached to a low negative pressure system. The sponge was changed every 3 to 5 days under local sedation.

Patients.—All 3 patients had giant omphaloceles. The first infant, a 34 week gestational age (WGA) male, was initially treated with silo reduction, which disrupted after 21 days. The large mass of bowel and liver made primary closure impossible. The VAC was applied for 45 days. The viscera was easily reduced and subsequently covered with acellular dermal matrix (AlloDerm). The VAC was reapplied, and the small remaining defect was skin-grafted. The second male infant was a 34 WGA male infant who became septic after failure of prosthetic mesh closure. The VAC was applied for 22 days after removal of the mesh. The infection resolved, and the defect size was reduced, allowing for skin flap closure. Mesh infection and development of an enterocutaneous fistula in the last patient, a 37 WGA female child, were treated by mesh removal and application of the VAC for 36 days. The VAC allowed for control of the fistula output and development of a healthy granulation bed.

Results.—Vacuum-assisted closure was associated with (1) rapid shrinkage and reduction of the viscera (22-45 days); (2) cleansing of the wound; (3) excellent granulation; (4) maintenance of a sterile environment; and (5) ease of use, with changes possible at the bedside.

Conclusion.—The VAC device should be considered a safe and effective alternative in treating complicated cases of giant omphalocele until a more definitive closure method can be used.

▶ The article under discussion is a brief case series of the authors' experience with VAC (KCI, San Antonio, Texas) for the treatment of giant omphalocele in 3 newborn infants. The authors used the VAC device in each of 3 infants as a secondary or salvage procedure, in that all 3 had failed previous attempts at closure/coverage of their large midline defects with the use of current standard-of-care procedures. The previous attempts at closure included silo reduction, nonabsorbable mesh placement, and the application of topical agents to induce epithelialization. As was seen in this case series, the failed omphalocele closure is complicated by the need for persistent mechanical ventilation, wound/skin infections, and enterocutaneous fistulae, among other morbidities. The related questions of how to optimally achieve durable primary biological coverage of a giant omphalocele and, as a related but separate problem, how to achieve effective treatment of failed primary reduction/coverage techniques before definitive skin and fascial closure remain significant unsolved problems. The latter issue was addressed in this case series by successfully applying the VAC device; the result was the appearance of a clean bed of granulation tissue over which re-epithelialization or skin grafting could occur. Obtaining initial biological coverage of a giant midline abdominal wall defect remains a challenging problem. In this case series, VAC was used as a secondary modality for cases that had already failed more traditional methods. Whether VAC could or should be applied as an alternative primary modality, as suggested in the discussion, cannot be adequately addressed from the data presented. Because current practice patterns are evolving to leave the giant omphalocele sac intact as a very durable primary biological dressing, any comparison of new methods to achieve primary biological closure (in preparation for staged fascial and skin repair) would be best studied in a prospective, randomized fashion. Despite the small case series and its inherent limitations, the observations do suggest that the VAC device can be safely applied over a modest time course (22-45 days) to achieve biological coverage (good granulation tissue and early re-epithelialization) in those cases that have failed other modalities.

K. G. Sylvester, MD

Ghrelin and cholecystokinin in term and preterm human breast milk
Kierson JA, Dimatteo DM, Locke RG, et al (Thomas Jefferson Univ, Philadelphia; Christiana Care Health Services, Newark, Del; Alfred I duPont Hosp for Children, Wilmington, Del)
Acta Paediatr 95:991-995, 2006   10–2

Aim.—To determine whether ghrelin and cholecystokinin (CCK) are present in significant quantities in term and preterm human breast milk, and to identify their source.

Methods.—Samples were collected from 10 mothers who delivered term infants and 10 mothers who delivered preterm infants. Estimated fat content was measured. Ghrelin and CCK levels were measured in whole and skim breast milk samples using radioimmunoassays (RIA). Reverse transcriptase-polymerase chain reaction (RT-PCR) was performed using RNA from human mammary epithelial cells (hMECs) and mammary gland with primers specific to ghrelin.

Results.—The median ghrelin level in whole breast milk was 2125 pg/ml, which is significantly higher than normal plasma levels. There was a direct correlation between whole milk ghrelin levels and estimated milk fat content ($r = 0.84$, $p < 0.001$). Both the mammary gland and hMECs produced ghrelin. While CCK was detected in some samples, levels were insignificant. Infant gestational age, birthweight, maternal age, and maternal pre-pregnancy body mass index did not significantly affect the results.

Conclusion.—Ghrelin, but not CCK, is present in breast milk. Since the mammary gland produces ghrelin message, and ghrelin levels in breast milk are higher than those found in plasma, we conclude that ghrelin is produced and secreted by the breast.

▶ This is just another example of the complex constituents in human milk. Ghrelin, a recently discovered hormone mainly secreted by the stomach, has several metabolic functions including regulation of food intake, energy homeostasis, and body weight. There are few studies on this hormone in healthy infants during the first year of life and even fewer in the immediate neonatal period. There does appear to be a negative correlation between ghrelin concentration and infant weight gain, which suggests that ghrelin, by modifying energy balance, might also play a role in the regulation of body weight in healthy infants. It is thus intriguing that Kierson et al remind us that there are significant amounts of ghrelin but not cholecystokinin (a modulator of appetite, too) in preterm and term milk.

Ghrelin and its mRNA have recently been found in numerous human tissues including breast. Aydin et al[1] compared the ghrelin levels in colostrum, mature and transitional milk, and plasma in lactating women with plasma samples from nonlactating women. They reported that the ghrelin levels in colostrum and transitional and mature milk were elevated concomitantly with increasing plasma ghrelin after delivery. The origin of milk ghrelin is not known, but it is probably derived from the plasma.

The possible long-term effects of prolonged breastfeeding in preventing obesity have, in light of the epidemic of obesity in the United States, led to the renewed interest in leptin, ghrelin, insulin-like growth factors, and other compounds, which may not only represent mediators involved in the metabolism of fat tissues, but may also potentially be able to explain the complex relationships between the gastrointestinal tract and the hypothalamic regulation of the sense of hunger and satiety.[2] Studies are needed to clarify how ghrelin might be involved in both short-term and long-term energy balance.

A. A. Fanaroff, MD

References

1. Aydin S, Aydin S, Ozkan Y, Kumru S. Ghrelin is present in human colostrum, transitional and mature milk. *Peptides.* 2006;27:878-882.
2. Agostoni C. Ghrelin, leptin and the neurometabolic axis of breastfed and formula-fed infants. *Acta Paediatr.* 2005;94:523-525.

Factors Influencing the Composition of the Intestinal Microbiota in Early Infancy
Penders J. Thijs C, Vink C, et al (Maastricht Univ, The Netherlands; Univ Hosp of Maastricht, The Netherlands)
Pediatrics 118:511-521, 2006   10–3

Objective.—The aim of this study was to examine the contribution of a broad range of external influences to the gut microbiotic composition in early infancy.

Methods.—Fecal samples from 1032 infants at 1 month of age, who were recruited from the KOALA Birth Cohort Study in the Netherlands, were subjected to quantitative real-time polymerase chain reaction assays for the enumeration of bifidobacteria, *Escherichia coli, Clostridium difficile, Bacteroides fragilis* group, lactobacilli, and total bacterial counts. Information on potential determinants of the gut microbiotic composition was collected with repeated questionnaires. The associations between these factors and the selected gut bacteria were analyzed with univariate and multivariate analyses.

Results.—Infants born through cesarean section had lower numbers of bifidobacteria and *Bacteroides*, whereas they were more often colonized with *C difficile*, compared with vaginally born infants. Exclusively formula-fed infants were more often colonized with *E coli, C difficile, Bacteroides*, and lactobacilli, compared with breastfed infants. Hospitalization and prematurity were associated with higher prevalence and counts of *C difficile*. Antibiotic use by the infant was associated with decreased numbers of bifidobacteria and *Bacteroides*. Infants with older siblings had slightly higher numbers of bifidobacteria, compared with infants without siblings.

Conclusions.—The most important determinants of the gut microbiotic composition in infants were the mode of delivery, type of infant feeding, gestational age, infant hospitalization, and antibiotic use by the infant. Term infants who were born vaginally at home and were breastfed exclusively seemed to have the most "beneficial" gut microbiota (highest numbers of bifidobacteria and lowest numbers of *C difficile* and *E coli*).

▶ A wise mentor once described intestinal colonization to me as, "People are 10% human and 90% bacterial." We have evolved this way over thousands of years, and recent data suggest it is beneficial for us to live in this symbiotic state. The factors that influence the development of the intestinal microbiota during infancy are the focus of this impressive research. Infant intestinal colonization has been previously studied in different types of newborns, from healthy babies to the tiniest neonatal ICU patients. The results are relatively consistent. The type of delivery, method of feeding, and hospitalization during infancy are important factors for colonization of the newborn gastrointestinal tract.

What is striking about this study is the number of patients prospectively studied and methods employed to obtain these results. A study of this magnitude would have been almost impossible if the labor-intensive and cumbersome technique of stool culture alone had been used. The stool analysis of 1032 patients was completed with the use of polymerase chain reaction to enumerate the bacteria. Now that this study has reaffirmed the reports that vaginal delivery and breastfeeding lead to the largest amounts of bifidobacteria making up the gastrointestinal flora, perhaps we can move forward from here to studies that will help us to understand why this is important. Future endeavors will, hopefully, focus on outcomes such as allergy development and immunity and enhance our understanding of the important relationship between man and bacteria. The authors have done great work; this is research that leads to more questions than answers.

C. Hoyen, MD

Prebiotic oligosaccharides reduce stool viscosity and accelerate gastrointestinal transport in preterm infants
Mihatsch WA, Hoegel J, Pohlandt F (Deaconry Hosp, Schwaebisch Hall, Germany; Ulm Univ, Germany)
Acta Paediatr 95:843-848, 2006   10–4

Aim.—To investigate whether a mixture of prebiotic non-digestible oligosaccharides (GosFos; referring to galacto- and fructo-oligosaccharides) would improve feeding tolerance in preterm infants on full enteral formula feeding. We hypothesized that GosFos would: (1) reduce stool viscosity and (2) accelerate gastrointestinal transport.

Methods.—In a placebo-controlled double-blind trial 20 preterm infants on full enteral nutrition (gestational age 27 (24–31) weeks, postnatal age 42 (11–84) days, and weight at study entry 1570 (1080–2300) g were randomly allocated to have their feedings supplemented with either GosFos (1 g/100 mL) or placebo for 14 days. Stool viscosity was measured by high-pressure capillary rheometry. Gastrointestinal transport time was assessed as the time from feeding carmine red to its appearance in the diaper. The hypotheses were tested as a priori ordered hypotheses. Data are shown as median (range).

Results.—Birth weight, gestational age, postnatal age, and weight at study entry did not differ between groups. GosFos significantly reduced both stool viscosity, as measured by extrusion force (32 (2–67) versus 158 (24–314) N), and gastrointestinal transit time (12 (4–33) versus 26 (5–52) h). No adverse effects were observed.

Conclusion.—Formula supplementation with GosFos reduced stool viscosity and accelerated gastrointestinal transport. Further trials are required to investigate whether GosFos facilitates enteral feeding advancement and early enteral nutrition thereby eventually reducing the incidence of catheter-related nosocomial infections and improving long-term outcome.

▶ To clarify the distinction between a prebiotic and a probiotic, I have included their definitions according to the *Physicians' Drug Reference*. "Prebiotics are defined as non digestible food ingredients that may beneficially affect the host by selectively stimulating the growth and/or the activity of a limited number of bacteria in the colon. Thus, to be effective, prebiotics must escape digestion in the upper gastrointestinal tract and be used by a limited number of the microorganisms comprising the colonic microflora. Prebiotics are principally oligosaccharides. They mainly stimulate the growth of bifidobacteria, for which reason they are referred to as bifidogenic factors. Probiotics are defined as live microorganisms, including *Lactobacillus* species, *Bifidobacterium* species and yeasts, that may beneficially affect the host upon ingestion by improving the balance of the intestinal microflora."[1]

Human milk contains 75% to 85% neutral and 15% to 25% acidic oligosaccharides. Fanaro et al,[2] in a prospective, randomized, double blind study, added a mixture of 80% neutral oligosaccharides (from long chain galacto- and long-chain fructo-oligosaccharides) with 20% acidic oligosaccharides derived from pectin hydrolysis and reported no difference in the intestinal microecology. Stool consistency was softest in infants fed the complete oligosaccharide mixture. There was no difference in growth, crying, vomiting, and regurgitation patterns between the groups. They concluded that acidic oligosaccharides from pectin hydrolysate are well tolerated as an ingredient in infant formulas without demonstrable effect on the intestinal microecology.

Preterm infants have major problems with motility and are at increased risk of systemic infections because increased intestinal permeability may result in bacterial translocation. It is thus encouraging that Mihatsch et al confirmed the reduction in stool viscosity as well as accelerated gastrointestinal transport in preterm infants. Furthermore, in a randomized trial, Moro et al[3] showed, for the first time, a beneficial effect of prebiotics on the development of atopic dermatitis in a high-risk population of infants. They postulated that the oligosaccharides modulate postnatal immune development by altering bowel flora and have a potential role in primary allergy prevention during infancy. The story on prebiotics is beginning to unfold, and it is set for a happy ending.

A. A. Fanaroff, MD

References

1. PDR*health* Web site. Available at: http://www.pdrhealth.com/drug_info/nmdrugprofiles. Accessed April 4, 2007.
2. Fanaro S, Jelinek J, Stahl B, Boehm G, Kock R, Vigi V. Acidic oligosaccharides from pectin hydrolysate as new component for infant formulae: effect on intestinal flora, stool characteristics, and pH. *J Pediatr Gastroenterol Nutr.* 2005;41:186-190.
3. Moro G, Arslanoglu S, Stahl B, Jelinek J, Wahn U, Boehm G. A mixture of prebiotic oligosaccharides reduces the incidence of atopic dermatitis during the first six months of age. *Arch Dis Child.* 2006;91:814-819.

Colour of bile vomiting in intestinal obstruction in the newborn: questionnaire study

Walker GM, Neilson A, Young D, et al (Royal Hosp for Sick Children, Glasgow, Scotland; Univ of Strathclyde, Glasgow, Scotland)
BMJ 332:1363-1365, 2006   10–5

Objectives.—To identify the colour that different groups of observers thought represented bile in a newborn's vomit.

Design.—Questionnaires displaying eight colours (pale yellow to dark green).

Setting.—General practices in Glasgow, postnatal ward and level III special care baby unit in a university teaching hospital, and mother and toddler groups in Glasgow.

Participants.—47 general practitioners, 29 nurses on the baby unit, 48 midwives, and 41 mothers of babies and infants.

Outcome Measures.—Participants indicated which colour would represent bile in a baby's vomit. More than one colour could be chosen. Respondents were also asked to indicate one colour that was the best match for bile.

Results.—When any colour could be chosen, 12 (25%) general practitioners, 1 (3%) nurse on the baby unit, 5 (10%) postnatal midwives, and 23 (56%) parents did not consider green an appropriate colour for a baby's vomit containing bile. Twenty three (49%) general practitioners, 7 (24%) neonatal nurses, 15 (31%) postnatal midwives, and 29 (71%) parents thought yellow was the best colour match.

Conclusions.—There is little agreement about the colour of bile vomit in a newborn. It is more pertinent to ask parents about the colour of vomit rather than whether it contained bile. Many general practitioners and parents do not recognise green as an appropriate colour for bile in the vomit of newborns, which may delay surgical referral. Though yellow vomit does not exclude intestinal obstruction, the presence of green vomiting in a baby is a surgical emergency and requires expeditious referral.

▶ This interesting little survey reports on the opinions of parents, general practitioners, special care baby unit nurses, and postnatal midwives about the color of baby vomit. What is instructive is not so much that opinions vary, but many individuals picked yellow as the most likely color representing bile in a baby's vomit. Of course, bile often appears green or some shade of green. The lesson is that it is better simply to ask about the color of the vomit and evaluate the rest of the clinical syndrome to make a determination as to whether investigative procedures are indicated or ultimately surgical intervention might be required. The authors correctly point out that yellow vomit may not exclude intestinal obstruction, but probably push the issue a little too far by claiming that the presence of green vomit in a baby is a surgical emergency and requires expeditious referral. It would be better to simply state that, in any case, vomiting in a baby should not be disregarded and the clinical state of the infant is paramount in determining the need for further investigation or surgical intervention.

D. K. Stevenson, MD

Killing the Messenger in the Nick of Time: Persistence of Breast Milk sCD14 in the Neonatal Gastrointestinal Tract
Blais DR, Harrold J, Altosaar I (Univ of Ottawa, Ont, Canada; Ottawa Hosp, Ont, Canada)
Pediatr Res 59:371-376, 2006   10–6

Human breast milk contains several proteins that supplement the newborn mucosal defense system and prevent gastrointestinal illnesses. One of these recently identified breast milk proteins is soluble CD14 (sCD14). By being an important component of the lipopolysaccharide (LPS) receptor complex, it has been suggested that breast milk sCD14 could stimulate the newborn immune system and help reduce gastrointestinal Gram-negative infections. However, to deliver its potential immune benefits to the neonate, sCD14 would have to survive the passage through the gastrointestinal tract and retain its biologic activity. We analyzed the presence of breast milk sCD14 in the neonatal digestive system and found breast milk sCD14 to be absent from the stools of breast-fed infants. *In vitro* digestion analysis with simulated gastric and pancreatic fluids revealed that sCD14 is likely to survive the pepsin digestion but is more prone to been nicked and digested by pancreatin. These findings suggest that the presence of intact breast milk sCD14 in the upper digestive system could promote innate immunity in this low bacteria density lumen. The low concentration of sCD14 in the LPS-rich environment of the distal gastrointestinal tract (*i.e.* commensal microflora) could prevent excessive inflammation.

▶ Considerable advances have occurred in recent years in the scientific knowledge of the benefits of breastfeeding, the mechanisms underlying these benefits, and in the clinical management of breastfeeding. The nutritional and bioactive aspects of human milk have been well summarized.[1-3] Breast-fed infants have improved general health, growth, and development, with fewer diarrheal disorders, or severity of diarrhea, fewer occurrences of sudden infant death syndrome (SIDS), fewer lower respiratory infections or otitis media, less bacteremia and bacterial meningitis, fewer urinary tract infections, and less necrotizing enterocolitis. Breastfeeding has also been related to possible enhancement of cognitive development. There are also considerable emotional and physical benefits for the mother. Long-term epidemiologic studies suggested a lower risk among breast-fed infants for later development of immunologically based diseases, such as type I diabetes,[4] childhood lymphoma,[5] and Crohn's disease.[6]

Blais et al have come up with a catchy title as they chronicle the saga of sCD14 as it traverses the gastrointestinal tract. They find that it survives the gastric acidity but "is prone to be nicked and digested by pancreatin." If, as they suggest, this prevents excessive inflammation in the distal gut, this is a good thing. The number of proteins in human milk is staggering and they each seem to play selected roles in nutrition and gut immunity. Nature conducts them all like the finest orchestra in the world and for that we are grateful. We can but recommend breast milk for all so that we can reach the World Health Organization targets for 2010, which are to initiate human milk feeding in 75% of the population and to have 50% still breast feeding at 6 months and 25% at 1 year. In the United States, the figures in 2003 were 71% initiation, 36% at 6 months, and 17% at 12 months, so the goal is attainable. Let's help accomplish this.

A. A. Fanaroff, MD

References

1. Wagner CL, Anderson DM, Pittard WB III. Special properties of human milk. *Clin Pediatr (Phila)*. 1996;35:283-293.
2. Lawrence R. *Breastfeeding: A Guide for the Medical Profession*. 4th ed. St. Louis, MO: Mosby-Year Book; 1994.
3. Gartner LM, Morton J, Lawrence RA, et al, for the American Academy of Pediatrics Section on Breastfeeding. Breastfeeding and the use of human milk. *Pediatrics*. 2005;115:496- 506.
4. Virtanen SM, Räsänen L, Ylönen K, et al. Early introduction of dairy products associated with increased risk of IDDM in Finnish children. The Childhood in Diabetes in Finland Study Group. *Diabetes*. 1993;42:1786-1790.
5. Davis MK, Savitz DA, Graubard BI. Infant feeding and childhood cancer. *Lancet*. 1988;2:365-368.
6. Koletzko S, Sherman P, Corey M, Griffiths A, Smith C. Role of infant feeding practices in development of Crohn's disease in childhood. *BMJ*. 1989;298:1617-1618.

Full Breastfeeding Duration and Associated Decrease in Respiratory Tract Infection in US Children

Chantry CJ, Howard CR, Auinger P (Univ of California, Sacramento; Univ of Rochester, NY; American Academy of Pediatrics Ctr for Child Health Research, Rochester, NY)
Pediatrics 117:425-432, 2006   10–7

Objective.—The American Academy of Pediatrics recommends exclusive breastfeeding for an infant's first 6 months of life. When compared with exclusive breastfeeding for 4 months, greater protection against gastrointestinal infection, but not respiratory tract infection, has been demonstrated for the 6-month duration. The objective of this study was to ascertain if full breastfeeding of ≥6 months compared with 4 to ≤6 months in the United States provides greater protection against respiratory tract infection.

Methods.—Secondary analysis of data from the National Health and Nutrition Examination Survey III, a nationally representative cross-sectional home survey conducted from 1988 to 1994, was performed Data from 2277 children aged 6 to <24 months, who were divided into 5 groups according to breastfeeding status, were compared. Children who required neonatal intensive care were excluded. SUDAAN software was used to account for the complex sampling design. Logistic regression adjusted for confounding factors. Outcome measures included adjusted odds of acquiring pneumonia, ≥3 episodes of cold/influenza, ≥3 episodes of otitis media (OM), or wheezing in the past year or acquiring first OM at <12 months of age.

Results.—In unadjusted analyses, infants who were fully breastfed for 4 to <6 months ($n = 223$) were at greater risk for pneumonia than those who were fully breastfed for ≥6 months ($n = 136$) (6.5% vs 1.6%). There were no statistically significant differences in ≥3 episodes of cold/influenza (45% vs 41%), wheezing (23% vs 24%), ≥3 episodes of OM (27% vs 20%), or first OM at <12 months of age (49% vs 47%). Adjusting for demographic variables, childcare, and smoke exposure revealed statistically significant increased risk for both pneumonia (odds ratio [OR]: 4.27; 95% confidence interval [CI]: 1.27–14.35) and ≥3 episodes of OM (OR: 1.95; 95% CI: 1.06–3.59) in those who were fully breastfed for 4 to <6 months compared with ≥6 months.

Conclusions.—This nationally representative study documents increased risk of respiratory tract infection including pneumonia and recurrent OM in children who were fully breastfed for 4 vs 6 months. These findings support current recommendations that infants receive only breast milk for the first 6 months of life.

▶ Whether to introduce solids at 4 months or 6 months to the exclusively breastfed infant has been controversial. A secondary analysis of an extensive national survey involving 2277 children between 6 and 24 months compared respiratory infection rates between those fully breastfed for 4 months versus 6 months. Adjustments were made for demographic variables, with the exception of pacifier use and number of day care attendees. Infants fully breastfed for 4 months were at greater risk for both pneumonia and recurrent OM. For the latter, the increased odds were assessed as greater than that associated with smoke exposure or day care attendance greater than 10 hours weekly.

The irony is that the most common reason given for discontinuing breastfeeding between 3 to 6 months is maternal employment, whereas the most common reason for maternal work absenteeism is illness of the child. This study not only supports the recommendation to exclusively breastfeed for 6 months, it also fuels the fire for legislation supporting improved maternity leave provisions and more flexible working conditions to facilitate breastfeeding and pumping for working mothers.

J. Morton, MD

Changes in Sucking Performance from Nonnutritive Sucking to Nutritive Sucking during Breast- and Bottle-Feeding

Mizuno K, Ueda A (Chiba Children's Hosp, Chiba City, Japan; Pigeon Co Ltd, Ibaraki, Japan)
Pediatr Res 59:728-731, 2006   10–8

Our aim was to obtain a better understanding of the differences between breast-feeding and bottle-feeding, particularly with regard to how sucking performance changes from nonnutritive sucking (NNS) to nutritive sucking (NS). Twenty-two normal term infants were studied while breast-feeding at 4 and 5 d postpartum. Five of the 22 infants were exclusively breast-fed, but we tested the other 17 infants while breast-feeding and while bottle-feeding. Before the milk ejection reflex (MER) occurs, little milk is available. As such, infants perform NNS before MER For bottle-feeding, a one-way valve was affixed between the teat and the bottle so that the infants needed to perform NNS until milk flowed into the teat chamber. At the breast, the sucking pressure (-93.1 ± 28.3 mm Hg) was higher during NNS compared with NS (-77.3 ± 27.0 mm Hg). With a bottle, the sucking pressure was lower during NNS (-27.5 ± 11.2 mm Hg) compared with NS (-87.5 ± 28.5 mm Hg). Sucking frequency was higher and sucking duration was shorter during NNS compared with that during NS both at the breast and with a bottle. There were significant differences in the changes of sucking pressure and duration from NNS to NS between breast- and bottle-feeding. The change in sucking pressure and duration from NNS to NS differed between breast-feeding and bottle-feeding. Even with a modified bottle and teats, bottle-feeding differs from breast-feeding.

▶ To understand the differences between the sucking performance changes from NNS to NS in breast- and bottle feeding, this study compares 17 term infants during both breastfeeding and then bottle feeding on postpartum days 4 and 5. To approximate the experience of the breastfed infant, who receives an insignificant volume of milk before the MER, a bottle was designed with a 1-way valve affixed between the nipple and bottle cavity. This required the infant to begin bottle feeding with NNS before drawing milk into the nipple. One of several noted differences between feeding patterns was that sucking pressures exerted with NS were lower with breastfeeding than with bottle feeding. Authors conclude that despite attempts to simulate breastfeeding with this bottle design, there remained significant differences between sucking behavior.

Is this a surprise? Consider the variables that could affect sucking behavior in breastfed infants: variations between mothers in breast/nipple anatomy, feed-to-feed volume changes, let-down to let-down intraductile pressure changes, and foremilk to hindmilk compositional changes, to name a few. Designing a bottle to resemble a breast is as impossible as designing formula to resemble breast milk. The variability and dynamic process of breastfeeding ensures artificial models can simulate neither the content nor the container. The conclusion is clear. They are completely different feeding methods.

J. Morton, MD

The Effect of Peer Counselors on Breastfeeding Rates in the Neonatal Intensive Care Unit: Results of a Randomized Controlled Trial
Merewood A, Chamberlina LB, Cook JT, et al (Boston Univ; Boston Med Ctr)
Arch Pediatr Adolesc Med 160:681-685, 2006   10–9

Objective.—To determine whether peer counselors impacted breastfeeding duration among premature infants in an urban population.

Design.—This was a randomized controlled clinical trial.

Setting.—The trial was conducted in the Newborn Intensive Care Unit at Boston Medical Center, an inner-city teaching hospital with approximately 2000 births per year.

Participants.—One hundred eight mother-infant pairs were enrolled between 2001 and 2004. Pairs were eligible if the mother intended and was eligible to breastfeed per the 1997 guidelines from the American Academy of Pediatrics and if the infant was 26 to 37 weeks' gestational age and otherwise healthy.

Intervention.—Subjects were randomized to either a peer counselor who saw the mother weekly for 6 weeks or to standard of care.

Main Outcome Measure.—The main outcome measure was any breast-milk feeding at 12 weeks postpartum.

Results.—Intervention and control groups were similar on all measured sociodemographic factors. The average gestational age of infants was 32 weeks (range, 26.3-37 weeks) with a mean birth weight of 1875 g (range, 682-3005 g). At 12 weeks postpartum, women with a peer counselor had odds of providing any amount of breast milk 181% greater than women without a peer counselor (odds ratio, 2.81 [95% confidence interval, 1.11-7.14]; $P=.01$).

Conclusions.—Peer counselors increased breastfeeding duration among premature infants born in an inner-city hospital and admitted to the neonatal intensive care unit. Peer counseling programs can help to increase breastfeeding in this vulnerable population.

▶ This study adds to a growing body of evidence about the effectiveness of breastfeeding peer counselors in increasing lactation rates for vulnerable population groups and is one of the first to detail this practice in the neonatal intensive care unit (NICU).[1-5] Breastfeeding peer counselors combine their own breastfeeding experiences with a 5-day educational program and translate breastfeeding knowledge into culturally sensitive mother-to-mother support mechanisms. In this randomized clinical trial, mothers of premature infants who received as little as 1 weekly visit from a breastfeeding peer counselor—who was not even a former NICU mother herself—were significantly more likely to be breastfeeding at 12 weeks after birth than mothers without this intervention.

This study had many methodologic limitations, most of which were acknowledged by the investigators. In particular, only 29% of potential mothers were eligible for sample inclusion, and definitions for the main outcome measure (duration of breastfeeding) included any breast milk feeding at 12 weeks, data which were largely self-reported by the mothers after NICU discharge. Nonetheless, in the African American subgroup analysis, mothers who received the breastfeeding peer counselor intervention were 3.59 times more likely than controls to provide any breast milk at 12 weeks after birth. These findings are especially relevant to NICU practice because prematurity rates are highest and breastfeeding rates are lowest for African American women in the United States.[6,7] Thus, the breastfeeding peer counselor intervention, already proven successful with other vulnerable population groups, holds promise and deserves further study in the NICU. Subsequent research in this area should address the cost effectiveness, quality, and satisfaction dimensions of this role in addition to breastfeeding rates.

P. P. Meier, RN, DNSc

References

1. Bronner Y, Barber T, Vogelhut J, Resnik AK. Breastfeeding peer counseling: results from the National WIC Survey. *J Hum Lact.* 2001;17:119-125.
2. Chapman D, Damio G, Young S, Pérez-Escamilla R. Effectiveness of breastfeeding peer counseling in a low-income, predominantly Latina population: a randomized controlled trial. *Arch Pediatr Adolesc Med.* 2004;158:897-902.
3. Kistin N, Abramson R, Dublin P. Effect of peer counselors on breastfeeding initiation, exclusivity, and duration among low-income urban women. *J Hum Lact.* 1994;10:11-15.
4. Meier PP, Engstrom JL, Mingolelli SS, Miracle DJ, Kiesling S. The Rush Mothers' Milk Club: breastfeeding interventions for mothers with very-low-birth-weight infants. *J Obstet Gynecol Neonatal Nurs.* 2004;33:164-174.
5. Rossman B. Breastfeeding peer counselors: review of literature and implications for practice and research. *J Midwifery Womens Health.* In press.
6. Centers for Disease Control and Prevention (CDC). Infant mortality and low birth weight among black and white infants—United States, 1980-2000. *MMWR Morb Mortal Wkly Rep.* 2002;51:589-592.
7. Li R, Grummer-Strawn L. Racial and ethnic disparities in breastfeeding among United States infants: Third National Health and Nutrition Examination Survey, 1988-1994. *Birth.* 2002;29:251-257.

Impact of standardised feeding regimens on incidence of neonatal necrotising enterocolitis: a systematic review and meta-analysis of observational studies

Patole SK, de Klerk N (Univ of Western Australia, Perth; Telethon Inst for Child Health Research, Perth, Western Australia)

Arch Dis Child Fetal Neonatal Ed 90:147-151, 2005   10–10

Background.—A significant and prolonged decline in the incidence of necrotising enterocolitis (NEC), nearing virtual elimination in some centres, has been observed consistently since implementation of a standardised feeding regimen.

Aim.—To systematically review the observational studies reporting incidence of NEC in preterm, low birth weight (LBW) neonates "before" and "after" implementation of a standardised feeding regimen.

Methods.—The Cochrane Central Register of Controlled Trials (CENTRAL, The Cochrane Library, Issue 4, 2002), Medline, Embase, Cinahl, and proceedings of the Pediatric Academic Societies (published in Pediatric Research from 1980) were searched in July and again in October 2003. The reference lists of identified observational studies, and personal files, were searched. No language restriction was applied. Key words were: standardised, enteral, feeding, neonates, necrotising enterocolitis. Authors were contacted for clarification of data.

Results.—Six eligible studies (1978–2003) were identified. A significant heterogeneity was noted between the studies indicating the variations in the population characteristics and feeding practices over a period of 25 years. Meta-analysis of the six studies using a random effects model revealed a pooled risk ratio of 0.13 (95% confidence interval 0.03 to 0.50)—that is, introduction of a standardised feeding regimen reduced the incidence of NEC by 87%.

Conclusion.—Standardised feeding regimens may provide the single most important global tool to prevent/minimise NEC in preterm neonates. Randomised controlled trials are needed.

▶ I will sponsor a huge celebration when I learn that necrotizing enterocolitis (NEC) is no longer the most common gastrointestinal emergency in newborn infants. Regrettably, that celebration is a long way off because we have made little progress in understanding the precipitating causes and underlying pathology of NEC. The interplay of the terrible triad, namely ischemia, inflammation, and ingestion of food, still dominate the pathogenetic landscape compounded by pharmacologic agents such as postnatal corticosteroids and indomethacin. Human milk has many protective factors but does not totally prevent NEC. We remain confused by the complexity of the precipitating events and challenged to come up with standardized therapy. Patole and de Klerk offer a glimmer of hope with their meta-analysis wherein they report that the use of standardized feeding regimens reduced the incidence of NEC by 87%. For a long time we have recognized that too rapidly advancing feeds and ignoring gastric residuals play a role in NEC. Standardizing feeding regimens, mandating gradual advances in volume, and paying attention to the gastric residuals help minimize the occurrence of NEC. When it occurs and the bowel perforates, we remain uncertain of the best approach to management. I am all in favor of a standardized feeding regimen, but I await with bated breath the trials on prebiotics and probiotics, and any other new strategies for prevention and treatment of NEC.[1]

A. A. Fanaroff, MD

Reference

1. Hammerman C, Kaplan M. Probiotics and neonatal intestinal infection. *Curr Opin Infect Dis*. 2006;19:277-282.

Coming full circle: an evidence-based definition of the timing and type of surgical management of very low-birth-weight (<1000 g) infants with signs of acute intestinal perforation
Tepas JJ III, Sharma R, Hudak ML, et al (Univ of Florida, Jacksonville)
J Pediatr Surg 41:418-422, 2006   10–11

Objective.—Gut disruption in very low birth weight follows 1 of 3 clinical pathways: isolated perforation with sudden free air, metabolic derangement (MD) complicated by appearance of free air, or progressive metabolic deterioration without evidence of free air. To refine evidence-based indications for peritoneal drainage (PD) vs laparotomy (LAP), we hypothesized that MD acuity is the determinant of outcome and should dictate choice of PD or LAP.

Methods.—Very low-birth-weight infants referred for surgical care because of free intraperitoneal air or MD associated with signs of enteritis were evaluated by univariate or multivariate logistic regression to investigate the effect on mortality of MD and initial surgical care (LAP vs PD). Metabolic derangement was scaled by assigning 1 point each for thrombocytopenia, metabolic acidosis, neutropenia, left shift of segmented neutrophils, hyponatremia, bacteremia, or hypotension. Laparotomy and PD were stratified by MD acuity, and odds of mortality were calculated for each surgical option.

Results.—From October 1991 to December 2003, 65 very low-birth-weight infants with suspected gut disruption were referred for surgical care. Peritoneal drainage and LAP infants had similar birth weight and gastrointestinal age, neither of which predicted mortality. Despite a higher incidence of isolated perforation with sudden free air in PD infants, the incidence of MD and overall mortality were similar for PD and LAP. Multivariate logistic regression demonstrated MD to be the best predictor of mortality (odds ratio [OR], 4.76; confidence interval [CI], 1.41-16.13, $P = .012$), which significantly increased with interval between diagnosis to surgical intervention ($P < .05$). Infants with MD receiving PD had a 4-fold increase in mortality (OR, 4.43; CI, 1.37-14.29; $P = .0126$). Conversely, those without MD and sudden free air who underwent LAP had a 3-fold increase in mortality (OR, 2.915; CI, 1.107-7.692; $P = .03$.) Of 5, 3 failed PD were "rescued" by LAP.

Conclusions.—The dramatic difference in mortality odds based on surgical option in the presence of MD defines the critical importance of a thorough assessment of physiological status to exclude MD. Absence of MD warrants consideration for PD, especially for sudden intraperitoneal free air. Overwhelming MD may limit options to PD; however, salvage of 3 of 5 infants with failed PD demonstrates the value of LAP, whenever possible, for infants with MD.

▶ A careful examination of this retrospective query of a neonatal database of 65 premature neonates who underwent surgical therapy for necrotizing enterocolitis (NEC) or isolated intestinal perforation (IP) at a single center over a 12-year period offers many insights into the surgical care of these patients. A point of clarification is that the study population is more appropriately categorized as extremely low birth weight based on a birth weight of less than 1000 g rather than very low birth weight (<1500 g). This detailed consideration may be useful when examining other published articles regarding either of these specific patient populations.

One merit of this case series is the fact that the data were prospectively collected, which places this study in the minority among studies that have examined the controversy of LAP versus drainage for premature neonates with either NEC or IP. A continuing controversy exists surrounding the reasons for choosing which surgical therapy (LAP or drainage) to apply to which patients. Prior literature suggests that this choice may be related to the suspected preoperative diagnosis (NEC vs IP), birth weight alone, the subjective assessment of the surgical risk, and other factors. This study presents the hypothesis that the "metabolic status" of the patient may be the most important patient characteristic to be used in deciding between initial LAP versus initial PD placement. The study also attempts to determine in which scenarios initial drainage might be more beneficial in reducing mortality (eg, sudden free air without MD) and in which scenarios LAP might be preferred (eg, with MD). This study does point out that patients without MD may have improved outcomes (lower mortality rates) after initial drainage. A remaining question is, which patients will survive with drainage only? The results of this study help to address this question.

The study also highlights and re-emphasizes many of the limitations of the evidence that is available to inform the decision of which therapy (LAP or drainage) is more beneficial as the initial surgical treatment. The vast majority of studies on this subject are single-center, retrospective reviews with the limitations therein. There is no apparent attempt to categorize the patients by specific disease process (NEC vs IP). Prior studies have shown that this distinction, which can reasonably be made preoperatively, is an important prognostic determinant. Patients in the article by Tepas et al that have "MD" may represent more commonly those with NEC, whereas those without MD more closely resemble those with "IP." In the study, no data are presented regarding the intraoperative findings that may predict outcome and help explain the cause of MD.

Although the title hints at an evaluation of the timing of surgical intervention, no data are presented to support that this was done. As this was a retrospective review of an established database, it does not appear that a critical evaluation of the timing of surgical intervention was done. Thus, whether it is better to operate early or only after definitive indications for operation occur (eg, clinical deterioration despite maximal medical therapy, pneumoperitoneum, or others) remains a question.

The information provided to the relevant audience (ie, pediatric surgeons, neonatologists, and families of relevant patients) of this publication should also be judged in the context of other publications occurring around the same time. One month before the presentation of the Tepas study and well before its publication, a prospective observational study[1] was published regarding the surgical management of the same patient population. This study showed that neonatal mortality after initial LAP or initial drainage was very similar after adjustment for differences between treatment groups with regard to known risk factors. Perhaps the most important finding from the prospective observational study was a trend toward a lower incidence of neurodevelopmental impairment (NDI) in the group of patients treated with initial LAP versus initial drainage. The adjusted odds ratio for death or NDI at 18 to 22 months postconceptual age was 0.55 (0.18-1.67), favoring LAP. A second prospective article, in fact, a randomized trial[2] comparing LAP versus drainage in infants weighing less than 1500 g also showed no difference in neonatal mortality rates. Thus, in the context of other articles published at similar times, it seems that the possibility of finding large differences in neonatal mortality rates in relation to the initial surgical choice is small. The finding that longer term NDIs may be more dramatically affected is of concern. The case for achieving a heightened awareness of longer term NDI is somewhat difficult to make in this disease process that has a mortality rate of 40% to 50%. Although difficult, it seems that it may be critically important.

Now that this case series by Tepas and the other prospective studies mentioned above have been published, it is time to "break out of the circle" and move forward to more formally explore longer term outcomes. The phrase "coming full circle" in the Tepas article title, if interpreted literally, implies coming back to the original starting point and, in a way, starting over again. A randomized trial of LAP versus drainage, stratified by preoperative diagnosis (NEC or IP) evaluating death and NDI well beyond discharge (eg, 18-22 months postconceptual age) appears to be needed. The Tepas article and the hypothesis that MD should be considered when choosing the initial surgical strategy should be utilized in the design of a trial.

M. L. Blakely, MD

References

1. Blakely ML, Lally KP, McDonald S, et al. Postoperative outcomes of extremely low birth-weight infants with necrotizing enterocolitis or isolated intestinal perforation: a prospective cohort study by the NICHD Neonatal Research Network. *Ann Surg.* 2005;241:984-994.
2. Moss RL, Dimmitt RA, Barnhart DC, et al. Laparotomy versus peritoneal drainage for necrotizing enterocolitis and perforation. *N Engl J Med.* 2006;354:2225-2234.

Portal vein thrombosis in the neonate: Risk factors, course, and outcome
Morag I, Epelman M, Daneman A, et al (Univ of Toronto)
J Pediatr 148:735-739, 2006   10–12

Objective.—To determine the risk factors, clinical features, and outcome of infants diagnosed with portal vein thrombosis (PVT).

Study Design.—A retrospective chart review was conducted of all consecutive infants admitted to the Hospital for Sick Children, Toronto, between January 1999 and December 2003 diagnosed with PVT.

Results.—PVT was diagnosed in 133 infants, all but 5 of whom were neonates, with a median age at time of diagnosis of 7 days (Table 1). An umbilical venous catheter (UVC) was inserted in 73% of the infants and was in an appropriate position in 46% of them (Table 2). Poor outcome, defined as portal hypertension or lobar atrophy, was diagnosed in 27% of the infants and was significantly more common in those with an initial diagnosis of grade 3 PVT and in those with a low or intrahepatically placed UVC (Fig 1 and Table 3). Anticoagulation treatment did not appear to have a significant effect on outcome.

Conclusions.—PVT occurs early in life; major risk factors in addition to the neonatal period are placement of UVC and severe neonatal sickness. Poor outcome is associated with an improperly placed UVC and with grade 3 thrombus (Table 4).

TABLE 1.—Primary Indication for Abdominal USG

Renal evaluation of hypertension	6
Thrombocytopenia	26
Inappropriate UVC placement	6
Elevated liver enzymes	9
Hepatosplenomegaly	5
Congenital anomalies	46
Abdominal distension	22
Sepsis	13

(Courtesy of Morag I, Epelman M, Daneman A, et al. Portal vein thrombosis in the neonate: risk factors, course, and outcome. *J Pediatr.* 148:735-739. Copyright 2006 by Elsevier.)

TABLE 2.—Characteristics of the Infants (n = 133)

	UVC (n = 95)	No UVC (n = 36)	Unknown UVC Placement (n = 2)
Female/male	36/59	19/17	2/0
>32 weeks gestational age	76	29	0
<32 weeks gestational age	19	7	2
Appropriately placed UVC	44	–	–
Inappropriate placed UVC	48	–	–
Unknown exact location of UVC tip	3	–	–

(Courtesy of Morag I, Epelman M, Daneman A, et al. Portal vein thrombosis in the neonate: risk factors, course, and outcome. *J Pediatr*. 148:735-739. Copyright 2006 by Elsevier.)

▶ It is not unusual in the transitional period after birth for infants, who have been depressed at birth and require admission to an intensive care nursery, to have a UVC placed, at least temporarily. This is often done in anticipation of clinical instability that would warrant central venous pressure monitoring, administration of crystalloid or colloid for intravascular volume support, treatment with various cardiotonic or vasoactive drugs, as well as easy access for blood sampling. However, many infants do not require such support or access and are rapidly weaned from various supportive therapies such that the UVC can be removed. Thus, there are some important lessons from this retrospective survey. First, most of the children afflicted with PVT are infants diagnosed within the first couple of weeks who have had UVC placement. Incorrect catheter placement, low or intrahepatic in location, is associated with PVT. Second, most infants do not have a thrombophilic disorder. Third, although the duration

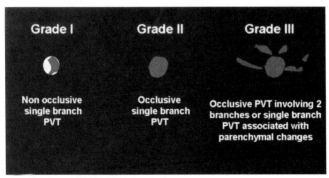

FIGURE 1.—Grading system for PVT. (Courtesy of Morag I, Epelman M, Daneman A, et al. Portal vein thrombosis in the neonate: risk factors, course, and outcome. *J Pediatr*. 148:735-739. Copyright 2006 by Elsevier.)

TABLE 3.—Outcome in Relation to UVC (n = 133)

	UVC (n = 95)	No UVC (n = 36)	Unknonw UVC Placement (n = 2)
PVT grade 1	41	18	1
PVT grade 2	33	10	1
PVT grade 3	21	8	–
Lobar atrophy	24	6	–
PHTN	2	4	–

(Courtesy of Morag I, Epelman M, Daneman A, et al. Portal vein thrombosis in the neonate: risk factors, course, and outcome. *J Pediatr.* 148:735-739. Copyright 2006 by Elsevier.)

of UVC placement has also been described as a risk factor, it is simply its use that sets the stage for complications. Portal hypertension is the most serious long-term complication but presents 5 to 6 years later and thus may not be apparent at the time of the original PVT diagnosis. Long-term follow-up is therefore indicated. Another clinical clue associated with poor outcome is atrophy of the left hepatic lobe, which also presents later. All neonatologists should consider the risks of inserting a UVC and reserve this intervention for those infants who are most likely to require it or, better yet, for those who actually do require it in order to ensure the safest transition after birth and, in particular, ensure that the risk that a baby faces with a UVC is not greater than the risk without it.

D. K. Stevenson, MD

TABLE 4.—Outcome in Relation to Grade of Thrombus

	Grade 1 (n = 60)	Grade II (n = 44)	Grade III (n = 29)	P
Complete or partial resolution	46 (77%)	25 (56%)	10 (34%)	.0005
No change	8	7	1	.2571
Progression to lobar atrophy or PHTN	6 (10%)	12 (27%)	18 (62%)	.0001

(Courtesy of Morag I, Epelman M, Daneman A, et al. Portal vein thrombosis in the neonate: risk factors, course, and outcome. *J Pediatr.* 148:735-739. Copyright 2006 by Elsevier.)

Intestinal O$_2$ Consumption in Necrotizing Enterocolitis: Role of Nitric Oxide

Nowicki PT, Reber KM, Giannone PJ, et al (Ohio State Univ, Columbus; Children's Hosp, Columbus, Ohio)
Pediatr Res 59:500-505, 2006
10–13

We tested the hypothesis that inducible isoform of nitric oxide synthase (iNOS)-derived nitric oxide (NO) inhibits oxygen consumption (Vo$_2$) in human intestine resected for necrotizing enterocolitis (NEC). Each NEC resection specimen was divided into two sections based on histologic appearance: healthy or diseased. Intestine removed from infants for reasons other than NEC was used as control. The tissue injury score (0–6, with 6 indicating complete necrosis) was 0.4 ± 0.2 in control tissue, 1.2 ± 0.4 in NEC-healthy tissue, and 4.6 ± 0.5 in NEC-diseased tissue. Prominent iNOS staining was present in villus enterocytes in NEC-healthy tissue but not in the other tissue types. Intestinal Vo$_2$ (per direct oximetry, in nM O$_2$/min/g) was significantly greater in control tissue than in NEC-healthy or NEC-diseased tissues. Accumulation of NO into buffer bathing intestinal slices (in nM NO/µL/g) was greater in NEC-healthy tissue than control or NEC-diseased tissues. The specific iNOS antagonist L-N$^{\omega}$-(1-iminoethyl)-lysine (L-NIL) reduced buffer NO concentration 76% and increased Vo$_2$ by 90% in NEC-healthy tissue; however, L-NIL had no effect on NO or Vo$_2$ in control or NEC-diseased tissue. Addition of exogenous NO *via* S-nitroso-N-acetylpenicillamine depressed Vo$_2$ in NEC-healthy and control tissues but not in NEC-diseased tissue. A significant correlation was present between buffer NO concentration and Vo$_2$ in NEC-healthy tissue. We conclude that iNOS-derived NO suppresses Vo$_2$ in intestine resected for NEC that demonstrates a relatively normal histology on light microscopy.

▶ The molecular pathogenesis of NEC has been the subject of several studies. iNOS expressed in villous enterocytes has been implicated in the etiology of the intestinal damage seen in NEC. However, the exact mechanism by which NO production results in tissue injury remains unknown. Nowicki et al conducted a series of experiments linking NO production in tissue resected for NEC with oxygen consumption. They measured iNOS expression, NO production, and oxygen consumption in 3 separate human intestinal tissue specimens: healthy tissue resected for reasons other than NEC (control), healthy tissue resected secondary to NEC but not necrotic (NEC-healthy), and NEC affected necrotic tissue (NEC-disease). iNOS expression and NO production were low to absent in both control and NEC-disease tissue. NEC-healthy tissue had the highest amount of iNOS expression as well as NO production. Oxygen consumption was closely correlated and inversely proportional to NO production in control tissue and NEC-healthy tissue. However, this relationship was altered in NEC-disease tissue in which both NO production and oxygen consumption were low. They next tested the effect of an iNOS-specific

antagonist and exogenous NO on oxygen consumption in each tissue specimen. Addition of the iNOS antagonist resulted in inhibiting NO production and
increasing oxygen consumption only in NEC-healthy tissue. No effect was
seen in control or NEC-disease tissue, possibly because neither of these specimens had much iNOS or NO production at baseline. Addition of exogenous
NO decreased oxygen consumption in control tissue and NEC-healthy tissue.
No effect was seen in NEC-disease tissue because baseline oxygen consumption was low. These experiments closely link increased expression of iNOS
and subsequent NO production with decreased oxygen consumption in the
early stages of NEC. Studies showing decreased injury in tissue specimens
treated with NO antagonist or increased injury in specimens treated with exogenous NO would have confirmed the etiology of NO in tissue damage in
NEC. However, until these studies are done, the role of NO in the pathogenesis of NEC remains unclear. It is possible that the increased expression of
iNOS and decreased oxygen consumption is an early protective mechanism in
the cascade of events that is set in place in response to tissue ischemia, or NO,
by decreasing oxygen consumption, may be contributing to the pathogenesis
of NEC.

A. Madan, MD

**C-Reactive Protein in the Diagnosis, Management, and Prognosis of Neo-
natal Necrotizing Enterocolitis**
Pourcyrous M, Korones SB, Yang W, et al (Univ of Tennessee, Memphis)
Pediatrics 116:1064-1069, 2005   10–14

Objective.—In this prospective, observational study, we determined
whether serum C-reactive protein (CRP) correlated with necrotizing enterocolitis (NEC) stages II and III. We hypothesized that serial CRP measurement if used as an adjunct to abdominal radiographs would improve the
identification of infants with NEC.

Methods.—Serum CRP level was measured every 12 hours for 3 measurements and, when abnormal, once daily. When clinical signs persisted and the
initial abdominal radiographs were abnormal, follow-up radiographs were
obtained.

Results.—Of 241 infants who were evaluated for gastrointestinal signs,
11 had ileus or benign pneumatosis intestinalis with persistently normal
CRP; gastrointestinal manifestations resolved within 48 hours, antibiotics
were discontinued in <48 hours, and feedings were restarted early without
complications. Fifty-five infants had NEC stages II and III; all had abnormal
CRP regardless of their blood culture results. In infants with stage II NEC,
CRP returned to normal at a mean of 9 days except in those who developed
complications such as stricture or abscess formation.

Conclusions.—In infants with suspected NEC, normal serial CRP values
would favor aborted antibiotic therapy and early resumption of feedings.
CRP becomes abnormal in both stage II and stage III NEC. In infants with

NEC, persistently elevated CRP after initiation of appropriate medical management suggests associated complications, which may require surgical intervention.

▶ Advanced NEC (Bell stage II or greater) develops in approximately 7% of very low birthweight (VLBW) infants and in 11% of infants with birth weights between 401 and 750 g.[1] Evaluations for possible NEC, or "NEC scares," are performed far more frequently, because of the nonspecific gastrointestinal and systemic signs, radiologic findings, and laboratory abnormalities associated with NEC. Even signs commonly used to assess feeding tolerance, such as the presence of gastric residuals and green gastric residuals, have uncertain predictive value.[2]

It would be a welcome clinical advance if serial CRPs could help determine which infants have significant bowel disease, as the authors suggest. In their study, among 66 patients with an abnormal abdominal radiograph, serial CRPs had 100% diagnostic accuracy. CRPs remained normal (<1.0 mg/dL) in all 11 patients who eventually were determined not to have NEC and became elevated within 24 hours in all 55 patients with advanced NEC.

These results are exciting, but should be interpreted with caution. Previous studies looking at the ability of CRPs to predict advanced NEC have not found this degree of accuracy.[3] Studies investigating the accuracy of CRPs in predicting neonatal sepsis have generally found a high negative predictive value, but "false-positive" tests have lead to a lower specificity and positive predictive value.[4] In the current study, diagnosis and management were not dictated but rather left to the discretion of the attending physicians, who were not blinded to CRP results. If CRP results played a large role in determining diagnoses, their high predictive value may have been partially preordained.

Aside from their diagnostic accuracy, serial CRPs appeared to actually help make an initial diagnosis only when they remained normal. This was particularly true in 5 patients who presented with pneumatosis, but by 48 hours their radiographs had normalized and they were determined to not have advanced NEC and were refed successfully. In patients who had advanced NEC develop, elevated CRPs did not appear to add to the diagnostic accuracy of radiographs. However, persistently elevated CRPs in patients with advanced NEC were helpful as indicators of an associated complication (all 7 such patients had either stricture or abscess and peritonitis). This observation has been made by previous investigators.[3]

Further experience with CRPs in the diagnosis and management of NEC is needed. CRP results must be interpreted in the context of other clinical, radiologic, and laboratory data, and how much additional data they provide is not well defined. Other biologic markers such as serum cytokines and fatty acid binding protein levels may also help in the diagnosis of NEC,[5] as may information obtained by abdominal US and Doppler flow studies.[6]

S. M. Peterec, MD

References

1. Guillet R, Stoll BJ, Cotton CM, et al. Association of H2-blocker therapy and higher incidence of necrotizing enterocolitis in very low birth weight infants. *Pediatrics.* 2006;117:e137-e142.
2. Cobb BA, Carlo WA, Ambalavanan N. Gastric residuals and their relationship to necrotizing enterocolitis in very low birth weight infants. *Pediatrics.* 2004;113: 50-53.
3. Isaacs D, North J, Lindsell D, Wilkinson AR. Serum acute phase reactants in necrotizing enterocolitis. *Acta Paediatr Scand.* 1987;76:923-927.
4. Benitz WE, Han MY, Madan A, Ramachandra P. Serial serum C-reactive protein levels in the diagnosis of neonatal infection. *Pediatrics.* 1998;102:e41.
5. Lin PW, Stoll BJ. Necrotising enterocolitis. *Lancet.* 2006;368:1271-1283.
6. Kim WY, Kim WS, Kim IO, Kwon TH, Chang W, Lee EK. Sonographic evaluation of neonates with early-stage necrotizing enterocolitis. *Pediatr Radiol.* 2005;35: 1056-1061.

Laparotomy versus Peritoneal Drainage for Necrotizing Enterocolitis and Perforation
Moss RL, Dimmitt RA, Barnhart DC, et al (Yale Univ, Hew Haven, Conn; Univ of Alabama, Birmingham; Stanford Univ, Calif; et al)
N Engl J Med 354:2225-2234, 2006   10–15

Background.—Perforated necrotizing enterocolitis is a major cause of morbidity and mortality in premature infants, and the optimal treatment is uncertain. We designed this multicenter randomized trial to compare outcomes of primary peritoneal drainage with laparotomy and bowel resection in preterm infants with perforated necrotizing enterocolitis.

Methods.—We randomly assigned 117 preterm infants (delivered before 34 weeks of gestation) with birth weights less than 1500 g and perforated necrotizing enterocolitis at 15 pediatric centers to undergo primary peritoneal drainage or laparotomy with bowel resection. Postoperative care was standardized. The primary outcome was survival at 90 days postoperatively. Secondary outcomes included dependence on parenteral nutrition 90 days postoperatively and length of hospital stay.

Results.—At 90 days postoperatively, 19 of 55 infants assigned to primary peritoneal drainage had died (34.5 percent), as compared with 22 of 62 infants assigned to laparotomy (35.5 percent, P=0.92). The percentages of infants who depended on total parenteral nutrition were 17 of 36 (47.2 percent) in the peritoneal-drainage group and 16 of 40 (40.0 percent) in the laparotomy group (P=0.53). The mean (±SD) length of hospitalization for the 76 infants who were alive 90 days after operation was similar in the primary peritoneal-drainage and laparotomy groups (126±58 days and 116±56 days, respectively; P=0.43) (Table 2). Subgroup analyses stratified according to the presence or absence of radiographic evidence of extensive necrotizing enterocolitis (pneumatosis intestinalis), gestational age of less than 25 weeks, and serum pH less than 7.30 at presentation showed no significant advantage of either treatment in any group (Table 3).

TABLE 2.—Comparison of Enrolled Patients and Eligible but Nonenrolled Patients Who Had Perforated Necrotizing Enterocolitis*

Variable	Enrolled Patients (N = 117)	Eligible Nonenrolled Patients (N = 121)	P Value	Eligible Nonenrolled Patients Who Underwent Laparotomy (N = 48)	Eligible Nonenrolled Patients Who Underwent Primary Peritoneal Drainage (N = 73)	P Value
Male sex — no. (%)	72 (61.5)	78 (64.5)	0.64	30 (62.5)	48 (65.8)	0.72
Race or ethnic group — no. (%)†			0.03‡			0.49‡
White	38 (32.5)	52 (43.0)		22 (45.8)	30 (41.1)	
Black	42 (35.9)	50 (41.3)		21 (43.8)	29 (39.7)	
Native American	21 (17.9)	7 (5.8)		3 (6.2)	4 (5.5)	
Asian	5 (4.3)	3 (2.5)		0	3 (4.1)	
Unknown	11 (9.4)	9 (7.4)		2 (4.2)	7 (9.6)	
Hispanic ethnic background — no. (%)	7 (6.0)	3 (2.5)	0.73	1 (2.1)	2 (2.7)	0.95
Birth weight — g	857±263	831±242	0.43	931±240	766±221	<0.001
Birth weight — no. (%)			0.99			0.009
<1000 g	90 (76.9)	93 (76.9)		31 (64.6)	62 (84.9)	
≥1000 g	27 (23.1)	28 (23.1)		17 (35.4)	11 (15.1)	
Gestational age — wk	27.8±2.5	27.8±2.4	0.96	26.8±2.1	25.5±2.0	<0.001
Gestational age — no. (%)			0.53‡			0.007‡
≤24 wk	29 (24.8)	37 (30.6)		7 (14.6)	30 (41.1)	
25 to 26 wk	49 (41.9)	40 (33.1)		17 (35.4)	23 (31.5)	
27 to 30 wk	29 (24.8)	34 (28.1)		17 (35.4)	17 (23.3)	
>30 wk	10 (8.5)	10 (8.3)		7 (14.6)	3 (4.1)	
Age at operation — days	13.6±11.6	15.2±12.0	0.32	15.8±13.5	14.7±11.0	0.64
Death within 90 days after intervention — no./total no. (%)	41/117 (35.0)	36/117 (30.8)	0.49	7/47 (14.9)	29/70 (41.4)	0.002

*Plus-minus values are means SD.
†Race or ethnic group was determined by the research team.
‡The P value was by analysis of variance.
(Reprinted by permission from Moss RL, Dimmitt RA, Barnhart DC, et al. Laparotomy versus peritoneal drainage for necrotizing enterocolitis and perforation. *N Engl J Med.* 354:2225-2234. Copyright 2006, Massachusetts Medical Society. All rights reserved.)

TABLE 3.—Mortality and Dependence on Total Parental Nutrition 90 Days after Intervention for Surviving Infants in Relation to Other Clinical Characteristics

Variable	Laparotomy	Primary Peritoneal Drainage	P Value	Relative Risk (95% CI)*
	number/total number (percent)			
Mortality				
All patients	22/62 (35.5)	19/55 (34.5)	0.92	1.03 (0.63-1.69)
<1000 g	15/45 (33.3)	16/45 (35.6)	0.82	0.94 (0.53-1.66)
≥1000 g	7/17 (41.2)	3/10 (30)	0.56	1.37 (0.46-4.14)
Pneumatosis on radiography	11/21 (52.4)	9/23 (39.1)	0.38	1.34 (0.70-2.57)
No pneumatosis on radiography	11/38 (28.9)	9/29 (31.0)	0.85	0.93 (0.45-1.95)
Gestational age				
<25 wk	9/30 (30.0)	10/31 (32.3)	0.85	0.93 (0.44-1.96)
≥25 wk	13/32 (40.6)	9/24 (37.5)	1.00†	1.08 (0.56-2.11)
pH				
<7.30	17/37 (45.9)	11/34 (32.4)	0.24	1.42 (0.78-2.58)
≥7.30	5/25 (20.0)	8/21 (38.1)	0.20†	0.53 (0.20-1.36)
Dependence on total parenteral nutrition 90 days after intervention				
All patients	16/40 (40.0)	17/36 (47.2)	0.53	0.85 (0.51-1.42)
<1000 g	12/30 (40.0)	15/29 (51.7)	0.37	0.77 (0.44-1.36)
≥1000 g	4/10 (40.0)	2/7 (28.6)	1.00†	1.40 (0.35-5.65)
Penumatosis on radiography	6/10 (60.0)	9/14 (64.3)	1.00†	0.93 (0.49-1.77)
No pneumatosis on radiography	10/27 (37.0)	8/20 (40.0)	0.84	0.93 (0.45-1.92)
Gestational age				
<25 wk	8/21 (38.1)	9/21 (42.9)	0.75	0.89 (0.43-1.85)
≥25 wk	8/19 (42.1)	8/15 (53.3)	0.73†	0.79 (0.39-1.60)
pH				
<7.30	8/20 (40.0)	10/23 (43.5)	0.82	0.92 (0.45-1.87)
≥7.30	8/20 (40.0)	7/13 (53.8)	0.49†	0.74 (0.36-1.55)

*The relative risk is reported as the risk of an event with laparotomy as compared with the risk of an event with peritoneal drainage. CI denotes confidence interval.
†The P value was determined with Fisher's exact test.
(Reprinted by permission from Moss RL, Dimmitt RA, Barnhart DC, et al. Laparotomy versus peritoneal drainage for necrotizing enterocolitis and perforation. *N Engl J Med*. 354:2225-2234. Copyright 2006, Massachusetts Medical Society. All rights reserved.)

Conclusions.—The type of operation performed for perforated necrotizing enterocolitis does not influence survival or other clinically important early outcomes in preterm infants.

▶ Neonatal-perinatal medicine has seen the introduction of a number of therapies, such as ECMO, without the benefit of rigorous, controlled evaluation. Primary peritoneal drainage for perforated necrotizing enterocolitis (NEC) was such a therapy. Since its introduction in the mid-1970s,[1] primary peritoneal drainage has had a checkered history and its use as the primary intervention for perforated NEC, instead of an exploratory laparotomy and resection, has remained controversial.[2] This multicenter, randomized, controlled trial conducted by Moss et al compared those procedures in very low birthweight (VLBW) infants with perforated NEC; they aimed to determine whether primary peritoneal drainage improved survival at 90 days postoperatively compared with laparotomy and resection. Secondary outcomes included dependence on total parenteral nutrition (TPN) 90 days after operation and length of hospital stay. The baseline characteristics of the 2 study groups were well-matched; in addition, of infants who were eligible but not enrolled, the baseline characteristics and mortality within 90 days of the intervention were similar to those of the study population (Table 2). As shown in Table 3, no significant differences were observed between the 2 study groups for any of the outcomes. Unfortunately, because the final sample size was smaller than originally planned, the actual power to detect a 50% relative reduction in the mortality rate (from 50% to 25%) was only 77% instead of 82%, and the relative risk (95% CI) was 1.03 (0.63-1.69). Therefore, clinically important reductions or increases in mortality with one approach or the other could not be excluded.

Although these results suggest that the choice of primary operation for perforated NEC in VLBW infants does not significantly influence survival, need for TPN at 90 days, or length of stay, this trial did not address whether one of these procedures was associated better long-term neurodevelopmental outcomes. Hintz et al[3] have reported that among extremely low birthweight (ELBW) infants, surgically managed NEC was associated with a significantly increased risk of neurodevelopmental impairments at 18 to 22 months corrected age compared with infants without NEC and medically managed NEC. Results of an observational study recently reported by Blakely et al[4] suggest that, compared with primary peritoneal drainage, laparotomy and resection may be associated with better neurodevelopmental outcomes. Therefore, although the short-term outcomes may be equivalent, the long-term outcomes may not be, and a trial powered to evaluate for significant differences in long-term neurodevelopmental outcomes should be considered.

R. A. Ehrenkranz, MD

References

1. Ein SH, Marshall DG, Girvan D. Peritoneal drainage under local anesthesia for perforations from necrotizing enterocolitis. *J Pediatr Surg.* 1977;12:963-967.
2. Moss RL, Dimmitt RA, Henry MC, Geraghty N, Efron B. A meta-analysis of peritoneal drainage versus laparotomy for perforated necrotizing enterocolitis. *J Pediatr Surg.* 2001;36:1210-1213.
3. Hintz SR, Kendrick DE, Stoll BJ, et al. Neurodevelopmental and growth outcomes of extremely low birth weight infants after necrotizing enterocolitis. *Pediatrics.* 2005;115:696-703.
4. Blakely ML, Tyson JE, Lally KP, et al. Laparotomy versus peritoneal drainage for necrotizing enterocolitis or isolated intestinal perforation in extremely low birth weight infants: outcomes through 18 months adjusted age. *Pediatrics.* 2006;117: e680-e687.

Ghrelin and motilin concentration in colicky infants
Savino F, Grassino EC, Guidi C, et al (Turin Univ, Italy)
Acta Paediatr 95:738-741, 2006   10–16

Aim.—To evaluate serum ghrelin and motilin concentration in infants with infantile colic.

Methods.—A case-control study was conducted on fasting blood venous samples obtained from 18 infants with infantile colic and 20 healthy infants to measure ghrelin (RIA test) and motilin (RIA test).

Results.—Colicky infants showed higher ghrelin serum levels (2534.2 ± 600.0 pg/ml; ln 7.8 ± 0.2) than controls (2126.1 ± 281.3 pg/ml; ln 7.6 ± 0.1) ($p = 0.011$). Serum motilin concentration was significantly higher in colicky infants (94.6 ± 23.2 pmol/l) than in controls (64.1 ± 30.1 pmol/l) ($p = 0.001$). Motilin concentrations were higher in formula-fed colicky infants (104.5 ± 20.4 pmol/l) than in breastfed ones (82.2 ± 21.3 pmol/l) ($p = 0.038$).

Conclusion.—Our finding shows that ghrelin and motilin concentrations are higher in infants with colic than in controls, supporting an organicistic aetiopathogenesis of this disorder. Furthermore, the role of ghrelin on gastrointestinal motility may open new doors to better understand the aetiology of infantile colic.

▶ To determine whether gut hormone peptides ghrelin and motilin that promote gastrointestinal motility are different in infants with colic, the authors performed case-controlled fasting venous blood assays in 18 colicky infants and 20 healthy control infants. Both ghrelin and motilin levels were significantly higher in the symptomatic infants compared with control infants. Also, motilin levels were higher in the colicky infants on breast milk compared with formula. A causal relationship was not established and correlative motility studies were not performed. Gastrointestinal hormone levels fluctuate throughout the day and it would be of interest to determine the pattern during and after a meal and in relationship to the peak time of discomfort, which is typically in the evening. The samples in this study were all drawn in the early morning. The relationship of elevated motilin in colicky infants on formula compared with breast milk remains unclear except that motilin is in breast milk and fails to explain the colic. Although the investigation draws focus on the potential role of ghrelin and motilin in infants with colic, more subjects and more samples throughout the day are necessary to link these hormones to colic.

W. Berquist, MD

Vitamin D Deficiency in Breastfed Infants in Iowa
Ziegler EE, Hollis BW, Nelson SE, et al (Univ of Iowa, Iowa City; Med Univ of South Carolina, Charleston)
Pediatrics 118:603-610, 2006   10–17

Objective.—The purpose of this work was to assess the vitamin D status of breastfed infants living in Iowa (latitude: 41° N).

Methods.—Blood samples and dietary records from 84 breastfed infants participating in another study were used for a survey of vitamin D status at 280 days of age. The vitamin D status of those (35 infants) who did not receive preformed vitamin D at 280 days of age (unsupplemented infants) was assessed longitudinally between 112 days and 15 months of age. Plasma 25-hydroxyvitamin D and, in most cases, parathyroid hormone and alkaline phosphatase were determined.

Results.—At 280 days of age, 10% of breastfed infants were vitamin D deficient (25-hydroxyvitamin D < 11 ng/mL). Deficiency was significantly more prevalent among dark-skinned infants and during winter and occurred exclusively in unsupplemented infants. During winter, 78% of unsupplemented infants were vitamin D deficient. During summer, only 1 infant who had dark skin pigmentation was vitamin D deficient. Longitudinal assessment of unsupplemented infants similarly showed that the majority of breastfed infants were vitamin D deficient during winter. Severe deficiency (25-hydroxyvitamin D < 5 ng/mL) was common and was accompanied by elevation of parathyroid hormone and alkaline phosphatase. The prevalence of vitamin D deficiency decreased with age but was still 12% at 15 months of age if no preformed vitamin D was received.

Conclusions.—Vitamin D deficiency, including severe deficiency, was common among breastfed infants in Iowa who did not receive preformed vitamin D. Deficiency occurred mostly during winter but was not completely absent during summer. It affected infants with light as well as dark skin pigmentation. Consumption of preformed vitamin D from vitamin supplements or formula is effective in preventing vitamin D deficiency. Vitamin D supplementation should be provided to all breastfed infants.

▶ The subject of this report, vitamin D deficiency, has historically been associated with rickets and hypocalcemia in the pediatric literature. However, as assays for the various metabolites of vitamin D and the other calciotropic hormones have become available in the last 30 years, it has been realized that infants and children are vitamin D "deficient" long before they develop clinical rickets or hypocalcemic seizures. This retrospective study looks at vitamin D deficiency in breastfed infants in Iowa as defined by serum 25-hydoxy vitamin D (25-OHD) concentrations, which are now used to define vitamin D "sufficiency," vitamin D "deficiency" and even vitamin D "insufficiency" states.[1] The specific cut-offs in infants for 25-OHD serum levels for defining these conditions have not been firmly established, but in the majority of reports including the present one, a value of less than 11 ng/mL (27.5 nmol/L) is considered deficient. In adults, vitamin D sufficiency is defined as 30 ng/mL or greater (75 nmol/L).[2] Part of the problem in defining the vitamin D state of the infant is that there is not a strong inverse correlation between decreasing serum 25-OH vitamin D level and increasing, serum parathyroid hormone levels in infants. This finding is demonstrated nicely in Figure 2 of the original article.

The issue specifically addressed in this article is the low vitamin D status of breastfed infants in Iowa who are not receiving the adequate intake of vitamin D (200 IU/day) recommended by the American Academy of Pediatrics.[3] Not surprisingly, the lowest levels of serum 25-OHD are seen during the winter months in Iowa in exclusively breastfed infants who are not receiving supplemental vitamins. Thus, 23 of 35 such infants (70%) had serum 25-OH levels below 11 ng/mL. The lowest levels are seen in black infants, though very few are included in this study. None of the 49 infants receiving supplemental vitamin D had low levels of serum 25-OHD. In fact, it has been shown that 400 IU of vitamin D a day given to exclusively breastfed infants will maintain mean serum 25-OHD concentrations 30 ng/mL or greater, the level associated with "sufficiency" in adults.

The authors emphasize that breast milk itself is a poor source of vitamin D, and that all exclusively breastfed infants living in temperate climates need supplemental vitamin D. This is important not only for bone health, but now that vitamin D receptors have been identified in most organs, and that vitamin D has been found to exert antiproliferative effects on cells, it is likely to play a role in the prevention of chronic diseases affecting many organs or organ systems.

F. R. Greer, MD

References

1. Greer FR. Issues in establishing vitamin D recommendations in infants and children. *Am J Clin Nutr.* 2004;80:1759S-1762S.
2. Bischoff-Ferrari HA, Giovannucci E, Willett WC, Dietrich T, Dawson-Hughes B. Estimation of optimal serum concentrations of 25-hydroxyvitamin D for multiple health outcomes. *Am J Clin Nutr.* 2006;84:18-28.
3. Gartner LM, Greer FR, for the Section on Breastfeeding and Committee on Nutrition. American Academy of Pediatrics. Prevention of rickets and vitamin D deficiency: new guidelines for vitamin D intake. 2003; *Pediatrics.* 111;908-910.

11 Hematology and Bilirubin

Incidence and causes of severe neonatal hyperbilirubinemia in Canada
Sgro M, Campbell D, Shah V (St Michael's Hosp, Toronto; Univ of Toronto)
CMAJ 175:587-590, 2006   11–1

Background.—Severe hyperbilirubinemia is the most common cause of neonatal readmission to hospital in Canada even though, in the majority of cases, risk factors can be identified before discharge. Severe neonatal hyperbilirubinemia and kernicterus continue to be reported worldwide in otherwise healthy term infants. We conducted this study to estimate the incidence of severe neonatal hyperbilirubinemia in Canada and to determine underlying causes, improved knowledge of which would be valuable to help identify strategies for risk reduction.

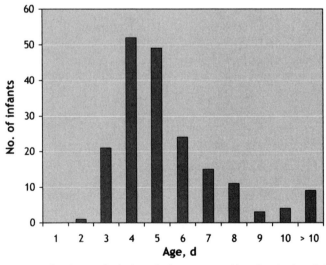

FIGURE 1.—Age of readmission for discharged infants. (Reprinted from Sgro M, Campbell D, Shah V. Incidence and causes of severe neonatal hyperbilirubinemia in Canada. *CMAJ*. 175:587-590. Copyright 2006, Canadian Medical Association.)

TABLE 1.—Baseline Demographic Characteristics

Characteristic	No. (%) of Infants* $n = 258$
Gestational age, wk, mean (SD)	38.5 (1.4)
Sex, male	162 (62.8)
Birth weight, g, mean (SD)	3360 (489)
Age at presentation, h, mean (SD)	111.6 (66)
Breast-feeding	210 (81.4)
Readmission	185 (71.7)
Peak total bilirubin level, µmol/L, mean (SD)	471 (76)
Weight loss† of 10%-15%	28 (10.9)
Weight loss† of > 15%	11 (4.3)

Note: SD = standard deviation.
*Unless stated otherwise.
†Calculated as $\frac{\text{birth weight} - \text{readmission weight}}{\text{birth weight}} \times 100$.

(Reprinted from Sgro M, Campbell D, Shah V. Incidence and causes of severe neonatal hyperbilirubinemiain Canada. *CMAJ*. 175:587-590. Copyright 2006, Canadian Medical Association.)

Methods.—Data on term infants 60 days of age and younger with unconjugated hyperbilirubinemia were collected prospectively through the Canadian Paediatric Surveillance Program from 2002 to 2004. Infants were included if they had a peak serum total bilirubin level of more than 425 µmol/L or underwent an exchange transfusion. Infants with rhesus isoimmunization or who were born at less than 36 weeks' gestation were excluded.

Results.—Of 367 cases reported, 258 were confirmed to be severe neonatal hyperbilirubinemia, for an estimated incidence of 1 in 2480 live births. Causes were identified in 93 cases and included ABO incompatibility ($n = 48$), glucose-6-phosphate dehydrogenase deficiency ($n = 20$), other antibody incompatibility ($n = 12$) and hereditary spherocytosis ($n = 7$). The mean peak bilirubin level reported was 471 µmol/L (standard deviation [SD] 76 µmol/L, range 156–841 µmol/L). Fifty-seven infants (22.1%) underwent

TABLE 2.—Causes of Severe Neonatal Hyperbilirubinemia

Cause	No. of Infants $n = 93$
ABO incompatibility	48
G6PD deficiency	20
Other antibody incompatibility	12
Hereditary spherocytosis	7
Urinary tract infection	2
Sepsis	1
Pyruvate kinase deficiency	1
Hypothyroidism	1
Unstable hemoglobin	1

(Reprinted from Sgro M, Campbell D, Shah V. Incidence and causes of severe neonatal hyperbilirubinemia in Canada. *CMAJ*. 175:587-590. Copyright 2006, Canadian MedicalAssociation.)

TABLE 3.—Characteristics of Infants With Severe Hyperbilirubinemia Identified Before and After Initial Discharge From Hospital

Characteristic	Identified Before Discharge n = 73	Identified After Discharge n = 185	p Value
Gestational age, wk, mean (SD)	38.6 (1.4)	38.4 (1.3)	0.26
Birth weight, g, mean (SD)	3369 (495)	3373 (488)	0.95
Sex, male, no. (%)	46 (63.0)	116 (62.7)	0.96
Peak total bilirubin level, μmol/L, mean (SD)	428 (77)	488 (68)	< 0.001
Age at presentation, d, mean (SD)	2.6 (2.2)	5.4 (2.6)	< 0.001
No. with diagnosis, no. (%)	30 (41.1)	63 (34.0)	0.29
Ethnicity, white, no. (%)	40 (54.8)	90 (48.6)	0.25
ABO incompatibility, no. (%)	15 (20.5)	34 (18.4)	0.69
G6PD deficiency, no. (%)	7 (9.6)	13 (7.0)	0.49
Other antibody incompatibility, no. (%)	6 (8.2)	6 (3.2)	0.10
Other diagnosis, no. (%)	3 (4.1)	10 (5.4)	0.67

Note: G6PD = Glucose-6-phosphate dehydrogenase.
(Reprinted from Sgro M, Campbell D, Shah V. Incidence and causes of severe neonatal hyperbilirubinemia in Canada.*CMAJ*. 175:587-590. Copyright 2006, Canadian Medical Association.)

an exchange transfusion. A total of 185 infants (71.7%) were readmitted to hospital, 121 (65.4%) of them within 5 days of age.

Interpretation.—Severe neonatal hyperbilirubinemia continues to occur frequently in Canada. In the majority of cases, the underlying cause was not identified. The high readmission rate within days after initial discharge indicates a need for a more thorough assessment of newborn infants and consideration of strategies to identify at-risk newborns, such as predischarge measurement of serum bilirubin levels (Fig 1 and Tables 1, 2, and 3).

▶ The authors report that severe hyperbilirubinemia (defined as a peak total bilirubin level > 425 μmol/L [roughly 25 mg/dL] or the need for a neonatal exchange transfusion, or both) continues to be a problem in Canada. Notably, infants who had rhesus isoimmunization were excluded in this study, as well as infants less than 36 weeks of gestational age. The latter criterion excludes a group of late preterm infants who are often, to their detriment, treated like term infants and, thus, are at higher risk of readmission for hyperbilirubinemia. Compared with term infants, late preterm infants may have both increased bilirubin production and impaired conjugation, which is sometimes exacerbated by breast-feeding failure and dehydration. Thus, the incidence of severe hyperbilirubinemia in this study population is clearly an underestimation. Also, the reliance on self-reported data limits interpretation. Nonetheless, some lessons can be reinforced based on the experience above the 49th parallel. A large proportion of the infants had diagnosed problems associated with increased bilirubin production, which is a major contributing cause of neonatal jaundice and is often found among those infants readmitted for treatment of hyperbilirubinemia, particularly in the first week of life. On the other hand, infants who present later may have impaired conjugation alone due to underlying genetic conditions, such as Gilbert syndrome, the G71R mutation, or other polymorphisms of the UGT1A1 gene promoter. What is also disturbing about this article is the fact that 51 infants (19.8%) of the 258 who met the criteria for inclusion had abnormal neurologic findings, some of which were quite serious. In addition, 13 infants had important neurologic abnormalities at final discharge, yet the incidence of kernicterus cannot be ascertained from the results of this survey. The Canadians do affirm the usefulness of the hour-specific bilirubin nomogram as a tool. However, if an inexpensive way were found to estimate bilirubin production and have information about the hour-specific bilirubin at the time of discharge, the causation of severe hyperbilirubinemia might be better understood on an individual basis, and anticipatory follow-up could be even more tailored. Moreover, unusual circumstances could also be identified, such as when an infant has a normal bilirubin production rate but is tracking in one of the higher risk zones of the nomogram or, more concerning, is crossing zones, which suggests a conjugating defect that might present later after the typical window for follow-up. Late causes of hemolysis, such as glucose-6-phosphate dehydrogenase deficiency, are also difficult to identify with the current screening approaches. The decision to screen for glucose-6-phosphate dehydrogenase deficiency could be based on a rationale for identifying infants at risk of later hemolysis or identifying infants who, if they were to have an impaired ability to conjugate the pigment (such as Gilbert syndrome), would be at extremely high risk of severe hyperbilirubinemia. For the record, increased bilirubin production is often present in infants with hyperbilirubinemia in the absence of a diagnosis.

D. K. Stevenson, MD

Transcutaneous Bilirubin Levels in the First 96 Hours in a Normal Newborn Population of ≥35 Weeks' Gestation

Maisels MJ, Kring E (William Beaumont Hosp, Royal Oak, Mich)
Pediatrics 117:1169-1173, 2006   11–2

Objective.—To obtain transcutaneous bilirubin (TcB) measurements, at 6-hour intervals, in the first 96 hours after birth in a normal newborn population (gestational age: ≥35 weeks).

Methods.—We performed 9397 TcB measurements on 3984 healthy newborn infants (gestational age: ≥35 weeks) from 6 to 96 hours of age. All measurements were performed in the well-infant nursery with a Draeger Air-Shields transcutaneous jaundice meter (model JM-103), within 2 hours of the designated time.

Results.—There was a distinct pattern to the velocity of the increase in TcB levels over different time periods. TcB levels increased in a linear manner most rapidly in the first 6 to 18 hours and then less rapidly from 18 to 42 hours, followed by a much slower increase until peak levels occurred. Decreasing gestational age was associated significantly with higher TcB levels.

Conclusions.—We provide data on neonatal bilirubinemia, based on TcB levels determined in a large, predominately white and breastfed, North American population. Infants who require closer evaluation and observation initially are those whose bilirubin levels are ≥95th percentile, ie, increasing more rapidly than 0.22 mg/dL per hour in the first 24 hours, 0.15 mg/dL per hour between 24 and 48 hours, and 0.06 mg/dL per hour after 48 hours. These data should be useful for detecting aberrant trends, identifying infants who need additional evaluation, and planning appropriate follow-up for jaundiced newborns.

▶ Maisels and Kring add to the ever-expanding database on neonatal hyperbilirubinemia. Their nomogram is different from that of Bhutani et al,[1] but then so again is their study population and the timing of their study. The Academy of Pediatrics is grappling with the lay public who are demanding bilirubin evaluations on all newborn infants to prevent kernicterus. As the arguments head toward the Congress, I have the feeling that PICK (Parents of Infants and Children with Kernicterus) will prevail. The data presented below will only strengthen PICK's cause.

Bhutani et al[2] modified hospital policy in order to manage newborn jaundice for safer outcomes. They authorized nurses to obtain a bilirubin (total serum/transcutaneous) measurement for clinical jaundice, mandated universal predischarge total serum bilirubin (at routine metabolic screening), and targeted follow-up (using the bilirubin nomogram).[1] They documented fewer adverse outcomes (exchange transfusion, intensive phototherapy, and readmission). Furthermore, during the study period no infant's bilirubin exceeded 30 mg/dl, while only 1 in 15,000 exceeded 25 mg/dl as compared with a reported incidence of 1 in 625. Eggert et al,[3] using a similar approach, was able to obtain similar results within a hospital system and noted a reduced proportion of neonates with significant hyperbilirubinemia and reduced rate of hospital readmissions with jaundice. Transcutaneous measurement of bilirubin has come of age and is used on a worldwide basis.[4,5]

A. A. Fanaroff, MD

References

1. Bhutani VK, Johnson L, Sivieri EM. Predictive ability of a predischarge hour-specific serum bilirubin for subsequent significant hyperbilirubinemia in healthy term and near-term newborns. *Pediatrics.* 1999;103:6-14.
2. Bhutani VK, Johnson LH, Schwoebel A, Gennaro S. A systems approach for neonatal hyperbilirubinemia in term and near-term newborns. *J Obstet Gynecol Neonatal Nurs.* 2006;35:444-455.
3. Eggert LD, Wiedmeier SE, Wilson J, Christensen RD. The effect of instituting a prehospital-discharge newborn bilirubin screening program in an 18-hospital health system. *Pediatrics.* 2006;117:e855-e862.

4. Sanpavat S, Nuchprayoon I. Comparison of two transcutaneous bilirubin-ometers—Minolta AirShields Jaundice Meter JM103 and Spectrx Bilicheck—in Thai neonates. *Southeast Asian J Trop Med Public Health*. 2005;36:1533-1537.
5. Ho EY, Lee SY, Chow CB, Chung JW. BiliCheck transcutaneous bilirubinometer: a screening tool for neonatal jaundice in the Chinese population. *Hong Kong Med J*. 2006;12:99-102.

Post-phototherapy neonatal bilirubin rebound: a potential cause of significant hyperbilirubinaemia

Kaplan M, Kaplan E, Hammerman C, et al (Shaare Zedek Med Ctr, Jerusalem)
Arch Dis Child 91:31-34, 2006   11–3

Aim.—To determine the incidence of post-phototherapy neonatal plasma total bilirubin (PTB) rebound.

Methods.—A prospective clinical survey was performed on 226 term and near-term neonates treated with phototherapy in the well baby nursery of the Shaare Zedek Medical Center from January 2001 to September 2002. Neonates were tested for PTB 24 hours (between 12 and 36 hours) after discontinuation of phototherapy, with additional testing as clinically indicated. The main outcome measure, significant bilirubin rebound, was defined as a post-phototherapy PTB ≥ 256 µmol/l. Phototherapy was not reinstituted in all cases of rebound, but rather according to clinical indications.

Results.—A total of 30 (13.3%) neonates developed significant rebound (mean (SD) PTB 287 (27) µmol/l, upper range 351 µmol/l). Twenty two of these (73%) were retreated with phototherapy at mean PTB 296 (29) µmol/l. Multiple logistic regression analysis showed significant risk for aetiological risk factors including positive direct Coombs test (odds ratio 2.44, 95% CI 1.25 to 4.74) and gestational age <37 weeks (odds ratio 3.21, 95% CI 1.29 to 7.96). A greater number of neonates rebounded among those in whom

TABLE 1.—Data Comparing Onset and Discontinuation of Phototherapy, and the Number of Neonates with Significant Bilirubin Rebound, Between the Two Subgroups Receiving Primary Phototherapy During Birth Hospitalization and Readmission Hospitalization, Respectively

	Primary Phototherapy During Birth Hospitalisation (n = 196)	Primary Phototherapy During Readmission (n = 30)	Significance
Age at onset (h)*	53 (29)	122 (38)	p < 0.001
PTB at onset (µmol/l)*	251 (53)	318 (22)	p < 0.001
Age at discontinuation*	96 (25)	152 (40)	p < 0.001
PTB at discontinuation*	182 (20)	182 (18)	NS
Duration of phototherapy (h)*	43 (23)	30 (9)	p = 0.002
Number of neonates rebounding to PTB ≥ 256 µmol/l	30 (15.3%)	0	p = 0.04

*Mean (SD).
(Courtesy of Kaplan M, Kaplan E, Hammerman C, et al. Post-phototherapy neonatal bilirubin rebound: a potential cause of significant hyperbilirubinaemia. *Arch Dis Child*. 2006;91:31-34. Reproduced with permission from the BMJ Publishing Group.)

phototherapy was commenced ≤72 hours (26/152, 17%) compared with >72 hours (4/74, 5.4%) (odds ratio 3.61, 95% CI 1.21 to 10.77).

Conclusion.—Post-phototherapy neonatal bilirubin rebound to clinically significant levels may occur, especially in cases of prematurity, direct Coombs test positivity, and those treated ≤72 hours. These risk factors should be taken into account when planning post-phototherapy follow up (Table 1).

▶ The finding that postphototherapy neonatal bilirubin rebound can occur in cases of prematurity, direct Coombs' test positivity, and infants treated at 72 hours or less suggests that increased bilirubin production is an important contributing cause to the jaundice encountered in these contexts. In particular, those infants who have no apparent risk factor but become jaundiced to an extent requiring intervention with phototherapy early in their postnatal course are most often high producers of the pigment. Notably, there are differences in HO-1 expression that may contribute to differences in bilirubin production depending on substrate (heme) availability independent of hemolysis. Of course, any increase bilirubin production, whether genetic or environmental in its causation, when combined with impaired elimination from any cause would further exacerbate neonatal jaundice. The converse of the reported observation is also true, that rebound is unlikely in infants who do not have increased bilirubin production, for example, those who are breastfeeding and only later develop hyperbilirubinemia requiring phototherapy. Such babies have most of their bilirubin in circulation bound to albumin, and with the application of phototherapy, bilirubin elimination will be enhanced with no rebound likely. It is only when the production of bilirubin exceeds the capacity to be bound in circulation by albumin, and thus moves into tissue, that the stage is set for a rebound. This most often occurs in the context of high production over time, leading to large amounts of bilirubin outside the circulation and a markedly increased total burden or load of the pigment in the particular baby. The same phenomenon is more often seen after exchange transfusion for infants with hemolytic jaundice.

D. K. Stevenson, MD

Efficacy of phototherapy for neonatal jaundice is increased by the use of low-cost white reflecting curtains
Djokomuljanto S, Quah BS, Surini Y, et al (Universiti Sains Malaysia, Kelantan; Univ of Oslo, Norway)
Arch Dis Child Fetal Neonatal Ed 91:F439-F442, 2006   11–4

Objective.—To determine whether the addition of low-cost reflecting curtains to a standard phototherapy unit could increase effectiveness of phototherapy for neonatal jaundice.

Design.—Randomised controlled clinical trial.

Setting.—Level-one nursery of the Hospital Universiti Sains Malaysia, Kelantan, Malaysia.

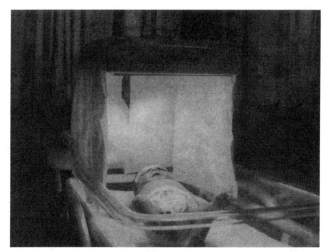

FIGURE 1.—Set-up for the intervention group using the white reflecting curtain hanging on both sides of the phototherapy unit. (Courtesy of Djokomuljanto S, Quah BS, Surini Y, et al. Efficacy of phototherapy for neonatal jaundice is increased by the use of low-cost white reflecting curtains. *Arch Dis Child Fetal Neonatal Ed*. 2006;91:F439-F442. Reproduced with permission from the BMJ Publishing Group.)

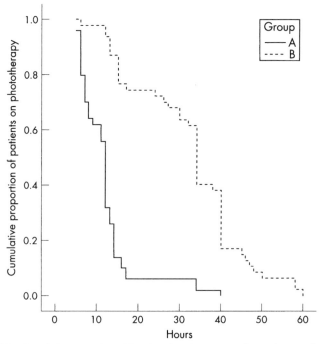

FIGURE 2.—Cumulative proportion of duration phototherapy according to the type of intervention. Group A, intervention group; group B, control group. (Courtesy of Djokomuljanto S, Quah BS, Surini Y, et al. Efficacy of phototherapy for neonatal jaundice is increased by the use of low-cost white reflecting curtains. *Arch Dis Child Fetal Neonatal Ed*. 2006;91:F439-F442. Reproduced with permission from the BMJ Publishing Group.)

Patients.—Term newborns with uncomplicated neonatal jaundice presenting in the first week of life.

Interventions.—Phototherapy with white curtains hanging from the sides of the phototherapy unit (study group, n = 50) was compared with single phototherapy without curtains (control group, n = 47).

Main Outcome Measures.—The primary outcome was the mean difference in total serum bilirubin measured at baseline and after 4 h of phototherapy. The secondary outcome was the duration of phototherapy.

Results.—The mean (standard deviation) decrease in total serum bilirubin levels after 4 h of phototherapy was significantly (p<0.001) higher in the study group (27.62 (25.24) µmol/l) than in the control group (4.04 (24.27) µmol/l). Cox proportional hazards regression analysis indicated that the median duration of phototherapy was significantly shorter in the study group (12 h) than in the control group (34 h; χ^2 change 45.2; p<0.001; hazards ratio 0.20; 95% confidence interval 0.12 to 0.32). No difference in adverse events was noted in terms of hyperthermia or hypothermia, weight loss, rash, loose stools or feeding intolerance.

Conclusion.—Hanging white curtains around phototherapy units significantly increases efficacy of phototherapy in the treatment of neonatal jaundice without evidence of increased adverse effects (Figs 1 and 2).

▶ It is good to know that hanging white curtains around phototherapy units can significantly increase the efficacy of phototherapy. This is an inexpensive fix using a very practical approach that avoids the need for purchasing more expensive equipment to increase the exposure of the jaundiced infant to therapeutic light. Foil has also been suggested for this purpose but may not be available everywhere. I like the application of simple physical principles to solve real problems in practical ways.

D. K. Stevenson, MD

Outcomes among Newborns with Total Serum Bilirubin Levels of 25 mg per Deciliter or More
Newman TB, for the Jaundice and Infant Feeding Study Team (Univ of California, San Francisco; et al)
N Engl J Med 354:1889-1800, 2006   11–5

Background.—The neurodevelopmental risks associated with high total serum bilirubin levels in newborns are not well defined.

Methods.—We identified 140 infants with neonatal total serum bilirubin levels of at least 25 mg per deciliter (428 µmol per liter) and 419 randomly selected controls from a cohort of 106,627 term and near-term infants born from 1995 through 1998 in Kaiser Permanente hospitals in northern California. Data on outcomes were obtained from electronic records, interviews, responses to questionnaires, and neurodevelopmental evaluations that had been performed in a blinded fashion.

TABLE 3.—Results of Testing With the Wechsler Preschool and Primary Scale of
Intelligence–Revised (WPPSI-R) Test and the Beery–Buktenica Developmental Test of
Visual-Motor Integration, 4th Edition (VMI-4)

Test	Control Group	Hyperbilirubinemia Group	Adjusted Difference (95% CI)*	P Value
WPPSI-R†				
Verbal IQ				0.18
No. of subjects	162	81		
Mean score	101.1	103.5	2.5 (−1.1 to 6.1)	
Performance IQ				0.29
No. of subjects	165	81		
Mean score	106.0	107.0	0.5 (−2.9 to 4.0)	
Full-scale IQ				0.42
No. of subjects	162	81		
Mean score	104.0	105.9	1.4 (−2.1 to 5.0)	
VMI-4‡				
Visual–motor integration				0.74
No. of subjects	165	81		
Mean score	102.1	103.3	0.6 (−2.8 to 3.9)	
Visual perception				0.60
No. of subjects	164	80		
Mean score	105.9	107.5	1.2 (−3.5 to 6.0)	
Motor coordination				0.54
No. of subjects	165	81		
Mean score	100.4	101.3	−1.3 (−5.6 to 2.9)	

*Adjusted differences were calculated with the use of multiple linear regression analysis. The models varied, but most models included paternal race or ethnic group and level of education. The covariates included in each model are given in the Supplementary Appendix, available with the full text of this article at www.nejm.org. CI denotes confidence interval.
†Scores on the WPPSI-R test are distributed with a mean of 100 and an SD of 15. Scores in this study ranged from 46 to 149.
‡Scores on the VMI-4 are distributed with a mean of 100 and an SD of 15. Scores in this study ranged from 45 to 150.
(Reprinted by permission from Newman TB, for the Jaundice and Infant Feeding Study Team. Outcomes among newborns with total serum bilirubin levels of 25 mg per deciliter or more. N Engl J Med.354:1889-1900. Copyright 2006, Massachusetts Medical Society. All rights reserved.)

Results.—Peak bilirubin levels were between 25 and 29.9 mg per deciliter (511 μmol per liter) in 130 of the newborns with hyperbilirubinemia and 30 mg per deciliter (513 μmol per liter) or more in 10 newborns; treatment involved phototherapy in 136 cases and exchange transfusion in 5. Follow-up data to the age of at least two years were available for 132 of 140 children with a history of hyperbilirubinemia (94 percent) and 372 of 419 controls (89 percent) and included formal evaluation at a mean (± SD) age of 5.1±0.12 years for 82 children (59 percent) and 168 children (40 percent), respectively. There were no cases of kernicterus. Neither crude nor adjusted scores on cognitive tests differed significantly between the two groups; on most tests, 95 percent confidence intervals excluded a 3-point (0.2 SD) decrease in adjusted scores in the hyperbilirubinemia group. There was no significant difference between groups in the proportion of children with abnormal neurologic findings on physical examination or with documented diagnoses of neurologic abnormalities. Fourteen of the children with hyperbilirubinemia (17 percent) had "questionable" or abnormal findings on neurologic examination, as compared with 48 controls (29 percent; P=0.05; adjusted odds ratio, 0.47; 95 percent confidence interval, 0.23 to 0.98; P=0.04). The frequencies of parental concern and reported behavioral problems also were not significantly different between the two groups.

TABLE 4.—Outcomes According to Neurological Examination, Motor-Performance Checklist, Parent Evaluation of Developmental Status (PEDS) Questionnaire, and Child Behavior Checklist (CBCL)*

Outcome	Control Group No./Total No. (%)	Hyperbilirubinemia Group No./Total No. (%)	Adjusted Odds Ratio (95% CI)	P Value
Neurologic examination				
Normal	120/168 (71)	67/81 (83)		
Normal or questionable	36/168 (21)	11/81 (14)		
Abnormal with minimal disability	10/168 (6)	3/81 (4)		
Abnormal with moderate disability	2/168 (1)	0		
Abnormal with severe disability	0	0		
Normal or questionable, or worse	48/168 (29)	14/81 (17)	0.47 (0.23-0.98)	0.04
Abnormal with minimal disability, or worse	12/168 (7)	3/81 (4)	0.50 (0.14-1.83)	0.29
Motor-performance checklist				
Score, ≥5†	58/165 (35)	30/81 (37)	0.99 (0.54-1.82)	0.98
PEDS questionnaire				
At least 1 answer of "yes"‡	56/239 (23)	26/96 (27)	1.2 (0.67-2.10)	0.56
CBCL preclinical or clinical total score§				
Internalizing behavior	24/227 (11)	9/95 (10)	0.75 (0.32-1.79)	0.52
Externalizing behavior	24/227 (11)	13/95 (14)	1.3 (0.60-2.63)	0.54
Outpatient follow-up to age of ≥2 yr	349/419 (83)	123/140 (88)	1.13 (0.62-2.05)	0.68
≥1 Neurologic diagnosis	18/419 (4)	5/140 (4)	0.78 (0.28-2.17)	0.63

*Odds ratios and P values were calculated with the use of multiple logistic-regression analysis. The covariates included in each model are given in the Supplementary Appendix. CI denotes confidence interval.
†Higher scores indicate worse functioning; a score of 4 or more was considered abnormal in slightly older children (mean age, 5.5 years).
‡A response of "yes" indicates a parent's concern regarding the child's development.
§The internalizing score summarizes the syndrome scales for "withdrawn," "somatic complaints," and "anxious/depressed." The externalizing score summarizes the syndrome scales for "delinquent behavior" and "aggressive behavior." A T score is classified as preclinical if it is at least 60 (approximately 1 SD above the mean) to 69 and clinical if it is at least 70 (approximately 2 SD above the mean).
(Reprinted by permission from Newman TB, for the Jaundice and Infant Feeding Study Team. Outcomes among newborns with total serum bilirubin levels of 25 mg per deciliter or more. N Engl J Med. 354:1889-1900. Copyright 2006, Massachusetts Medical Society. All rights reserved.)

Within the hyperbilirubinemia group, those with positive direct antiglobulin tests had lower scores on cognitive testing but not more neurologic or behavioral problems.

Conclusions.—When treated with phototherapy or exchange transfusion, total serum bilirubin levels in the range included in this study were not associated with adverse neurodevelopmental outcomes in infants born at or near term (Tables 3 and 4).

▶ The long-term developmental outcome of newborns with significant hyperbilirubinemia has been a source of concern and clinical investigation for more than 50 years and, when Rh erythroblastosis fetalis was prevalent, the indications for intervention with exchange transfusion were more or less standardized. If the infant had hemolytic disease and the serum bilirubin was rising at a rate that predicted it would reach 20 mg/dL, an exchange transfusion was preformed. The administration of Rh immune globulin to Rh-negative mothers was introduced in the late 1960s at about the same time that phototherapy made its debut in the United States. Rh disease more or less disappeared, and phototherapy for hyperbilirubinemia—now mainly for very low birth weight infants in neonatal ICUs (NICUs) or term and near-term infants with non-hemolytic jaundice became the primary intervention. The risk of kernicterus in these infants is extremely small, but questions were raised about whether moderate hyperbilirubinemia might, nevertheless, lead to subtle neurodevelopmental defects manifesting as abnormalities of cognition, behavior, or motor development.

The results of long-term follow-up of these infants have been conflicting but, more recently, relatively small studies in Germany[1] and Holland[2] have suggested an increase in subtle neurologic dysfunction in infants exposed to moderate degrees of nonhemolytic hyperbilirubinemia.

After grappling with the published data,[3] the committee charged with developing the most recent American Academy of Pediatrics' (AAP) guidelines for the management of hyperbilirubinemia, provided guidelines for intervention with phototherapy and exchange transfusion for infants of 35 weeks of gestation. But the committee, recognizing the uncertainty of the data on which its recommendations were based, noted that "these guidelines are based on limited evidence and levels shown are approximations."[3]

The study by Newman et al has several important strengths. Very few previous studies included infants with total serum bilirubin (TSB) levels of 25 mg/dL or more, and none have included as many as 140 such infants. Infants were followed up for at least 2 years and formal, blinded neurodevelopmental and cognitive evaluations were performed on the majority of those in the hyperbilirubinemia group at the age of 5 years. The main limitation was the fact that formal evaluations could not be performed on all eligible subjects. It should also be noted that, although all study infants with hyperbilirubinemia had a TSB of at least 25 mg/dL, 135 of 140 infants were effectively treated with phototherapy and the duration of TSB more than 25 mg/dL was less than 6 hours in almost three quarters of the hyperbilirubinemia group.

Nevertheless, the results are reassuring. There was no significant difference between the hyperbilirubinemia or control infants with regard to their cognitive performance or the presence of abnormal neurologic findings. On the other hand, "questionable" or abnormal findings on neurologic examination occurred significantly more frequently in the control infants (29%) than the hyperbilirubinemic infants (17%, odds ratio 0.47, *P* = .04).

It is interesting that 9 children in the hyperbilirubinemia group with peak TSB levels of 25.1 27.9 mg/dL, had significantly lower intelligence quotient (IQ) scores than the control group. It has long been believed and taught that isoimmune hemolytic disease is a risk factor for bilirubin-induced brain damage although it has never been clear why this should be so. Nevertheless, the AAP recommends that infants with hemolysis should be treated more aggressively,[4] and these findings support that recommendation.

Finally, as a member of the committee that drafted the most recent AAP guidelines,[4] it is reassuring to know that the possibility of mild cognitive, behavioral or motor impairment in children who have been exposed to severe hyperbilirubinemia but treated promptly is quite remote. The AAP recommends performing an exchange transfusion on a term, healthy newborn who is at least 4 days old if the TSB is 25 mg/dL or more and does not respond promptly to phototherapy.[4] This important study supports that recommendation.

M. J. Maisels, MB, BCh

References

1. Grimmer I, Berger-Jones K, Bührer C, Brandl U, Obladen M. Late neurological sequelae of non-hemolytic hyperbilirubinemia of healthy term neonates. *Acta Paediatr.* 1999;88:661- 663.
2. Soorani-Lunsing I, Woltil H, Hadders-Algra M. Are moderate degrees of hyperbilirubinemia in healthy term neonates really safe for the brain? *Pediatr Res.* 2001;50:701-705.
3. Ip S, Chung M, Kulig J, et al, for the American Academy of Pediatrics Subcommittee on Hyperbilirubinemia. An evidence based review of important issues concerning neonatal hyperbilirubinemia. *Pediatrics.* 2004;114:e130-e153.
4. Maisels MJ, Baltz RD, Bhutani V, et al, for the American Academy of Pediatrics Subcommittee on Hyperbilirubinemia. Management of hyperbilirubinemia in the newborn infant 35 or more weeks of gestation. *Pediatrics.* 2004;114:297-316.

Toward Understanding Kernicterus: A Challenge to Improve the Management of Jaundiced Newborns
Wennberg RP, Ahlfors CE, Bhutani VK, et al (Univ of Washington, Seattle; LW Ligand, LLC, Vashon, Wash; Stanford Univ, Calif; et al)
Pediatrics 117:474-485, 2006   11–6

Purpose.—We sought to evaluate the sensitivity and specificity of total serum bilirubin concentration (TSB) and free (unbound) bilirubin concentration (B$_f$) as predictors of risk for bilirubin toxicity and kernicterus and to examine consistency between these findings and proposed mechanisms of bilirubin transport and brain uptake

Methods.—A review of literature was undertaken to define basic principles of bilirubin transport and brain uptake leading to neurotoxicity. We then reviewed experimental and clinical evidence that relate TSB or B_f to risk for bilirubin toxicity and kernicterus.

Results.—There are insufficient published data to precisely define sensitivity and specificity of either TSB or B_f in determining risk for acute bilirubin neurotoxicity or chronic sequelae (kernicterus). However, available laboratory and clinical evidence indicate that B_f is better than TSB in discriminating risk for bilirubin toxicity in patients with severe hyperbilirubinemia. These findings are consistent with basic pharmacokinetic principles involved in bilirubin transport and tissue uptake.

Conclusions.—Experimental and clinical data strongly suggest that measurement of B_f in newborns with hyperbilirubinemia will improve risk assessment for neurotoxicity, which emphasizes the need for additional clinical evaluation relating B_f and TSB to acute bilirubin toxicity and long-term outcome. We speculate that establishing risk thresholds for neurotoxicity by using newer methods for measuring Bf in minimally diluted serum samples will improve the sensitivity and specificity of serum indicators for treating hyperbilirubinemia, thus reducing unnecessary aggressive intervention and associated cost and morbidity.

▶ My esteemed colleagues have made another effort to approach the management of newborn jaundice from a scientific perspective. The article begins with a primer on bilirubin biochemistry, which can be summarized in the following equation, where B_f is the "free" bilirubin concentration, A is the albumin concentration, TSB is the total serum bilirubin concentration, and K is the albumin-bilirubin binding constant:

$$B_f = \frac{TSB}{(A-TSB) \times K}$$

They point out that the albumin-bilirubin binding constant (K), which is important in the relationship, is not "constant" but varies considerably among newborns, being lower in sick ones and increasing with postnatal age. They also point out that various drugs administered to infants can alter the effective concentration of albumin by binding with it. The bottom line of the article is that assessing risk for neurotoxicity and kernicterus is difficult at best, even using B_f, but it is nearly impossible by simply measuring the TSB. However, the causal link between B_f, acute bilirubin-induced neurologic dysfunction, and long-term neurodevelopmental outcome has not been established to everyone's satisfaction. If such a relationship were affirmed convincingly, there should be a rapid change to using B_f as a surrogate for risk of bilirubin toxicity in the newborn under the various conditions encountered and recommending commensurate preventive and therapeutic maneuvers.

D. K. Stevenson, MD

Neonatal Subgaleal Hematoma: Presentation and Outcome—Radiological Findings and Factors Associated with Mortality

Kilani RA, Wetmore J (Washington Univ, St Louis)
Am J Perinatol 23:41-48, 2006   11–7

To describe the presentation and outcome of infants who develop subgaleal hematoma (SGH), we compared perinatal factors, clinical and head imaging findings, and outcome in a cohort (N = 34) of all infants admitted to Saint Louis Children's Hospital neonatal intensive care unit with SGH from January 1991 to June 2003. All except three of the infants admitted with SGH had instrumental deliveries (31 of 34; 91.2%): 21 vacuum, eight vacuum followed by forceps, two forceps). There was also a high frequency of occurrence of associated intracranial hemorrhage (17 of 34; 50%: subarachnoid hemorrhage, n = 4; intraventricular hemorrhage, n = 4; intraparenchymal hemorrhage, n = 4; subdural hemorrhage, n = 11), and skull fracture (six of 34; 19.4%; three of six [50%] of them depressed fractures). There was mortality associated with SGH (four of 34, 11.8%); those who died had significant volume loss with anemia, coagulopathy, and shock requiring large volumes of blood and blood products transfusions. The presence of ICH did not correlate with the severity of SGH or mortality, but the severity of SGH correlates with mortality. Minor neurological abnormalities were noted in only four infants at discharge. In conclusion, SGH is an uncommon type of birth trauma, and is associated with delivery or attempted delivery by instrumentation (vacuum and/or forceps). Severe hypovolemia and coagulopathy, but not intracranial hemorrhage, were the most commonly associated clinical problems with mortality. ICH does not correlate with severity of SGH. A brain computed tomography or magnetic resonance imaging should be considered in evaluating a clinically symptomatic SGH. There is associated mortality in severe cases but short-term outcome in survivors is good.

▶ The birth process has been described as a blend of compression, contractions, torques, and traction. It is surprising, given the magnitude of the forces applied to the fetus, that tissue damage, edema, hemorrhage, or fracture in the neonate is not more common.

SGHs are rare, but potentially fatal, accumulations of blood beneath the galea aponeurotica of the scalp in the newborn. SGH is caused by rupture of the emissary veins between the dural sinuses and the scalp veins. The subgaleal (subaponeurotic) space is extensive and can accommodate a significant amount of blood estimated to be as much as 260 mL in term neonates, which represents the total blood volume in a 3-kg infant. Blood accumulates between the epicranial aponeurosis of the scalp and the periosteum. In contrast to the cephalohematoma, which is limited by the periosteum, this potential space extends forward to the orbital margins, backward to the nuchal ridge, and laterally to the temporal fascia at the ears, crossing sutures. As noted by Kilani and Wetmore, the condition is uncommon. Their series is the largest published in the past 3 years and provides some insight into the precipitating events and prognostic features.

SGH is seen most often after repeated applications of the vacuum extractor or other instrumental-assisted deliveries, but may also be anticipated with co-agulation disorders. Other risk factors include prematurity, macrosomia, pro-longed labor, cephalopelvic disproportion, primiparity, male sex, and African lineage.[1,2] Pitting edema of the scalp (which has a boggy feel), accompanied by periorbital or auricular bleeding, are the characteristic local features, and the infants may rapidly become anemic, hypovolemic and hypotensive. Therapy is directed at restoring blood volume; correcting any coagulopathy and treating hyperbilirubinemia, which follows the large extravascular blood load. The use of imaging studies is suggested to rule out associated intracranial injury.

A. A. Fanaroff, MD

References

1. Plauché WC. Subgaleal hematoma. A complication of instrumental delivery. *JAMA*. 1980;244:1597-1598.
2. Davis DJ. Neonatal subgaleal hemorrhage: diagnosis and management. *CMAJ*. 2001;164:1452-1453.

Formation of photoproducts and cytotoxicity of bilirubin irradiated with turquoise and blue phototherapy light

Roll EB, Christensen T (Norwegian Radiation Protection Authority, Østerås, Norway; Norwegian Univ of Science and Technology, Trondheim, Norway)
Acta Paediatr 94:1448-1454, 2005   11–8

Aim.—To compare a new turquoise ("green") fluorescent phototherapy lamp (490 nm) with a conventional blue phototherapy lamp (450 nm) with respect to cytotoxicity and photochemical effects of bilirubin.

Methods.—Mouse lymphoma cells (L5178Y-R) in the presence of bilirubin solutions were exposed to phototherapy light. Occurrence of ne-crosis and apoptosis, reduction of mitotic index and inhibited cell growth was assayed by appropriate methods. The presence of bilirubin and its photoisomers was measured by high-pressure liquid chromatography analysis and absorption spectroscopy.

Results.—At constant and equal light irradiances, the cytotoxic effects in the presence of bilirubin bound to human serum albumin showed that the green lamp caused significantly less necrosis ($n = 4$, $p < 0.05$) and less inhi-bition of cell multiplication ($n = 3$, $p < 0.05$) than the blue lamp. A slightly lower apoptotic fraction, although not statistically significant, was observed in cells exposed to the blue lamp. Photo-oxidation of bilirubin was more prominent with blue light irradiation. The photoequilibria between geomet-ric isomers of bilirubin were different for the two lamps; more geometric photoisomers were formed by blue irradiation ($n = 6$, $p < 0.05$). The amounts of the most water-soluble isomers (presumably mainly lumirubin) were rather similar for the two lamps.

Conclusion.—The two lamps were similar in the formation of therapeutically relevant photoproducts, but the blue lamp showed potential in forming more photo-oxidation products and in causing more severe cellular damage in the presence of bilirubin.

▶ This provocative *in vitro* study compared the ability of a new turquoise (blue-green) lamp with a conventional blue fluorescent lamp (TL20W/52, Philips, Eindhoven, The Netherlands) to degrade bilirubin and to produce wavelength-dependent cell damage. It has been hypothesized that blue-green light, with its longer wavelength (490 vs 450 nm for blue light), can penetrate deeper into the skin and also can lead to the increased formation of easily excreted lumirubin. The authors exposed cell suspensions in the presence of bilirubin to turquoise or blue fluorescent light at an equivalent irradiance for various exposure times. The study used a propidium iodide staining and fluorescence technique to measure apoptosis and cell morphology as indexes of cytotoxicity. The results showed that the shorter wavelength (ie, blue) light caused more cell damage and also inhibited cell multiplication more than turquoise light. To compare efficacy, the production of bilirubin photoproducts after light exposures was measured by HPLC. The authors found that blue light was more effective in degrading the native 4Z,15Z bilirubin to more water-soluble compounds, such as the geometric isomers (4Z,15E; 4E,15Z, and 4E,15E bilirubin), and lumirubin than turquoise light. They also speculated that through this mechanism, blue light may cause the formation of photo-oxidation products and increased cellular damage and growth retardation.

This is an interesting study, but because it lacks a number of important technical details and adequate controls, interpretation of the results is somewhat limited. For example, there is no mention of the temperature at which the relatively long (24 hours) light exposures were performed, what the cell viability rates were when the cells were exposed to light in the absence of bilirubin, how the cells were adversely affected by blue light more than by turquoise due to the presence of bilirubin (a known photosensitizer), or if the appearance and distribution of bilirubin isomers were affected by the presence of the cells (and their antioxidant mechanisms). The authors stated that longitudinal heterogeneity of the irradiance was controlled for by moving the flasks periodically during light exposure; however, the outer diameters for the two types of lamps differ by 50% (38 vs 26 mm for the TL52 and turquoise, respectively). This fact and the unreported spacing between the 2 lamps could also have resulted in a lateral heterogeneity of flask exposure. It is conceivable that the cells exposed to the narrow blue-green tubes received relatively less irradiance and, therefore, could account for the lesser cell damage.

Most interesting and provocative was that the authors appear to demonstrate the importance of the much-debated role of photo-oxidation in the process of bilirubin photoalteration. Although the results of photo-oxidation to colorless, relative small molecules could not be determined with the HPLC methodology used, the Z,Z-bilirubin isomer was shown to be almost exclusively converted to nonmeasurable products by 4 hours. The authors cautiously state in the discussion that "the data in Figures 3 and 4 (see original article) strengthen the assumption that the discrepancy between the reduction in Z,Z-bilirubin and the formation of photoisomers was due to generation of photo-oxidation products. Therefore, it cannot be excluded that photo-oxidative reactions can take place *in vivo*, but the relative potency of blue and green light cannot be determined." In fact, Figure 3 appears to show clearly, and not surprisingly, that blue is more potent in photo-oxidizing Z,Z-bilirubin than turquoise light. Whether this phenomenon occurs *in vivo* in neonates undergoing phototherapy still remains to be investigated. In general, the study does gives credence to the hypothesis that turquoise light may be safer than blue light phototherapy, but it is less effective in degrading bilirubin. The results of this work merit rigorously designed follow-up studies to determine the relative importance of the mechanism of photo-oxidation to photodegrade bilirubin *in vitro* and *in vivo*, possibly using the narrow wavelength band blue or blue-green (turquoise) light-emitting diodes.

R. J. Wong, MD

H. J. Vreman, PhD

The Effect of Blue Light Exposure on the Expression of Circadian Genes: *Bmal1* and *Cryptochrome 1* in Peripheral Blood Mononuclear Cells of Jaundiced Neonates
Chen A, Du L, Xu Y, et al (Zhejiang Univ, Hangzhou, PR China)
Pediatr Res 58:1180-1184, 2005   11–9

The purpose of this study was to investigate the effect of blue light phototherapy on the expression of circadian genes in peripheral blood mononuclear cells (PBMC) and plasma melatonin levels in neonates. Real-time reverse-transcriptase polymerase chain reaction (RT-PCR) was used to determine the expression of *Bmal1* and *Cry1* in PBMC, and an enzyme-linked immunosorbent assay was used to determine plasma melatonin levels in 32 breast-milk jaundiced neonates before and after phototherapy, compared with 29 control neonates. The results showed that the expression of *Bmal1* was decreased and *Cry1* increased significantly after phototherapy. Plasma melatonin levels were decreased after phototherapy. There was no statistical difference in *Bmal1* and *Cry1* gene expression and plasma melatonin levels in the control group. In conclusion, phototherapy does affect the expression of the circadian genes *Bmal1* and *Cry1* in PBMC and plasma melatonin concentration in jaundiced neonates. Our results suggest that phototherapy should be timed according to circadian rhythms when treating jaundiced neonates.

▶ Throughout most of its history, genetic testing (apart from chromosome analysis) in clinical practice has concerned itself primarily with the DNA sequence of individual genes considered in isolation. It is difficult to overstate the importance of such testing in clinical practice. Diagnoses such as fragile X syndrome, cystic fibrosis, familial adenomatous polyposis, and dozens of others that once could be made only after extensive clinical investigation and often only with a relatively modest degree of certainty, can now be made quickly, objectively, accurately, and reliably. Early and reliable diagnosis, in turn, often permits early detection of and intervention for complications of these disorders, leading to greatly improved outcomes; objective and reliable diagnosis also often permits specific and accurate genetic counseling for people with these conditions and the families of these people.

Recently, however, medical science has slowly acquired the ability to look not only at the structure and function of an individual gene considered in isolation, but also at genes and genetic processes considered as a whole and at greater and greater levels of complexity. Thus, genomics (the study of the genome, the entire complement of a person's genes) and proteomics (the study of the proteome, the protein complement of the genome) seek to better understand the workings of genes and their products in a manner that more closely resembles the actions and interactions of those genes and their products as they actually occur within the person. These newer ways of looking at genetic processes will gradually provide medical researchers with an increasingly accurate and sophisticated understanding of how genes work "in the real world."

Although the term "genomics" is now familiar to most clinicians, and although the term "proteomics" is rapidly gaining familiarity, other related areas of endeavor are only just beginning to enter the general clinical vocabulary. Among these less familiar areas is transcriptomics, the genome-wide study of messenger RNA (mRNA) expression levels. Analysis of the DNA sequence of a gene may provide insight into whether the gene is capable of specifying the production of a normal mRNA transcript and, hence, a normal protein product, but it does not give insight into whether the gene is, in fact, "turned on" and actively specifying the production of its protein. By analyzing the levels of various mRNA transcripts within a cell, one may infer which genes within the cell are active, and by correlating this information with carefully selected clinical observations, one may begin to understand the interactions that occur between the individual patient, his or her genes, and his or her environment.

Journal articles that relate levels of gene expression to specific behaviors, diseases, and so forth will undoubtedly be commonplace in the not-too-distant future; they remain fairly rare today, however, even within the genetic literature. The article by Chen and colleagues represents an early example of a clinical investigation into the effect of a specific environmental factor upon the expression of a specific set of genes.

Stimulated by the observation that neonates undergoing phototherapy often present with an increased rate of crying and jitteriness, the authors sought to investigate whether nonocular exposure to blue light during phototherapy for breast milk jaundice could influence the expression of the circadian rhythm in such neonates and how that exposure may be related to behavioral changes. They did so by examining the expression of 2 genes known to be involved in regulating the circadian rhythm, *Bmal1*, a positive regulator of the interacting transcriptional translational feedback loops that are thought to be the mechanism underlying the circadian rhythm, and *CRY1*, a negative regulator in a group of infants undergoing phototherapy and in a control group of infants. They found that the expression of *BMAL1* was decreased and that the expression of *CRY1* was increased after phototherapy. They concluded that phototherapy affects the expression of the 2 circadian genes studied (as well as plasma melatonin levels, which were found to be decreased after phototherapy), and noted that their results suggest that phototherapy should be timed according to circadian rhythms.

The study is imperfect. For example, infants in the experimental group underwent phototherapy while unclothed, apart from black cloth covering the eyes and perineum, whereas infants in the control group remained clothed in addition to the black cloth that covered their eyes. The authors presumed that the differences in gene expression levels observed between the experimental and control infants were attributable to the experimental, but not control, infants' nonocular exposure to blue light. This presumption is probably correct; however, it is at least conceivable that the differences may have owed at least in part to, for example, differences in the tactile stimulation provided by the control infants' clothing. Similarly, although the authors acknowledge that their inability to continuously record the infants' behaviors was a significant limitation of the study, they nevertheless suggest that phototherapy should be timed according to circadian rhythms, presumably because of the presumed, but undemonstrated, association between changes in circadian gene expression and increased crying and jitteriness of the infants. In addition, the authors chose to normalize their measurements of *BMAL1* and *CRY1* transcript against measurements of mRNA transcribed from glyceraldehyde-3-phosphate dehydrogenase (GAPDH); although it is understood that GAPDH mRNA is a commonly used internal control for the accurate quantitation of RNA levels, there is evidence that GAPDH is, itself, subject to regulation by the circadian clock.[1] Although this physician reviewer is not a molecular geneticist, and does not have the training and experience that might be required to formally criticize the laboratory methods, it is odd, and perhaps, a potential confounding factor that the expression of a gene that is, itself, regulated by the circadian cycle was used to assess the circadian expression of genes involved in the regulation of that cycle.

For all this, however, the study remains a very interesting early example of applied clinical transcriptomics. Minor refinements in the experimental design would, in fact, permit an accurate assessment of the effect, if any, of nonocular blue light exposure during phototherapy upon the expression of 2 (or potentially even more) genes involved in the regulation of the circadian rhythm, and to evaluate the relationship, if any, between that effect and changes in infant behaviors during phototherapy. Such information, in turn, could permit neonatologists to design more sophisticated phototherapy regimens that would maximize the therapeutic effect of the light exposure while minimizing the potential adverse impact of phototherapy on patient comfort and well being. The potential power of transcriptomics to improve patient care is obvious even in this early example, and it is anticipated that clinicians will be seeing, and relying upon, many more such articles over time.

D. J. Aughton, MD

Reference

1. Katagiri S, Onai K, Nakashima H. Spermidine determines the sensitivityto the calmodulin antagonist, chlorpromazine, for the circadian conidiation rhythm but not for mycelial growth in Neurospora crassa. *J Biol Rhythms.* 1998;13:452-460.

Effects of Phototherapy on the Growth Plate in Newborn Rats
Atabek ME, Pirgon O, Kurtoglu S, et al (Selcuk Univ, Konya, Turkey; Erciyes Univ, Kayseri, Turkey)
J Pediatr Orthop 26:144-147, 2006   11–10

The aim of the present study was to evaluate the effect of phototherapy and oxidative stress on the growth plate of newborn rats. Forty newborn Sprague-Dawley rats were randomized into a phototherapy group and a control group. Twenty of the rats received phototherapy for 7 days. All zones of the growth plate were assessed with quantitative histomorphometric analysis. Individual zonal lengths were measured for the reserve zone (RZ), the proliferative zone (PZ), the hypertrophic zone (HZ), ossifying cartilage (OC), and total zone (TZ) of the growth plate. Levels of plasma malondialdehyde (MDA), an index of oxidative stress, were also evaluated. Compared with zonal lengths on day 7 after phototherapy between the two groups, the phototherapy group had significantly lower values than those of controls for RZ (5.13 ± 0.36 vs. 6.4 ± 0.85 mm $\times 10^{-2}$; $P < 0.001$), PZ (20.6 ± 3.0 vs. 29.25 ± 1.68 mm $\times 10^{-2}$; $P < 0.001$), HZ (15.4 ± 1.44 vs. 20.87 ± 1.12 mm $\times 10^{-2}$; $P < 0.001$), OC (47.08 ± 4.25 vs. 62.06 ± 3.7 mm $\times 10^{-2}$; $P < 0.001$), and TZ (88.15 ± 6.56 vs. 118.48 ± 4.50 mm $\times 10^{-2}$; $P < 0.001$). Plasma MDA levels were correlated with the size of the PZ in the phototherapy group ($r = -0.53, P = 0.01$). In a multivariate regression model for all rats, being in the phototherapy group was the best predictor of the size of the TZ ($\beta = -0.94, P < 0.001$), with the total variance explained being 88%. These results suggest that in newborn rats, receiving phototherapy is associated with early impairment of growth plate structure, and oxidative stress may be the main risk factor for growth plate injury.

▶ In this randomized, controlled trial, the investigators show that phototherapy can impair the growth plate structure in the tibia of newborn rats. They suggest that this is the result of oxidative stress manifested by higher plasma malondialdehyde levels and a negative correlation between these levels and the size of the proliferative zone of the tibial growth plate. Could these findings be extrapolated to the human newborn? Newborn rats are tiny creatures, and they grow very rapidly. They were exposed to phototherapy for 7 days, and the authors point out that, even if the effect on linear growth is real, it is likely to be temporary.

In our nursery, term and near-term newborns who require phototherapy seldom require it for more than 24 hours and, in the neonatal ICU (NICU), it is rarely used for more than 3 days. Furthermore, sick infants in the NICU do not grow while they are acutely ill, and exposure to phototherapy in well infants is so brief that any effect that phototherapy could possibly have on the growth plates is more than likely trivial.

M. J. Maisels, MB, BCh

The premature infants in need of transfusion (PINT) study: A randomized, controlled trial of a restrictive (low) versus liberal (high) transfusion threshold for extremely low birth weight infants
Kirpalani H, for the PINT Investigators (McMaster Univ, Hamilton, Ont, Canada; et al)
J Pediatr 149:301-307, 2006   11–11

Objective.—To determine whether extremely low birth weight infants (ELBW) transfused at lower hemoglobin thresholds versus higher thresholds have different rates of survival or morbidity at discharge.

Study Design.—Infants weighing <1000 g birth weight were randomly assigned within 48 hours of birth to a transfusion algorithm of either low or high hemoglobin transfusion thresholds. The composite primary outcome was death before home discharge or survival with any of either severe retinopathy, bronchopulmonary dysplasia, or brain injury on cranial ultrasound. Morbidity outcomes were assessed, blinded to allocation.

Results.—Four hundred fifty-one infants were randomly assigned to low (n = 223) or high (n = 228) hemoglobin thresholds. Groups were similar, with mean birth weight of 770 g and gestational age of 26 weeks. Fewer infants received one or more transfusions in the low threshold group (89% low versus 95% high, P = .037). Rates of the primary outcome were 74.0% in the low threshold group and 69.7% in the high (P = .25; risk difference, 2.7%; 95% CI −3.7% to 9.2%). There were no statistically significant differences between groups in any secondary outcome.

Conclusions.—In extremely low birth weight infants, maintaining a higher hemoglobin level results in more infants receiving transfusions but confers little evidence of benefit.

▶ Failure to take into consideration the infant's birth weight, postnatal age, and the site of blood sampling when attempting to define anemia in the neonatal period can lead to diagnostic mistakes and unnecessary laboratory tests. Preterm infants, even if healthy, have lower hemoglobin (Hb) levels than term infants at birth and for the first 2 to 3 months of life. Whereas all infants have a decreased level of hematocrit after birth, this phenomenon is more pronounced and prolonged in preterm infants and even more so in extremely preterm infants who are subjected to repeated blood draws. Low plasma levels of erythropoietin (EPO) in preterm infants provide a rationale for the use of EPO to prevent or treat anemia. However, Aher and Ohlsson, in their 2006 *Cochrane Review*,[1] noted that early administration of EPO reduced the number and volume of transfusions and donor exposure but concluded, "The small reductions are of limited clinical importance." Furthermore, there was a significant increase in the rate of retinopathy of prematurity (ROP) (stage >3), but not other major neonatal adverse outcomes including mortality. Their final comment reflects the current approach in most nurseries: "Due to the limited benefits and the increased risk of ROP, early administration of EPO is not recommended."

Without the use of EPO, Kirpalani and colleagues, in a well-designed and executed randomized trial ,with what has become the inevitable cool acronym (PINT Study) were unable to demonstrate any benefits from an aggressive versus a conservative transfusion policy. This should not be surprising as 89% of the conservative group were transfused. The aggressively treated group received more blood but did not have fewer adverse outcomes. Coming from a unit where every effort is made to avoid transfusion, the data are reassuring. We can all agree that we should limit the number and volume of blood draws to a minimum in ELBW infants.

A. A. Fanaroff, MD

Reference

1. Aher SM, Ohlsson A. Early versus late erythropoietin for preventing red blood cell transfusion in preterm and/or low birth weight infants. *Cochrane Database Syst Rev.* 2006;3:CD004865.

Effects of timing of umbilical cord clamping on iron status in Mexican infants: a randomised controlled trial
Chaparro CM, Neufeld LM, Alavez GT, et al (Univ of California, Davis; Natl Inst of Public Health, Cuernavaca, Mexico; Instituto Mexicano de Seguro Social, México DF)
Lancet 367:1997-2004, 2006   11–12

Background.—Delayed clamping of the umbilical cord increases the infant's iron endowment at birth and haemoglobin concentration at 2 months of age. We aimed to assess whether a 2-minute delay in the clamping of the umbilical cord of normal-weight, full-term infants improved iron and haematological status up to 6 months of age.

Methods.—476 mother-infant pairs were recruited at a large obstetrics hospital in Mexico City, Mexico, randomly assigned to delayed clamping (2 min after delivery of the infant's shoulders) or early clamping (around 10 s after delivery), and followed up until 6 months postpartum. Primary outcomes were infant haematological status and iron status at 6 months of age, and analysis was by intention-to-treat.

Findings.—358 (75%) mother-infant pairs completed the trial. At 6 months of age, infants who had delayed clamping had significantly higher mean corpuscular volume (81.0 fL *vs* 79.5 fL 95% CI −2.5 to −0.6, p=0.001), ferritin (50.7 µg/L *vs* 34.4 µg/L 95% CI −30.7 to −1.9, p=0.0002), and total body iron. The effect of delayed clamping was significantly greater for infants born to mothers with low ferritin at delivery, breastfed infants not receiving iron-fortified milk or formula, and infants born with birthweight between 2500 g and 3000 g. A cord clamping delay of 2 minutes increased 6-month iron stores by about 27–47 mg.

Interpretation.—Delay in cord clamping of 2 minutes could help prevent iron deficiency from developing before 6 months of age, when iron-fortified complementary foods could be introduced.

▶ The adverse consequences of iron deficiency on long-term developmental outcome have been appreciated for a number of years.[1] The prevention of iron deficiency anemia during the first several years of life, especially in developing countries where poverty and undernutrition are common, continues to be a challenge. This report by Chaparro et al convincingly demonstrates that a simple intervention at the time of delivery, a delay in umbilical cord clamping of 2 minutes, improves iron status for up to 6 months of age and could help prevent the development of iron deficiency. The effect of delayed cord clamping on an infant's hematologic and iron status has been known for years. In addition, compared with preterm infants 27 to 33 weeks' gestation who had their cords clamped immediately, a 30-second delay of cord clamping has been shown to result in a significantly higher hematocrit at birth and a significant reduction in transfusion requirements.[2]

Given the worldwide acceptance and dissemination of the Neonatal Resuscitation Program, one wonders why that infrastructure could not be used in developing countries to teach the personnel responsible for the delivery and care of the newborn infant about the benefit of delayed cord clamping. As Chaparro et al point out, clamping the cord once cord pulsations stop (between 1 and 3 minutes), even if the infant is maintained at the level of the mother's uterus, allows for transfer of most of the placental blood to the infant and ensures an improved iron status.

R. A. Ehrenkranz, MD

References

1. Lozoff B, Jimenez E, Wolf AW. Long-term developmental outcome of infants with iron deficiency. *N Engl J Med.* 1991;325:687-694.
2. Kinmond S, Aitchison TC, Holland BM, Jones JG, Turner TL, Wardrop CA. Umbilical cord clamping and preterm infants: a randomised trial. *BMJ.* 1993;306:172-175.

Platelet Dysfunction in Asphyxiated Newborn Piglets Resuscitated with 21% and 100% Oxygen
Cheung P-Y, Stevens JP, Haase E, et al (Univ of Alberta, Edmonton, Canada; Inst of Molecular Medicine, Houston)
Pediatr Res 59:636-640, 2006   11–13

Hemostatic disturbances are common in asphyxiated newborns after resuscitation. We compared platelet function in hypoxic newborn piglets reoxygenated with 21% or 100% oxygen. Piglets (1–3 d, 1.5–2.1 kg) were anesthetized and acutely instrumented for hemodynamic monitoring. After stabilization, normocapnic hypoxia was induced with an inspired oxygen concentration of 10–15% for 2 h. Piglets were then resuscitated for 1 h with 21% or 100% oxygen, followed by 3 h with 21% oxygen. Platelet counts and collagen (2, 5, and 10 µg/mL)-stimulated whole blood aggregation were studied before hypoxia and at 4 h of post-hypoxia/reoxygenation. Platelet function was studied using transmission electron microscopy and by measuring plasma thromboxane B_2 (TxB_2) and matrix metalloproteinase (MMP)-2 and -9 levels. Control piglets were sham-operated without hypoxia/reoxygenation. The hypoxemic (PaO_2 33 mm Hg) piglets developed hypotension with metabolic acidosis (pH 7.02–7.05). Upon reoxygenation, piglets recovered and blood gases gradually normalized. At 4 h reoxygenation, platelet aggregation *ex vivo* was impaired as evidenced by a rightward-downward shifting of the concentration-response curves. Electron microscopy showed features of platelet activation. Plasma MMP-9 but not MMP-2 activity significantly increased. Resuscitation with 100% but not 21% oxygen increased plasma TxB_2 levels. Platelet counts decreased after hypoxia/reoxygenation but were not different between groups during the experiment. Resuscitation of hypoxic newborn piglets caused platelet activation with significant deterioration of platelet aggregation *ex vivo* and increased plasma MMP-9 levels. High oxygen concentrations may aggravate the activation of prostaglandin-thromboxane mechanistic pathway.

▶ The authors found increased markers of platelet activation in 100% oxygen resuscitated piglets compared with those resuscitated with room air. The methods used here for modeling hypoxic injury involved a 2-hour period of hypoxemia with arterial oxygen saturation goals of 30% to 40% (PaO_2 of 20 to 40 mm Hg), followed by a 1-hour period of resuscitation with oxygen. It is worth noting that varying models are used for research in asphyxia/reoxygenation injury. Acid-base balance and blood pressure were similar in both groups after resuscitation, whereas PaO_2 differed greatly, as would be expected, with the 100% group having a mean PaO_2 of 367 mm Hg and the room air group 82 mm Hg. Although platelet counts did not differ significantly between the 2 groups after resuscitation and remained normal, both groups had a reduction in levels over time. Collagen-induced platelet aggregation remained the same during the hypoxic episode but was impaired somewhat more in the 100% group after resuscitation compared with the room air group, although both were impaired compared with controls. Similarly, MMP-9 levels were higher in the 100% and room air groups compared with controls. The authors note that a larger sample size may have been able to differentiate more between the 2 study groups.

It is possible that the initial injury itself may have set in motion a sequence of events that overwhelms any of the subsequent potential harm from therapies. If we do eventually find an optimal strategy for oxygen concentration, it will likely only confer slight benefits beyond the baseline resuscitative efforts regardless of oxygen concentration. However, with the often devastating consequences of asphyxia, slight benefits may be the best that we can achieve.

H. C. Lee, MD

12 Renal, Metabolism, and Endocrine Disorders

Long-term Follow-up of Neonatal Mitochondrial Cytopathies: A Study of 57 Patients
García-Cazorla A, De Lonlay P, Nassogne MC, et al (Centre Hospitalier Universitaire Necker Enfants-Malades, Paris; Institut Natl de la Santé, Paris)
Pediatrics 116:1170-1177, 2005   12–1

Objectives.—We sought to determine the long-term clinical and biochemical outcome of newborns with mitochondrial cytopathies (MCs) and to identify possible prognostic factors that may modify the course of these diseases.

Material and Methods.—Fifty-seven newborns with MCs were identified in a retrospective review (1983–2002). We defined 2 different outcome categories: clinical (neurologic, hepatic, myopathic, and multiorganic) and biochemical (lactate level normalization or initially normal remaining unchanged, decreased but not normalized, and persistently high). We used 2 different statistical approaches: (1) survival studies depending on the initial symptoms and lactate and enzymatic deficiencies using the Kaplan-Meier method; and (2) the same variables compared with different survival age groups and clinical and biochemical outcome categories using the χ^2 test.

Results.—Thirty-three patients died (57.8%), 12 remain alive (21%), and 12 were lost in the follow-up; 6 of them are currently older than 4 years. Most of the patients manifested multiorganic disease (64.8%) and high lactate level (77.1%) over time. Children surviving to 2.5 to 3 years of age were more likely to survive for a long period of time. Initial neurologic and hepatic presentation increased the risk to develop neurologic disease and severe persistent hyperlactacidemia, respectively. Initial severe hyperlactacidemia and combined enzyme deficiencies were significant risk factors for higher mortality and multiorganic disorders. Two patients with exclusively myopathic outcome are alive and cognitively normal at 12 years of life.

Conclusions.—Children with neonatal-onset MCs have very high mortality and poor prospects. However, some with life-threatening presentations may gradually improve, giving rise to less severe diseases. Those with exclusively myopathic symptoms have a better prognosis.

▶ Life is the interplay between structure and energy, yet the role of energy deficiency in human disease has until recently been poorly understood. Mitochondrial cytopathies are multisystem disorders of extremely variable expression due to a deficiency in oxidative phosphorylation. Mitochondrial cytopathies are metabolic diseases, expressing mutations in nuclear DNA, punctiform mutations or depletions in mitochondrial DNA. These genetic lesions alter mitochondrial oxidative phosphorylation, with a reduction in energy produced for cell activity.

Mitochondrial disorders occur infrequently, but have come into prominence and, according to Van Coster in 2000,[1] "Since 1988, more then 70 different mutations were reported in the mitochondrial DNA. Some point mutations are associated with a specific phenotype; others have a wide range of clinical symptoms. We expect that many more mitochondrial DNA mutations will be identified in the future. The number of mutations in nuclear genes will also increase, especially since progress has been made in techniques used for identification of nuclear genes (microcell transfer)."

This series of 57 patients from García-Cazorla et al from Paris took two decades to accumulate, but their experience provides valuable insights into the variable clinical presentations, therapeutic options, and prognosis. This is the first study showing data on the long-term outcome of various types of neonatal onset mitochondrial cytopathies (MCs). Not surprisingly, perhaps those infants with myopathy alone do better. Management of these patients should really be reserved for our colleagues with expertise in metabolic derangements, and I was interested to learn that "All the patients were initially treated with different cofactors (thiamin, riboflavin, carnitine, most of them with bicarbonate (40 of 57 [70.1%]), some of them with a ketogenic diet (3 of 57 [5.2%]), and some others more recently with coenzyme Q_{10} (3 of 57 [5.2%])." In the discussion the authors emphasized three major points. First, the high mortality (57.8%) in the first 3 months of life. Second, multiple health handicaps in 68% of survivors, so that not only is mortality high, but the chances of intact survival are low. Third, in contrast to the late-onset mitochondrial disorders where lactate levels are lower and tend to normalize, the neonatal mitochondrial disorders have persistent hyperlactic academia. Increased awareness of these disorders will, no doubt, result in earlier diagnosis and the opportunity to develop alternative therapies so that the outcomes can be improved.

A. A. Fanaroff, MD

Reference

1. Van Coster R, De Meirleir L. Mitochondrial cytopathies and neuromuscular disorders. *Acta Neurol Belg.* 2000;100:156-161.

Hyperinsulinemia in Cord Blood in Mothers With Type 2 Diabetes and Gestational Diabetes Mellitus in New Zealand

Westgate JA, Gamble G, Lindsay RS, et al (Univ of Auckland, New Zealand; Univ of Glasgow, England; Middlemore Hosp, Auckland, New Zealand)
Diabetes Care 29:1345-1350, 2006   12–2

Objective.—In genetically diabetes-prone populations, maternal diabetes during pregnancy increases the risk of their children developing diabetes and obesity (the vicious cycle of type 2 diabetes). Fetal hyperinsulinemia at birth acts as a marker of this risk. We therefore examined whether cord insulin and leptin concentrations are increased in offspring of Maori and Pacific Island mothers with type 2 and gestational diabetes mellitus (GDM) and varying degrees of glycemic control (HbA_{1c}).

Research Designs and Methods.—Maori and Pacific Island mothers were prospectively recruited at Middlemore Hospital, South Auckland. Cord blood was taken from umbilical vein at birth from singleton babies born after 32 weeks of gestation to 138 mothers with GDM, 39 mothers with type 2 diabetes, and 95 control mothers.

Results.—Babies born to mothers with both type 2 diabetes and GDM had higher birth weight and skinfold thickness and markedly higher concentrations of insulin (median [interquartile range] type 2 diabetes 77 pmol/l [42–143], GDM 67 pmol/l [42–235], and control subjects 33 pmol/l [18–62]; $P < 0.001$) and leptin (type 2 diabetes 39 ng/ml [18–75], GDM 31 ng/ml [17–58], and control subjects 13 ng/ml [8–22]; $P < 0.001$) in cord blood. Cord insulin concentrations >120 pmol/l were found in 29% of offspring of mothers with GDM and 31% of mothers with type 2 diabetes. Many mothers with GDM had abnormalities of glucose tolerance postpartum (20% type 2 diabetes, 34% impaired glucose tolerance or impaired fasting glucose). Higher cord insulin (57 pmol/l [40–94]) and leptin (26 ng/ml [17–39]) concentrations were found even in offspring of GDM mothers with normal glucose tolerance postpartum.

Conclusions.—Raised cord insulin and leptin concentrations are a common finding in offspring of mothers with type 2 diabetes and GDM in this population.

Lipid Profile, Glucose Homeostasis, Blood Pressure, and Obesity-Anthropometric Markers in Macrosomic Offspring of Nondiabetic Mothers

Evagelidou EN, Cholevas VK, Kiortsis DN, et al (Univ of Ioannina, Greece)
Diabetes Care 29:1197-1201, 2006   12–3

Objective.—The study was to determine whether being the macrosomic offspring of a mother without detected glucose intolerance during pregnancy has an impact on lipid profile, glucose homeostasis, and blood pressure during childhood.

Research Design and Methods.—Plasma total, HDL, and LDL cholesterol; triglycerides; apolipoprotein (Apo) A-1, -B, and -E; lipoprotein (a); fasting glucose and insulin; homeostasis model assessment of insulin resistance (HOMA-IR) index; blood pressure; BMI; and detailed anthropometry were evaluated in 85 children aged 3–10 years old, born appropriate for gestational age (AGA; $n = 48$) and large for gestational age (LGA; $n = 37$) of healthy mothers.

Results.—At the time of the assessment, body weight, height, skinfold thickness, BMI, waist circumference, and blood pressure did not differ between the LGA and AGA groups with the exception of head circumference ($P < 0.01$). There were no significant differences in plasma total or LDL cholesterol; triglycerides; Apo A-1, -B, or -E; lipoprotein (a); Apo B–to–Apo A-1 ratio; or glucose levels between the groups. The LGA group had significantly higher HDL cholesterol levels ($P < 0.01$), fasting insulin levels ($P < 0.01$), and HOMA-IR index ($P < 0.01$) but lower values of the glucose-to-insulin ratio ($P < 0.01$) as compared with the AGA group.

Conclusions.—Children born LGA of mothers without confirmed impaired glucose tolerance during pregnancy show higher insulin concentrations than AGAs.

Serum Ghrelin Concentration and Weight Gain in Healthy Term Infants in the First Year of Life

Savino F, Liguori SA, Fissore MF, et al (Univ of Turin, Italy)
J Pediatr Gastroenterol Nutr 41:653-659, 2005   12–4

Objectives.—Ghrelin, a recently discovered hormone mainly secreted by the stomach, has several metabolic functions including regulation of food intake, energy homeostasis and body weight. There are few studies on this hormone in healthy infants during the first year of life. The aim of this study was to examine the correlations between ghrelin and weight gain in healthy term infants in the first year of life.

Methods.—104 healthy term infants aged 0 to 12 months were included in a cross-sectional study. Anthropometric measurements were assessed and mean weight gain was calculated. Serum ghrelin concentrations have been determined at least 3 hours after feeding by radioimmunoassay test.

Results.—Ghrelin concentrations were correlated negatively to weight gain (r = −0.302; $P = 0.003$) and positively to age (r = 0.412; $P < 0.001$), weight (r = 0.374; $P < 0.001$) and length (r = 0.387; $P < 0.001$). In breastfed infants a statistically significant negative correlation between ghrelin concentration and infant weight gain (r = −0.407; $P = 0.001$) was observed, whereas in formula-fed infants this correlation was not statistically significant (r = −0.067; $P = 0.719$).

Conclusions.—The negative correlation observed between ghrelin concentration and infant weight gain suggests that ghrelin might also play a role in the regulation of body weight in healthy infants with a physiologic energy balance. Further studies are needed to clarify how ghrelin might be involved in both short-term and long-term energy balance.

▶ Both intrauterine and early postnatal life are considered important windows during which risks for long-term health may be influenced. The concept of developmental programming has been developed to explain the relationship between adverse intrauterine environment and long-term metabolic consequences, in particular obesity, insulin resistance, and type 2 diabetes mellitus. The World Health Organization estimates that 1.1 million people died as a result of diabetes in 2005, and this is almost certainly an underestimate. Moreover, the figure is expected to increase by 50% during the next 10 years.[1] This escalation is due in part to the increasing rate of obesity among adults and children. Metabolic regulation is clearly very redundant and robust. Many pathways seem to be independently regulated by similar stimuli to provide a safety network to prevent dysregulation.

Several studies have investigated the effects of abnormalities in carbohydrate or lipid metabolism in diabetic, gestational diabetic (GDM) or obese mothers on their offspring. Epigenetic modification of gene expression by the maternal metabolic milieu and synergistic interaction between prenatal and postnatal energy homeostasis are etiologic factors.

Fetal growth and development is to a great extent controlled by the action of insulin. Data presented by Westgate et al (Abstract 12–2) demonstrate that maternal diabetes commonly results in fetal hyperinsulinism at birth in a population genetically prone to obesity and diabetes. The higher birth weight offspring of type 2 diabetic and GDM mothers have increased cord blood levels of insulin, proinsulin, and leptin. They suggest that elevated cord blood insulin and leptin levels are markers of fetal exposure to abnormal in utero environment. Measurements of insulin propeptides are useful indicators of overall fetal insulinemia and better predictors of fetal outcomes.

Hyperinsulinemia/insulin resistance is an independent predictor for later development of metabolic abnormalities regardless of the birth weight. The study by Evagelidou et al (Abstract 12–3) further supports this notion, and demonstrates that macrosomic offspring of healthy, nondiabetic, mothers without detected glucose intolerance during pregnancy (tested at 24-28 weeks' gestation) exhibit higher insulin levels, insulin resistance determined by HOMA-IR index, and significantly higher HDL cholesterol levels between age 3 and 10 years. Although the distinction between LGA and AGA infants is somewhat arbitrary as intrauterine growth is a continuous process, it seems that children at the upper end of the weight range may need more careful attention because of the possible development of metabolic aberration during early childhood.

Many metabolic changes once thought to be caused by insulin might only coincide with insulin signaling and may actually have other regulatory stimuli.[2,3] The hypothalamus and brainstem receive neural and hormonal signals from the periphery, including adipose tissue and the intestinal tract that encode information about the state of nutrition. The interrelationships between these systems are extensively studied in adults in contrast to the few studies published on infant subjects.

Ghrelin is a peptide hormone released into circulation from the stomach; it is a potent stimulator of growth hormone release and a regulator of food intake in humans. In a cross-sectional study, Savino et al (Abstract 12–4) correlate anthropometric measurements and ghrelin levels in healthy term infants during their first year of life. They observed a negative correlation between plasma ghrelin concentrations and infant weight gain. It is an important finding, defining ghrelin as a hormonal modulator of physiologic regulation of growth and energy balance during infancy. This observation raises the question about whether, in healthy infants, ghrelin concentration responds to changes in body weight in a compensatory manner or if ghrelin has a causative role in the determination of the body weight.[4] Diet-related differences in the circulating concentration of ghrelin were also observed. Breastfed infants did have a significant negative correlation between weight gain and ghrelin levels in the first 4 months of life, whereas greater weight gain correlated with lower ghrelin levels in formula-fed infants at 8 to 12 months of life.

These studies underlie the need to conduct longitudinal studies on mothers and infants as a unit to identify biologic markers of the energy status. Determination of the biomarker profile of the pregnant mother and her infant might aid in the development of strategies to modify prenatal and perinatal determinants of adverse neonatal outcomes leading to adult health hazards. From a public health perspective, the hope for breakthrough therapies for obesity and diabetes are as high as they have ever been. Obesity during pregnancy represents an important, modifiable risk factor for adverse pregnancy outcome. At the current time there are no evidence-based management strategies for maternal obesity and/or for early detection of metabolic abnormalities in their offspring.

E. Pinter, MD

References

1. Nath D, Heemels M, Anson L. Obesity and diabetes. *Nature.* 2006;444:839.
2. Rosen ED, Spiegelman BM. Adipocytes as regulators of energy balance and glucose homeostasis. *Nature.* 2006;444:847-853.
3. Murphy KG, Bloom SR. Gut hormones and the regulation of energy homeostasis. *Nature.* 2006;444:854-859.
4. Savino F, Grassino EC, Fissore MF, et al. Ghrelin, motilin, insulin concentration in healthy infants in the first month of life: relation to fasting time and anthropometry. *Clin Endocrinol (Oxf).* 2006;65:158-162.

Neonatal Screening for Very Long-Chain Acyl-CoA Dehydrogenase Deficiency: Enzymatic and Molecular Evaluation of Neonates With Elevated C14:1-Carnitine Levels
Liebig M, Schymik I, Mueller M, et al (Univ Children's Hosp, Duesseldorf, Germany; Univ of Amsterdam; Vanderbilt Univ, Nashville, Tenn)
Pediatrics 118:1065-1069, 2006   12–5

Objective.—Neonatal screening programs for very long-chain acyl-coenzyme A dehydrogenase deficiency have been implemented recently in various countries. Mildly elevated C14:1-carnitine on day 3 of life strongly suggests very long-chain acyl-coenzyme A dehydrogenase deficiency.

Design.—We characterized 11 neonates with elevated C14:1-carnitine by enzyme and molecular analyses. Palmitoyl-coenzyme A oxidation was measured in lymphocytes. Sequencing of all 20 exons of the VLCAD gene was performed from genomic DNA.

Results.—Palmitoyl-coenzyme A oxidation revealed significantly decreased residual activities consistent with very long-chain acyl-coenzyme A dehydrogenase deficiency in 7 neonates. In 2 individuals, residual activities of 48% and 44%, respectively, suggested heterozygosity. Two disease-causing mutations were detected in 6 of 7 neonates with very long-chain acyl-coenzyme A dehydrogenase deficiency; in the remaining 1 patient, only 1 mutation was identified. Of 2 individuals with residual activities consistent with heterozygosity, 1 was heterozygous for a VLCAD mutation. The other child and both individuals with normal palmitoyl-coenzyme A oxidation had normal genotypes.

Conclusions.—In 4 of 11 neonates identified with elevated C14:1-carnitine, very long-chain acyl-coenzyme A dehydrogenase deficiency was excluded. A C14:1-carnitine level > 1 µmol/L strongly suggests very long-chain acyl-coenzyme A dehydrogenase deficiency, whereas concentrations ≤ 1 µmol/L do not allow a clear discrimination among affected patients, carriers, and healthy individuals. Further diagnostic evaluation, including enzyme and molecular analyses, is essential to identify very long-chain acyl-coenzyme A dehydrogenase deficiency correctly.

▶ Expanded newborn screening by tandem mass spectrometry continues to be adopted by developed countries throughout the world. Fatty acid oxidation disorders are an important type of metabolic disorder detected by such programs. VLCAD is the most commonly detected defect of long-chain fat metabolism, with an incidence estimated at 1:50,000 to 1:120,000. Considerable clinical heterogeneity is present in VLCAD deficiency; affected individuals have clinical features ranging from hypoketotic hypoglycemia to life-threatening cardiomyopathy, arrhythmias, or symptoms similar to Reye's syndrome. Liebig and colleagues describe their experience in screening for VLCAD deficiency using tandem mass spectrometry to screen for elevated C14:1-carnitine levels in an estimated 1 million German neonates. Although 11 neonates were found to have elevated C14:1-carnitine levels, VLCAD deficiency was ultimately confirmed in 7 children. Of the remaining 4 children, 2 were likely heterozygous carriers of VLCAD deficiency, and 2 were healthy. An elevated C14:1-carnitine level more than 1 µmol/L correlated with the presence of VLCAD deficiency. However, elevated C14:1-carnitine concentrations of 1 µmol/L or less did not discriminate between affected and healthy children. Furthermore, individuals affected with VLCAD deficiency may normalize C14:1-carntine levels as caloric intake increases after birth. Therefore, the authors recommend that an elevated C14:1-carnitine level on newborn screening should *always* result in a further, detailed diagnostic evaluation, including measurement of palmitoyl-CoA oxidation in skin fibroblasts and molecular genetic analysis, even if the second, confirmatory plasma acylcarnitine profile is normal. This is clearly sound advice, given the potential for cata-strophic outcomes in patients with VLCAD deficiency. However, at present, it is still unclear which patients with diagnoses by newborn screening will become symptomatic later in life. Further longitudinal studies documenting clinical, biochemical, and molecular features of affected individuals in a variety of ethnic groups are required to address this question. Nevertheless, this well-considered study certainly has immediate practical implications.

G. M. Enns, MB, ChB

The natural history of medium-chain acyl CoA dehydrogenase deficiency in The Netherlands: Clinical presentation and outcome

Derks TGJ; Reijngoud D-J, Waterham HR, et al (Univ Med Ctr Groningen, The Netherlands; Academic Med Ctr Amsterdam; Univ of Maastricht, The Netherlands)

J Pediatr 148:665-670, 2006   12–6

Objectives.—To describe the clinical presentation and long-term follow-up of a large cohort of patients with medium-chain acyl-CoA dehydrogenase (MCAD) deficiency.

Study Design.—A nationwide, retrospective analysis of clinical presentation and follow-up in 155 Dutch patients with MCAD deficiency.

Results.—Most patients presented between 3 months and 5.1 years of age; 13% had symptoms as neonates not exclusively related to breast-feeding. An acute presentation before the diagnosis was made resulted in a mortality of 22% (25/114), whereas 21% (19/89) developed disabilities after the diagnosis. On follow-up, a total of 44 patients reported fatigue (35%; 28/80), muscle pain (31%; 25/80), and/or reduced exercise tolerance (39%; 31/80). Cardiac evaluation in 11 adult patients revealed no abnormalities in cardiac function explaining these complaints. Children with MCAD deficiency readily become overweight.

Conclusions.—Mortality and morbidity were high in undiagnosed children with MCAD deficiency; establishment of the diagnosis significantly improves outcome. Strikingly, after the diagnosis and initiation of treatment, overweight and chronic complaints (fatigue, muscle pain, and reduced exercise tolerance) were prominent.

▶ MCAD deficiency has been the "poster child" for expanded newborn screening by tandem mass spectrometry. Previous articles have shown that children with MCAD deficiency detected and treated presymptomatically typically have an excellent prognosis. On the other hand, if children first come to medical attention at the time of acute metabolic derangement, the risk of severe neurologic impairment and mortality is high. Derks and colleagues present clinical, biochemical, and molecular data on 155 Dutch patients with MCAD deficiency so that the natural history of this disorder can be further understood. This article provides further support for the institution of expanded newborn screening for MCAD deficiency by tandem mass spectrometry and is particularly useful because of the size of the cohort studied and the follow-up in 32 patients until adulthood. Patients were given diagnoses both before (n = 35) and after (n = 120) the appearance of clinical symptoms. Although most children presented between ages 3 months and 5 years, 13% (n = 18) had symptoms as neonates. A previous study[1] suggested that patients with MCAD deficiency become symptomatic as neonates if breastfed because of inadequate caloric intake. However, 5 of 15 symptomatic neonates in the current article had been bottle-fed since birth and presumably had adequate caloric intake. In the group of patients given diagnoses based on clinical signs and symptoms, nearly all (n = 114) had at least 1 acute metabolic crisis before the diagnosis was established, and 25 (22%) died during such an episode. Disabilities were present in 19% of surviving patients. No additional mortality occurred in affected children after the diagnosis of MCAD deficiency had been established. Interestingly, chronic problems, including fatigue, muscle pain, exercise intolerance, and dietary fat intolerance were frequently reported in older patients and adults. Unlike long-chain fatty acid oxidation disorders, cardiac involvement does not appear to be typical of MCAD deficiency; a detailed cardiac evaluation was performed in 11 adult patients, and the findings in all evaluations were normal. Because symptoms of MCAD deficiency may appear before the results of newborn screening are known, an awareness of this condition is important for all clinicians caring for neonates so that appropriate management can begin without delay.

G. M. Enns, MB, ChB

Reference

1. Wilcken B, Carpenter KH, Hammond J. Neonatal symptoms in medium-chain acyl conenzyme A dehydrogenase deficiency. *Arch Dis Child.* 1993;69:292-294.

Hormonal Changes in 3-Month-Old Cryptorchid Boys
Suomi A-M, Main KM, Kaleva M, et al (Univ of Turku, Finland; GR-5064 Rigshospitalet, Copenhagen)
J Clin Endocrinol Metab 91:953-958, 2006   12–7

Context.—Hormonal dysregulation has been suggested to be one of many etiological factors of cryptorchidism.

Objectives.—The objective of this study was to assess the hypothalamic-pituitary-testicular axis in cryptorchid boys during the postnatal hormonal surge.

Design.—This was a prospective, longitudinal, population-based study.

Setting.—The study was performed at two primary obstetric centers.

Participants.—Study participants included 388 Finnish and 433 Danish boys (88 and 34 with cryptorchidism, respectively).

Interventions.—Clinical examinations were performed at 0 and 3 months. Blood samples were taken at 3 months.

Main Outcome Measures.—The main outcome measures were testis position and reproductive hormone levels.

Results.—Finnish cryptorchid boys had significantly higher FSH [1.59 (0.50–3.53) *vs.* 1.30 (0.49–2.92) IU/liter; $P < 0.0001$] and lower inhibin B [426 (254–770) *vs.* 459 (266–742) pg/ml; $P < 0.015$] levels than Finnish control boys [median (2.5th–97.5th percentiles)]. Danish cryptorchid boys had higher FSH levels than controls [1.47 (0.54-3.89) *vs.* 1.18 (0.41–3.04) IU/liter; $P = 0.018$]. Inhibin B levels in healthy Danish boys were lower than those in Finnish boys [380 (233–637) pg/ml; $P < 0.0001$] and were not reduced in Danish cryptorchid boys [392 (236–672) pg/ml; $P = 0.851$]. Changes in hormone levels were strongest in boys with severe, persistent cryptorchidism, but were also detectable in mild and transient cryptorchidism. Effects on Leydig cell function were subtle, with an increase in LH in Finnish (but not Danish) cryptorchid boys *vs.* controls [1.97 (0.77–5.91) *vs.* 1.75 (0.58–4.04) IU/liter; $P < 0.021$], but testosterone levels remained within the normal range.

Conclusions.—Our results support the hypothesis that cryptorchidism is associated with a primary testicular disorder, which could be a cause or a consequence of cryptorchidism. This malfunction is reflected by low inhibin B production in the Finnish cohort and high gonadotropin drive in both the Finnish and Danish cohorts.

▶ This series is a continuation of a theme on hypospadias by the same group of investigators.[1,2] In prior reports we were informed that the incidence of cryptorchidism was higher in Denmark than Finland[1] and that the incidence of hypospadias was 4% amongst males in Denmark. Hypospadias was associated with elevated serum follicle-stimulating hormone (FSH) levels at 3 months.[2] The present cohort documents higher FSH levels in Danish boys with cryptorchidism, and the authors present data to support the concept that cryptorchidism is associated with a primary testicular disorder. We will watch with interest as these cohorts are followed to school and beyond.

The same investigators, in a manuscript by Main et al,[3] identified phthalates in human milk and concluded that there was incomplete virilization in infant boys exposed to phthalates prenatally.

A. A. Fanaroff, MD

References

1. Boisen KA, Kaleva M, Main KM, et al. Difference in prevalence of congenital cryptorchidism in infants between two Nordic countries. *Lancet.* 2004;363:1264-1269.
2. Boisen KA, Chellakooty M, Schmidt IM, et al. Hypospadias in a cohort of 1072 Danish newborn boys: prevalence and relationship to placental weight, anthropometrical measurements at birth, and reproductive hormone levels at three months of age. *J Clin Endocrinol Metab.* 2005;90:4041-4046.
3. Main KM, Mortensen GK, Kaleva MM, et al. Human breast milk contamination with phthalates and alterations of endogenous reproductive hormones in infants three months of age. *Environ Health Perspect.* 2006;114:270-276.

Longitudinal Changes in Insulin-Like Growth Factor-I, Insulin Sensitivity, and Secretion from Birth to Age Three Years in Small-for-Gestational-Age Children

Iñiguez G, Ong K, Bazaes R, et al (Univ of Chile, Santiago; Univ of Cambridge, England; Med Research Council Epidemiology Unit, Cambridge, England)
J Clin Endocrinol Metab 91:4645-4649, 2006   12–8

Introduction.—Insulin resistance (IR) develops as early as age 1 to 3 yr in small for gestational age (SGA) infants who show rapid catch-up postnatal weight gain. In contrast, greater insulin secretion is related to infancy height gains. We hypothesized that IGF-I levels could be differentially related to gains in length and weight and also differentially related to IR and insulin secretion.

Methods.—In a prospective study of 50 SGA (birth weight < 5th percentile) and 14 normal birth weight [appropriate for gestational age (AGA)] newborns, we measured serum IGF-I levels at birth, 1 yr, and 3 yr. IR (by homeostasis model assessment) and insulin secretion (by short iv glucose tolerance test) were also measured at 1 yr and 3 yr.

Results.—SGA infants had similar mean length and weight at 3 yr compared with AGA infants. SGA infants had lower IGF-I levels at birth ($P < 0.0001$), but conversely they had higher IGF-I levels at 3 yr ($P = 0.003$) than AGA infants. Within the SGA group, at 1 yr IGF-I was associated with length gain from birth and insulin secretion ($P < 0.0001$); in contrast at 3 yr IGF-I was positively related to weight, body mass index, and IR.

Conclusions.—IGF-I levels increased rapidly from birth in SGA, but not AGA children. During the key first-year growth period, IGF-I levels were related to beta-cell function and longitudinal growth. In contrast, by 3 yr, when catch-up growth was completed, IGF-I levels were related to body mass index and IR, and these higher IGF-I levels in SGA infants might indicate the presence of relative IGF-I resistance.

▶ It is remarkable that there is a already a difference in insulin resistance seen at 1 and 3 years between the SGA and AGA groups despite the children having similar sizes. The clinical significance of this difference for long-term cardiovascular health and type 2 diabetes mellitus is an intriguing question.

Is insulin resistance already preprogrammed at birth for SGA babies or is it a consequence of promoting catch-up growth? Although catch-up growth has been implicated as a cause for later metabolic syndrome, it may be possible that the growth itself is just a manifestation of the underlying physiology as indicated by markers such as IGF-I early in life and continuing throughout childhood, although this may be less likely when one considers that an association has not been established for IGF-I levels at birth with a relationship to levels at 1 and 3 years. The important question here is whether anything can be done to prevent the progression to disease. The SGA population was the focus of the study here. But, it may also be informative to look at AGA infants closer to see whether there are relationships of IGF-I level and growth parameters similar to that of the SGA population.

The children studied here were exclusively breast-fed for a mean of 3.7 months (range 0-8 months). It would be interesting to see whether there was any impact of a longer duration of breast-feeding on any of the parameters studied.

H. C. Lee, MD

Antenatal Hydronephrosis as a Predictor of Postnatal Outcome: A Meta-analysis
Lee RS, Cendron M, Kinnamon DD, et al (Children's Hosp Boston; Univ of Miami, Fla)
Pediatrics 118:586-593, 2006   12–9

Objective.—Antenatal hydronephrosis is diagnosed in 1% to 5% of all pregnancies; however, the antenatal and postnatal management of hydronephrosis varies widely. No previous studies define the risk of postnatal pathology in infants with antenatal hydronephrosis. Our objective was to review the current literature to determine whether the degree of antenatal hydronephrosis and related antenatal ultrasound findings are associated with postnatal outcome.

Methods.—We searched Medline (1966–2005), Embase (1991–2004), and the Cochrane Library databases for articles on antenatal hydronephrosis. We required studies to have subjects selected on the basis of documented measurements of antenatal hydronephrosis and followed to a postnatal diagnosis. We excluded case reports, review articles, and editorials. Two independent investigators extracted data.

Results.—We screened 1645 citations, of which 17 studies met inclusion criteria. We created a data set of 1308 subjects. The risk of any postnatal pathology per degree of antenatal hydronephrosis was 11.9% for mild, 45.1% for moderate, and 88.3% for severe. There was a significant increase in risk per increasing degree of hydronephrosis. The risk of vesicoureteral reflux was similar for all degrees of antenatal hydronephrosis.

Conclusions.—The findings of this meta-analysis can potentially be used for prenatal counseling and may alter current postnatal management of children with antenatal hydronephrosis. Overall, children with any degree of antenatal hydronephrosis are at greater risk of postnatal pathology as compared with the normal population. Moderate and severe antenatal hydronephrosis have a significant risk of postnatal pathology, indicating that comprehensive postnatal diagnostic management should be performed. Mild antenatal hydronephrosis may carry a risk for postnatal pathology, but additional prospective studies are needed to determine the optimal management of these children. A well-defined prospective analysis is needed to further define the risk of pathology and the appropriate management protocols.

▶ In light of the lack of comprehensive, prospective studies on the postnatal implications of antenatal hydronephrosis (ANH), this meta-analysis of case series is a laudable attempt to uncover the predictive value of these antenatal findings. ANH was classified as mild, moderate, or severe by the anterior posterior diameter, with specific ranges defined for the second and third trimester. The authors noted marked variability in prenatal and postnatal imaging protocols, making interpretation of results difficult.

A total of 36% of patients with any degree of ANH had pathology noted on postnatal investigation, with ureteropelvic junction obstruction and vesicoureteral reflux being the most common findings in all degrees of ANH. As noted by the authors, the finding of a high percentage of postnatal pathology in the severe ANH group (88.3%) was not surprising. However, the finding of postnatal pathology in 11.9% of those with mild ANH and 45.1% of those with moderate ANH were higher than expected and may have significant implications in terms of ensuring adequate postnatal follow-up for these infants. Therefore, the most important take-home message from this article is that well-designed, prospective studies, with standardized prenatal and postnatal imaging, are desperately needed to further delineate the appropriate follow-up for this large group of neonates.

R. L. Chapman, MD

Perinatal renal venous thrombosis: presenting renal length predicts outcome
Winyard PJD, Bharucha T, De Bruyn R, et al (Great Ormond Street Hosp for Children NHS Trust, London; Univ College London; Inst of Child Health, England)
Arch Dis Child Fetal Neonatal Ed 91:F273-F278, 2006   12–10

Background.—Renal venous thrombosis (RVT) is the most common form of venous thrombosis in neonates, causing both acute and long term kidney dysfunction. Historical predisposing factors include dehydration, maternal diabetes, and umbilical catheters, but recent reports highlight associations with prothrombotic abnormalities.

Study.—Twenty three patients with neonatal RVT were analysed over 15 years. Predisposing factors, presentation, and procoagulant status were compared with renal outcome using multilevel modelling.

Results.—Median presentation was on day 1: 19/23 (83%) had pre/perinatal problems, including fetal distress (14), intrauterine growth retardation (five), and pre-identified renal abnormalities (two); 8/18 (44%) had procoagulant abnormalities, particularly factor V Leiden mutations (4/18). Long term abnormalities were detected in 28/34 (82%) affected kidneys; mean glomerular filtration rate was 93.6 versus 70.2 ml/min/1.73 m^2 in unilateral versus bilateral cases (difference 23.4; 95% confidence interval 6.4 to 40.4; p = 0.01). No correlation was observed between procoagulant tendencies and outcome, but presenting renal length had a significant negative correlation: mean fall in estimated single kidney glomerular filtration rate was 3 ml/min/1.73 m^2 (95% confidence interval 3.7 to −2.2; p = 0.001) per 1 mm increase, and kidneys larger than 6 cm at presentation never had a normal outcome.

Conclusions.—This subgroup of neonatal RVT would be better termed perinatal RVT to reflect antenatal and birth related antecedents. Prothrombotic defects should be considered in all patients with perinatal RVT. Kidney length at presentation correlated negatively with renal outcome. The latter, novel observation raises the question of whether larger organs should be treated more aggressively in future.

▶ Renal vein thrombosis (RVT) is the most common cause of spontaneous, non-catheter-related thromboembolic disease in the neonate. It is a rare occurrence with an incidence of approximately 2 to 5 per 100,000 live births. Our knowledge of RVT comes primarily from case reports and retrospective studies such as this report by Winyard et al from Great Ormond Street.[1-4] Typical presentation includes hematuria, oliguria, palpable abdominal mass, hypertension, and thrombocytopenia. RVT is more common on the left, and approximately 10% to 20% of cases are bilateral. Associated conditions include maternal diabetes, preeclampsia, fetal distress, asphyxia, prematurity, cyanotic congenital heart disease, sepsis, dehydration, hyperviscosity, and hemoconcentration. In their 23 cases, Winyard et al[1] found most cases presented on day of life one, with 2 presenting prenatally.

Ultrasonographic findings include an enlarged, echogenic kidney with loss of corticomedullary differentiation as well as the renal vein thrombus in most cases. Doppler studies demonstrate decreased or absent venous signal, abnormal flow patterns in renal vessels, or development of venous collaterals. Concomitant adrenal hemorrhage and extension of the clot into the inferior vena cava are also sometimes found.

Inherited prothrombotic risk factors associated with RVT have included factor V Leiden G1691A, prothrombin gene G20210A, and methylenetetrahydrofolate reductase C677T genotypes, elevated lipoprotein Lp(a), protein C or S deficiency, antithrombin deficiency, antiphospholipid antibodies, lupus anticoagulant, and hyperhomocysteinemia. In the Winyard report, approximately half of the patients with RVT had at least 1 inherited risk factor for thrombosis.[1] These data emphasize several important points. First, inherited prothrombotic risk factors should be sought in neonates with RVT. Second, when these factors are detected, patients need monitoring for recurrent thromboembolism throughout life, especially when subjected to acquired thromboembolic risks such as surgery, prolonged travel, immobilization, pregnancy, and oral contraceptive use. Finally, genetic counseling of family members is also indicated.

Management of RVT is controversial, with many advocating supportive care while others prescribe low molecular weight or unfractionated heparin. IV thrombolytic therapy has been described in a few cases, with the suggestion that bilateral cases are most likely to benefit.[4] However, no clear indications for treatment are currently available.

Sequelae include chronic renal disease, hypertension, and real failure. Using multilevel modeling, Winyard et al found that absolute kidney length at presentation had a highly significant negative correlation with outcome (ie, larger kidneys had worse outcome). This is the most noteworthy association of a neonatal finding with long-term outcome. If this observation holds up in future clinical investigations, it may be a potential indicator of the need for aggressive treatment.

P. G. Gallagher, MD

References

1. Winyard PJD, Bharucha T, De Bruyn R, et al. Perinatal renal venous thrombosis: presenting renal length predicts outcome. *Arch Dis Child Fetal Neonatal Ed.* 2006;91:F273-F278.
2. Kosch A, Kuwertz-Bröking E, Heller C, Kurnik K, Schobess R, Nowak-Göttl U. Renal venous thrombosis in neonates: prothrombotic risk factors and long-term follow-up. *Blood.* 2004;104:1356-1360.
3. Marks SD, Massicotte MP, Steele BT, et al. Neonatal renal venous thrombosis. clinical outcomes and prevalence of prothrombotic disorders. *J Pediatr.* 2005;146:811-816.
4. Messinger Y, Sheaffer JW, Mrozek J, Smith CM, Sinaiko AR. Renal outcome of neonatal renal venous thrombosis: review of 28 patients and effectiveness of fibrinolytics and heparin in 10 patients. *Pediatrics.* 2006;118:e1478-e1484.

Renal Tubular Dysgenesis, a Not Uncommon Autosomal Recessive Disorder Leading to Oligohydramnios: Role of the Renin-Angiotensin System

Lacoste M, Cai Y, Guicharnaud L, et al (Université René Descartes, Paris; Institut Natl de la Santé, Paris; Hôpital Edouard Herriot, Lyon, France; et al)
J Am Soc Nephrol 17:2253-2263, 2006   12–11

Renal tubular dysgenesis is a clinical disorder that is observed in fetuses and characterized by the absence or poor development of proximal tubules, early onset and persistent oligohydramnios that leads to the Potter sequence, and skull ossification defects. It may be acquired during fetal development or inherited as an autosomal recessive disease. It was shown recently that autosomal recessive renal tubular dysgenesis is genetically heterogeneous and linked to mutations in the genes that encode components of the renin-angiotensin system. This study analyzed the clinical expression of the disease in 29 fetus/neonates from 18 unrelated families and evaluated changes in renal morphology and expression of the renin-angiotensin system. The disease was uniformly severe, with perinatal death in all cases as a result of persistent anuria and hypoxia related to pulmonary hypoplasia. Severe defects in proximal tubules were observed in all fetuses from 18 gestational weeks onward, and lesions also involved other tubular segments. They were associated with thickening of the renal arterial vasculature, from the arcuate to the afferent arteries. Renal renin expression was strikingly increased in 19 of 24 patients studied, from 13 families, whereas no renal renin was detected in four patients from three families. Angiotensinogen and angiotensin-converting enzyme were absent or present in only small amounts in the proximal tubule, in correlation with the severity of tubular abnormalities. No specific changes were detected in angiotensin II receptor expression. The severity and the early onset of the clinical and pathologic expression of the disease underline the major importance of this system in fetal kidney function and development in humans. The identification of the disease on the basis of precise histologic analysis and the research of the genetic defect now allow genetic counseling and early prenatal diagnosis.

▶ Renal tubular dysgenesis (RTD), alternatively called primitive renal tubule syndrome, is an autosomal recessive disorder characterized by severe and persistent oligohydramnios and skull ossification defects.[1,2] The absence of fetal urine production leads to the development of the Potter sequence (oligohydramnios sequence), characterized by facial anomalies, arthrogryposis, and severe pulmonary hypoplasia. Perinatal death is common, primarily due to the severe pulmonary disease. In addition, neonates with this condition may exhibit severe hypotension that is refractory to therapy.

In contrast to other inherited and sporadic causes of early oligohydramnios, such as autosomal recessive kidney disease (ARPKD), in which kidneys are usually massively enlarged, and bilateral renal dysplasia, in which kidneys are typically small, kidneys of patients with RTD generally appear normal in size with minimal or no echogenicity by ultrasonography. Similarly, kidneys typically appear normal by gross pathologic examination. Histologically, however, the kidneys exhibit profound tubular dysgenesis, with complete absence of proximal tubule development, thus explaining the basis for the absent fetal urine.[1,2]

The clinical features of RTD are similar to those of fetuses with in utero exposure to angiotensin-converting enzyme inhibitors (ACEIs)[3] or angiotensin receptor blockers (ARBs),[4] two classes of antihypertensive medications that target the renin-angiotensin system (RAS). Renal dysfunction and open fontanelles are well-recognized complications of ACE/ARB fetopathy, which occurs with exposure to these medications in the second or third trimester. Although first-trimester exposure has been shown recently to be teratogenic, renal anomalies are not reported in those exposed at this earlier stage of gestation.[5] The recognition that RTD clinically resembles medication-induced abnormalities resulting from RAS disruption led to the hypothesis that abnormalities of one or more of the RAS genes could underlie the pathogenesis of RTD. Subsequently, marked up-regulation of renin was reported in kidneys of 3 RTD patients.[6] In 2005, mutations in the genes encoding the major RAS proteins, including renin, angiotensinogen, ACE, and angiotensin II receptor type I were identified in affected kindreds.[7]

In this study by Lacoste et al, who described the RAS mutation abnormalities in RTD, RAS protein expression is characterized in kidneys from 29 fetuses/infants with known or suspected RTD mutations. The disease in this patient group was severe and all patients studied died in the perinatal period. In histologic studies, the authors confirm the universal finding of absent proximal tubule development. They report two patterns of RAS expression abnormalities in the kidneys studied: (1) low or undetectable renin; or (2) markedly up-regulated renin. In either case, expression of the downstream proteins (ie, angiotensinogen or ACE) was low or undetectable. No abnormalities in angiotensin II receptor expression were found.

This study demonstrates the importance of the RA in the development of the fetal kidney. It also highlights the importance of recognizing RTD in fetuses and neonates with early and severe oligohydramnios, particularly those in whom radiographic evidence or history may not suggest an underlying etiology. The recognition of the causative role of RAS gene mutations in this disorder also permits more informed genetic counseling and testing in affected kindreds.

K. M. Dell, MD

References

1. Allanson JE, Hunter AG, Mettler GS, Jimenez C. Renal tubular dysgenesis: a not uncommon autosomal recessive syndrome. a review. *Am J Med Genet.* 1992;43:811-814.
2. Online Mendelian Inheritance in Man, OMIM™. Johns Hopkins University, Baltimore, MD. MIM Number: 267430. Date last edited: January 22, 2007. Available at: http://www.ncbi.nlm.nih.gov/omim/. Accessed March 5, 2007.
3. Pryde PG, Sedman AB, Nugent CE, Barr M Jr. Angiotensin-converting enzyme inhibitor fetopathy. *J Am Soc Nephrol.* 1993;3:1575-1582.
4. Martinovic J, Benachi A, Laurent N, Daikha-Dahmane F, Gubler MC. Fetal toxic effects of angiotensin-II-receptor antagonists. *Lancet.* 2001;358:241-242.
5. Cooper WO, Hernandez-Diaz S, Arbogast PG, et al. Major congenital malformations after first trimester exposure to ACE inhibitors. *N Engl J Med.* 2006;354:2443-2451.
6. Bernstein J, Barajas L. Renal tubular dysgenesis: evidence of abnormality in the renin-angiotensin system. *J Am Soc Nephrol.* 1994;5:224-227.
7. Gribouval O, Gonzales M, Neuhaus T, et al. Mutations in genes in the renin-angiotensin system are associated with autosomal recessive renal tubular dysgenesis. *Nat Genet.* 2005;37:964-968.

Increased Echogenicity as a Predictor of Poor Renal Function in Children With Grade 3 to 4 Hydronephrosis
Chi T, Feldstein VA, Nguyen HT (Univ of California, San Francisco)
J Urol 175:1898-1901, 2006   12–12

Purpose.—Prenatally diagnosed hydronephrosis is a common finding that often requires further radiological evaluation to determine whether it is associated with compromised renal function. We hypothesize that findings on postnatal renal sonography may help determine which patients require more extensive evaluation of renal function in the assessment for prenatal hydronephrosis. We show that increased renal parenchymal echogenicity on postnatal US is a strong predictor of compromised renal function.

Materials and Methods.—A total of 97 patients diagnosed with prenatal hydronephrosis presented to our institution for furoscmide ^{99m}technetium MAG3 renogram evaluation of renal function between January 2000 and December 2001. All patients had SFU grade 3 to 4 hydronephrosis noted on postnatal US before age 6 months. For these 97 patients (178 renal units), we correlated the degree of renal parenchymal echogenicity and parenchymal

TABLE 3.—Performance of Echogenicity and Parenchymal Thinning in Predicting Renal Function

Renal Function	% Echogenicity		2% Parenchymal Thinning	
	20 or Less	40 or Less	20 or Less	40 or Less
Sensitivity	100	48	29	22
Specificity	99	100	90	90
Pos predictive value	89	96	9	23
Neg predictive value	100	93	97	90
p Value	<0.001	<0.001	0.38	0.170

(Reprinted from Chi T, Feldstein VA, Nguyen HT. Increased echogenicity as a predictor of poor renal function in children with grade 3 to 4 hydronephrosis. *J Urol.* 175:1898-1901. Copyright 2006, with permission from the American Urological Association.)

thinning on the first postnatal sonogram with the differential renal function as determined by furosemide MAG3 renography.

Results.—Among 97 patients diagnosed with prenatal hydronephrosis 10 of 20 renal units (50%) with markedly increased echogenicity had severely decreased relative renal function of less than 10%, while 136 of 151 (90%) with normal echogenicity exhibited normal relative renal function of 40% or greater. Increased echogenicity on US yielded a sensitivity of 100% and specificity of 99% for predicting relative renal function of 20% or greater. In predicting relative renal function of 40% or less sensitivity and specificity were 48% and 100%, respectively.

Conclusions.—Increased renal parenchymal echogenicity found on the first postnatal ultrasound can be used as a predictor of impaired relative renal function as measured on furosemide MAG3 renogram (Table 3).

▶ Hydronephrosis is the most common renal anomaly detected by antenatal US and is reported to occur in up to 1% of pregnancies.[1,2] Between 25% and 50% of those fetuses have "physiologic hydronephrosis," which does not represent underlying disease but rather is a reflection of several factors, including a large fetal urine output.[3,4] Physiologic hydronephrosis typically resolves at or soon after birth.

Hydronephrosis is graded on a scale of 0 to 4 (absent to severe), based on criteria established by the SFU.[3] The differential diagnosis of antenatal hydronephrosis that persists after birth includes a spectrum of disorders including obstructive uropathies (eg, posterior urethral valves [PUVs] and ureteropelvic junction [UPJ] obstruction), vesicoureteral reflux (VUR), and isolated hydronephrosis without evidence of obstruction or VUR. Oligohydramnios, prematurity, and persistently depressed renal function (glomerular filtration rate [GFR], <20mL/min) in the postnatal period are poor prognostic factors for antenatal hydronephrosis.[4] Evaluation of patients with a history of antenatal hydronephrosis typically includes 1 or more of the following diagnostic imaging studies:

1. US is recommended for all patients with a history of antenatal hydronephrosis so that the presence and severity of hydronephrosis can be confirmed

postnatally. In addition, postnatal US can assess kidney size and the presence of other abnormalities, such as renal cysts. However, the timing of the US is important, as US scans in the first 72 hours of life may underestimate or overestimate the severity of the hydronephrosis. Thus, it is recommended that patients who have a US performed in the first 72 hours of life have a follow-up study performed at 10 to 14 days of age to more accurately assess the severity of the hydronephrosis.[3]

2. Voiding cystourethrography (VCUG) is performed to evaluate for the presence of VUR and to evaluate for urethral obstruction (such as PUVs) and bladder pathology. VCUG is typically recommended for patients with confirmed hydronephrosis on postnatal US. VCUG should be performed while the patient is still in the nursery if the hydronephrosis is severe and/or bilateral. For patients with mild, unilateral hydronephrosis, VCUG can be performed after discharge. Patients with confirmed hydronephrosis are typically given prophylactic antibiotics (amoxicillin) pending the results of the VCUG.

3. Diuretic renal scans (DTPA or MAG3 lasix renogram) are nuclear medicine studies that examine the relative contribution of each kidney ("differential" or "split" renal function) to the overall renal function. They are typically used to determine relative function in the case of unilateral renal disease and are specifically used to determine the presence or absence of obstruction due to UPJ or ureterovesical junction obstruction. Several factors can affect the interpretation of MAG3 studies. These include the presence of bilateral disease and impaired renal function, which can give the appearance of "normal" split function because both kidneys are similarly affected. Because newborn kidneys are immature, MAG3 scans should generally be done after the first month of life.[3]

Chi et al retrospectively studied 97 patients with a history of antenatal hydronephrosis and grade 3 or 4 hydronephrosis on postnatal US scans obtained within the first 6 months of life (mean, 2.1 ± 2 months) who underwent MAG3 renograms at their institution. Specifically, they examined 2 US features: echogenicity and parenchymal thickness. Renal echogenicity is generally defined as kidneys that are as bright or brighter than the liver and is often considered an indicator of so-called medical renal disease. These 2 criteria were then correlated with the renal function as determined by MAG3 renogram studies. The authors report that increased echogenicity is a predictor of poor renal function (ie, a poorly functioning kidney) in children with more severe grades (ie, grade 3 or 4) of hydronephrosis.

The results of this study are not surprising, given that echogenicity is often associated with abnormal kidney structure (eg, renal dysplasia), function, or both. Unfortunately, the study has significant limitations. First, significant selection bias exists because only those patients who presented for MAG3 renograms were studied. Second, the timing of the postnatal US was highly variable (mean, 2.1 months ± 2 months). Given that hydronephrosis severity can change significantly over the first several weeks and months of life, this variability makes data interpretation difficult. Third, all patients, regardless of the underlying diagnosis, were included. Because the natural histories of UPJ,

VUR, PUVs, and multicystic dysplastic kidney may differ significantly, the results of this study may not be applicable to each individual disease. Finally, MAG3 studies examine relative function. Thus, the presence of impaired renal function can significantly affect interpretation of the results, as the authors note.

Two other recent studies have examined some of these issues in a more systematic, prospective fashion in subjects with the same underlying disease and provide important insights into the natural history of these disorders:

1. Vesicoureteral reflux. Ismaili et al[5] prospectively followed up 43 infants with VUR with postnatal renal US scans at 5 days and at 1, 3, 6, 12, and 24 months; with VCUG within 1 month and at 12 and 24 months; and with MAG3 renograms and plasma clearance of chromium-51 EDTA (a measure of GFR) in patients with high grade (grades IV and V) VUR. They found that the US appearance of renal dysplasia (small and/or echogenic kidneys) and loss of corticomedullary differentiation strongly correlated with the severity of VUR. Despite the fact that 88% of kidneys with high-grade reflux showed abnormalities on US (eg, hydronephrosis, dysplasia, and loss of corticomedullary differentiation) at 1 year of age, the majority of kidneys with high-grade reflux (13 of 17) showed improvement in single-kidney GFR in the interval between ages 3 months and 24 months. The authors conclude that, although high-grade VUR generally does not resolve by itself, persistence of reflux rarely impairs normal maturation of kidney function.

2. Isolated antenatal hydronephrosis. Cheng et al[6] prospectively examined the outcomes of 63 patients with a history of antenatal hydronephrosis and no evidence of VUR or urinary tract obstruction. Twenty-five percent of patients showed resolution of the antenatal hydronephrosis on the first postnatal US, obtained at a mean age of 18 days. Fifty-four percent had mild and 21% had moderate to severe hydronephrosis. By 2 years of age, hydronephrosis had decreased in severity in the majority of patients; only 3 patients showed a worsening of hydronephrosis. In all 3 cases, the patients had mild hydronephrosis that progressed to moderate hydronephrosis. Renal growth in all patients was normal. Taken as a whole, these findings suggest a very favorable outcome in patients with isolated antenatal hydronephrosis.

Unfortunately, similar prospective studies for patients with obstructive uropathies (eg, UPJ or ureterovesical junction obstruction or PUVs) have not been performed. However, a retrospective study[7] of patients with PUVs suggests that the likelihood of deterioration of renal function to the point of requiring dialysis or transplantation by age 15 years is 13%.

The overall variability in outcome among these different causes of antenatal hydronephrosis highlights the importance of establishing the underlying cause of the hydronephrosis through postnatal imaging studies. This will allow for more informed counseling of parents about the predicted outcomes for their infants.

K. M. Dell, MD

References

1. Blyth B, Snyder HM, Duckett JW. Antenatal diagnosis and subsequent management of hydronephrosis. *J Urol.* 1993;149:693-698.
2. Rosendahl H. Ultrasound screening for fetal urinary tract malformations: a prospective study in general population. *Eur J Obstet Gynecol Reprod Biol.* 1990; 36:27-33.
3. Elder JS. Antenatal hydronephrosis: Fetal and neonatal management. *Pediatr Clin North Am.* 1997;44:1299-1321.
4. Oliveira EA, Diniz JS, Cabral AC, et al. Prognostic factors in fetal hydronephrosis: a multivariate analysis. *Pediatr Nephrol.* 1999;13:859-864.
5. Ismaili K, Hall M, Piepsz A, et al. Primary vesicoureteral reflux detected in neonates with a history of fetal renal pelvis dilatation: a prospective clinical and imaging study. *J Pediatr.* 2006;148:222-227.
6. Cheng AM, Phan V, Geary DF, Rosenblum ND. Outcome of isolated antenatal hydronephrosis. *Arch Pediatr Adolesc Med.* 2004;158:38-40.
7. Smith GH, Canning DA, Schulman SL, Snyder HM III, Duckett JW. The long term outcome of posterior urethral valves treated with primary valve ablation and observation. *J Urol.* 1996;155:1730-1734.

13 Pharmacology

Empiric Use of Ampicillin and Cefotaxime, Compared With Ampicillin and Gentamicin, for Neonates at Risk for Sepsis Is Associated With an Increased Risk of Neonatal Death
Clark RH, Bloom BT, Spitzer AR, et al (Pediatrix-Obstetrix Ctr for Research and Education, Sunrise, Fla)
Pediatrics 117:67-74, 2006   13–1

Background.—We reported previously that the use of cephalosporin among premature neonates increased the risk of subsequent fungal sepsis. As a result, we recommended that ampicillin and gentamicin be used as empiric coverage for early-onset neonatal sepsis while culture results are awaited.

Objectives.—To describe antibiotic use during the first 3 days after birth for neonates admitted to the NICU and to evaluate the outcomes for neonates treated with 2 different antibiotic regimens.

Methods.—We assembled a cohort of inborn neonates, from our deidentified administrative database, who had documented exposure to ampicillin during the first 3 days after birth. Infants treated concurrently with cefotaxime or gentamicin were evaluated, to identify the factors that were associated independently with death before discharge, with both univariate and multivariate analyses.

Results.—There were 128,914 neonates selected as the study cohort; 24,111 were treated concurrently with ampicillin and cefotaxime and 104,803 were treated concurrently with ampicillin and gentamicin. Logistic modeling showed that neonates treated with ampicillin/cefotaxime were more likely to die (adjusted odds ratio: 1.5; 95% confidence interval: 1.4–1.7) and were less likely to be discharged to home or foster care than were neonates treated with ampicillin/gentamicin. This observation was true across all estimated gestational ages. Other factors that were associated independently with death included immature gestational age, need for assisted ventilation on the day of admission to the NICU, indications of perinatal asphyxia or major congenital anomaly, and reported use of ampicillin/cefotaxime.

Conclusions.—For patients receiving ampicillin, the concurrent use of cefotaxime during the first 3 days after birth either is a surrogate for an unrecognized factor or is itself associated with an increased risk of death, compared with the concurrent use of gentamicin (Fig 2).

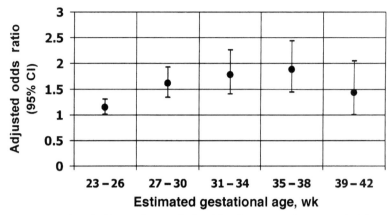

FIGURE 2.—Adjusted odds ratio (based on final model) within gestational-age groups (logistic regression [odds of death] adjusted for need for assisted ventilation, anomalies, birth depression, and estimated gestational age within each estimated gestational-age group). (Reproduced with permission from Clark RH, Bloom BT, Spitzer AR, et al. Empiric use of ampicillin and cefotaxime, compared with ampicillin and gentamicin, for neonates at risk for sepsis is associated with an increased risk of neonatal death. *Pediatrics.* 2006;117:67-74.)

▶ The study by Clark and colleagues offers the intriguing possibility that empirical treatment with cefotaxime in the first 3 days of life is associated with a greater risk of neonatal mortality compared with treatment with gentamicin. For infectious disease specialists, particularly those engaged in hospital infection control, the use of the third-generation cephalosporins in critically ill patients has been falling out of favor for some time. This prejudice is based on the observation that the third-generation cephalosporins have a particularly strong propensity to select gram-negative bacilli expressing extended-spectrum β-lactamases and AmpC-β-lactamase[1] (as well as vancomycin-resistant enterococci[2]) compared with other drugs. An ever-increasing proportion of ICU–acquired infections in adult patients are caused by gram-negative bacilli expressing these enzymes,[3] both of which render the organism resistant to virtually all β-lactam agents except for the carbapenems and, to a lesser extent, the fourth-generation cephalosporin cefepime. Some published data suggest that NICU populations share this risk. In the study by de Man and colleagues,[4] for example, investigators measured the incidence of colonization by an antibiotic-resistant gram-negative organism in infants initially given penicillin–gentamicin versus ampicillin–cefotaxime, employing 2 NICUs in a crossover design. The incidence of colonization by an antibiotic-resistant gram-negative bacillus in the ampicillin–cefotaxime group proved significantly higher.

The outcome of the study by Clark et al is not acquisition of an antibiotic-resistant organism but all-cause mortality. Their conclusion is provocative because, in contrast to studies examining the emergence of resistant bacteria, a biological reason to explain this observation is not immediately apparent. The study is retrospective, drawn from a large multicenter database, which raises the possibility that receipt of cefotaxime is a confounder for a more explanatory variable (eg, practitioners may have been inclined to treat sicker neonates with the "stronger" antibiotic cefotaxime as opposed to the "more conventional" gentamicin). The authors readily recognize this weakness in their study design and go to considerable lengths to address it, most notably by entering other variables potentially contributing to neonatal mortality in a regression model to establish the independent contribution of antecedent cefotaxime administration on mortality. Regression models are only as strong as the variables used to construct them, however, and in the end, one is still left wondering, at least from the biological standpoint, why cefotaxime exposure immediately after birth should cause a statistically detectable disproportionate mortality later on. With that said, the evidence generated by other investigators that the third-generation cephalosporins select antibiotic-resistant gram-negative bacilli and enterococci more readily than comparator agents is compelling. In the absence of a clear requirement for their use, they should be administered with caution in long-term ICU residents of all ages.

P. H. Toltzis, MD

References

1. Paterson DL, Bonomo RA. Extended-spectrum beta-lactamases: a clinical update. *Clin Microbiol Rev.* 2005;18:657-686.
2. Fridkin SK, Edwards JR, Courval JM, et al. The effect of vancomycin and third-generation cephalosporins on prevalence of vancomycin-resistant enterococci in 126 U.S. adult intensive care units. *Ann Intern Med.* 2001;135:175-183.
3. Moland ES, Hanson ND, Black JA, Hossain A, Song W, Thomson KS. Prevalence of newer beta-lactamases in gram-negative clinical isolates collected in the United States from 2001 to 2002. *J Clin Microbiol.* 2006;44:3318-3324.
4. de Man P, Verhoeven BA, Verbrugh HA, Vos MC, van den Anker JN. An antibiotic policy to prevent emergence of resistant bacilli. *Lancet.* 2000;355:973-978.

Theophylline for renal function in term neonates with perinatal asphyxia: A randomized, placebo-controlled trial
Bhat MA, Shah ZA, Makhoomi MS, et al (Shere-Kashmir Inst of Med Sciences, India)
J Pediatr 149:180-184, 2006   13–2

Objective.—To study whether prophylactic theophylline can reduce the incidence and/or severity of renal failure in term infants with perinatal asphyxia.

Study Design.—Term neonates with severe perinatal asphyxia were randomized to receive a single dose of either theophylline (study group, n = 40) or placebo (control group, n = 30) during the first hour of life. Daily weight, output/input ratio, 24-hour fluid intake, and urine volumes were recorded during the first 5 days of life. Those infants with asphyxial renal failure were followed up for 1 year.

Results.—The incidence of severe renal dysfunction was increased in the control group. Creatinine clearance was higher and excretion of beta 2 microglobulin (β2M) was lower in the theophylline group. Conversely, the glomerular filtration rate was lower in the control group. In infants with renal failure, serum creatinine and creatinine clearance returned to normal in the neonatal period, and the increased β2M excretion normalized by age 6 weeks.

Conclusions.—A single dose of theophylline within the first hour of birth in term neonates with perinatal asphyxia results in a significant decrease in serum creatinine level and urinary excretion of β2M, along with an increase in creatinine clearance.

▶ In this well-designed and meticulously executed randomized, controlled, masked trial, these authors demonstrate that a single dose of theophylline, administered intravenously within the first hour after birth, can significantly alter the course of renal dysfunction following an episode of presumed intrapartum asphyxia. The salutary effects of treatment, particularly the improved urine output and the more appropriate postnatal weight loss, may make management of these at-risk infants easier over the first several days after birth. However, long-term outcomes did not differ between treatment and control groups: rates of mortality and recovery of apparently normal renal function within 6 weeks were comparable in all subjects. Theophylline did not have apparent effects on signs of CNS injury in the perinatal period, and no data on long-term CNS outcomes are provided; thus, it is not clear whether this intervention should be routinely recommended. Nonetheless, this study exemplifies the principle that thoughtful design of therapies based on an understanding of the pathophysiology of asphyxia can ameliorate the adverse effects of that insult. We can hope that application of this principle will pay similar dividends in the management of cerebral hypoxic–ischemic injuries.

W. E. Benitz, MD

Selective Serotonin-Reputake Inhibitors and Risk of Persistent Pulmonary Hypertension of the Newborn
Chambers CD, Hernandez-Diaz S, Van Marter LJ, et al (Univ of California, San Diego; Boston Univ; Harvard Med School)
N Engl J Med 354:579-587, 2006   13–3

Background.—Persistent pulmonary hypertension of the newborn (PPHN) is associated with substantial infant mortality and morbidity. A previous cohort study suggested a possible association between maternal use of the selective serotonin-reuptake inhibitor (SSRI) fluoxetine late in the third trimester of pregnancy and the risk of PPHN in the infant. We performed a case–control study to assess whether PPHN is associated with exposure to SSRIs during late pregnancy.

Methods.—Between 1998 and 2003, we enrolled 377 women whose infants had PPHN and 836 matched control women and their infants. Maternal interviews were conducted by nurses, who were blinded to the study hypothesis, regarding medication use in pregnancy and potential confounders, including demographic variables and health history.

Results.—Fourteen infants with PPHN had been exposed to an SSRI after the completion of the 20th week of gestation, as compared with six control infants (adjusted odds ratio, 6.1; 95 percent confidence interval, 2.2 to 16.8). In contrast, neither the use of SSRIs before the 20th week of gestation nor the use of non-SSRI antidepressant drugs at any time during pregnancy was associated with an increased risk of PPHN.

Conclusions.—These data support an association between the maternal use of SSRIs in late pregnancy and PPHN in the offspring; further study of this association is warranted. These findings should be taken into account in decisions as to whether to continue the use of SSRIs during pregnancy.

▶ It has long been the suspicion of clinicians that infants born following in utero exposure to selective serotonin-reuptake inhibitor (SSRI) exhibit subtle cardiorespiratory symptoms at birth. It has been unclear whether these symptoms reflect in utero exposure at postnatal withdrawal to the ever-increasing number of these agents. Disordered respiratory control was considered a possible etiology of respiratory symptoms in SSRI-exposed neonates as serotonergic neurons in the brainstem project extensively to autonomic and respiratory nuclei and help regulate homeostatic function. In fact, abnormalities in serotonergic neurons and their receptor bind sites in the medulla and have recently been implicated in sudden infant death syndrome.[1]

Chambers and colleagues now report an association between maternal use of SSRIs in late pregnancy and persistent pulmonary hypertension in the offspring of such pregnancies. This could certainly explain the reported episodes of tachypnea and cyanosis described in this population. However, because the SSRIs (as inhibitors of serotonin uptake) increase the postsynaptic concentration of serotonin, resultant effects may well extend beyond the cardiorespiratory system. Such adverse effects have been proposed to include neurobehavioral consequences and an increased risk for necrotizing enterocolitis.[2]

Unfortunately, progress in this area is hampered by the diversity of SSRIs available to mothers and the subtlety of proposed adverse effects. The decision as to whether to continue SSRI therapy during gestation is clearly not an easy one for our obstetric colleagues.

R. J. Martin, MD

References

1. Paterson DS, Trachtenberg FL, Thompson EG, et al. Multiple serotonergic brainstem abnormalities in sudden infant death syndrome. *JAMA*. 2006;296:2124-2132.
2. Potts A, Young KL, Carter BS, Shenai JP. Necrotizing enterocolitis associated with in utero and breast milk exposure to the selective serotonin reuptake inhibitor, escitalopram. *J Perinatol*. 2007;27:120-122.

Premedication for Nonemergent Neonatal Intubations: A Randomized, Controlled Trial Comparing Atropine and Fentanyl to Atropine, Fentanyl, and Mivacurium

Roberts KD, Leone TA, Edwards WH, et al (Dartmouth-Hitchcock Med Ctr, Lebanon, NH; Univ of California San Diego)
Pediatrics 118:1583-1591, 2006   13–4

Objective.—The purpose of this work was to investigate whether using a muscle relaxant would improve intubation conditions in infants, thereby decreasing the incidence and duration of hypoxia and time and number of attempts needed to successfully complete the intubation procedure.

Patients/Methods.—This was a prospective, randomized, controlled, 2-center trial. Infants requiring nonemergent intubation were randomly assigned to receive atropine and fentanyl or atropine, fentanyl, and mivacurium before intubation. Incidence and duration of hypoxia were determined at oxygen saturation thresholds of $\leq 85\%$, $\leq 75\%$, $\leq 60\%$, and $\leq 40\%$. Videotape was reviewed to determine the time and number of intubation attempts and duration of action of mivacurium.

Results.—Analysis of 41 infants showed that incidence of oxygen saturation $\leq 60\%$ of any duration was significantly less in the mivacurium group (55% vs 24%). The incidence of saturation level of any duration $\leq 85\%$, 75%, and 40%; cumulative time ≥ 30 seconds; and time below the thresholds were not significantly different. Total procedure time (472 vs 144 seconds) and total laryngoscope time (148 vs 61 seconds) were shorter in the mivacurium group. Successful intubation was achieved in ≤ 2 attempts significantly more often in the mivacurium group (35% vs 71%).

Conclusions.—Premedication with atropine, fentanyl, and mivacurium compared with atropine and fentanyl without a muscle relaxant decreases the time and number of attempts needed to successfully intubate while significantly reducing the incidence of severe desaturation. Premedication including a short-acting muscle relaxant should be considered for all nonemergent intubations in the NICU.

▶ This controlled trial of alternative premedication regimens for nonemergent neonatal intubations addresses the important question of optimal management of this common clinical circumstance. Because the chosen primary end point (ie, desaturation detected by pulse oximetry) turned out to be infelicitous, the trial was abandoned after a preliminary analysis indicated that a much larger than anticipated sample size would be required to detect a clinically significant difference. After the Bonferroni correction, no significant difference was found in various measures of desaturation or other vital signs between the groups managed with or without mivacurium before the intubation attempt. However, both the duration of the procedure and laryngoscopy time (secondary end points) were significantly greater in the group not given mivacurium ($P < .005$ for both measures), and intubation was more frequently achieved in 2 or fewer attempts after mivacurium. No statistical analysis is provided, but it is essentially certain that the duration of neuromuscular paralysis and the concomitant requirement for positive pressure ventilation was significantly greater in the mivacurium group (mean of at least 11.5 minutes) than in control subjects (mean likely close to 0 minutes). It is not clear whether the benefits of more rapid completion of the procedure are outweighed by potential adverse effects of assisted ventilation during recovery from neuromuscular blockade. This preliminary report suggests that this question will be very difficult to answer.

W. E. Benitz, MD

Prospective Evaluation of Postnatal Steroid Administration: A 1-Year Experience From the California Perinatal Quality Care Collaborative
Finer NN, for the California Perinatal Quality Care Collaborative Executive Committee (Univ of California San Diego; et al)
Pediatrics 117:704-713, 2006   13–5

Objective.—Postnatal steroids (PNSs) are used frequently to prevent or treat chronic lung disease (CLD) in the very low birth weight (VLBW) infant, and their use continues despite concerns regarding an increased incidence of longer-term neurodevelopmental abnormalities in such infants. More recently, there has been a suggestion that corticosteroids may be a useful alternative therapy for hypotension in VLBW infants, but there have been no prospective reports of such use for a current cohort of VLBW infants.

Methods.—The California Perinatal Quality Care Collaborative (CPQCC) requested members to supplement their routine Vermont Oxford Network data collection with additional information on any VLBW infant treated during their hospital course with PNS, for any indication. The indication, actual agent used, total initial daily dose, age at treatment, type of respiratory support, mean airway pressure, fraction of inspired oxygen, and duration of first dosing were recorded.

Results.—From April 2002 to March 2003 in California, 22 of the 62 CPQCC hospitals reported supplemental data, if applicable, from a cohort of 1401 VLBW infants (expanded data group [EDG]), representing 33.2% of the VLBW infants registered with the CPQCC during the 12-month period. PNSs for CLD were administered to 8.2% of all VLBW infants in 2003, 8.6% of infants in the 42 hospitals that did not submit supplemental data (routine data-set group, compared with 7.6% in EDG hospitals). Of the 1401 VLBW infants in the EDG, 19.3% received PNSs; 3.6% received PNSs for only CLD, 11.8% for only non-CLD indications, and 4.0% for both indications. At all birth weight categories, non-CLD use was significantly greater than CLD use. The most common non-CLD indication was hypotension, followed by extubation stridor, for which 36 (16.3%) infants were treated. For hypotension, medications used were hydrocortisone followed by dexamethasone. Infants treated with PNSs exclusively for hypotension had a significantly higher incidence of intraventricular hemorrhage, periventricular leukomalacia, and death when compared with infants treated only for CLD or those who did not receive PNSs.

Conclusions.—The common early use of hydrocortisone for hypotension and the high morbidity and mortality in children receiving such treatment has not been recognized previously and prospective trials evaluating the short- and long-term risk/benefit of such treatment are urgently required.

▶ This study reports on the frequent use of PNSs for the management of refractory hypotension in premature neonates in California during the period April 2002 to March 2003. In this cohort, the use of steroids for non-chronic lung disease (CLD) indications, primarily hypotension, far exceeded use for CLD. The authors conclude that prospective trials evaluating the risks and benefits of such steroid use are urgently needed.

Glucocorticoid therapy for hypotension is usually started in the first few days after birth. In this report, the first dose was begun at a median age of 2 days and treatment was continued for a median of 3 days. The need for further study of the potential toxicity of this therapy is strongly supported by the analysis of postnatal glucocorticoid therapy for CLD in the Cochrane database. The Cochrane reviews indicate that the incidence of cerebral palsy (CP), or CP or death, was significantly increased only when glucocorticoids were initiated within the first 96 hours after birth.[1] There was no significant increase in CP, or CP or death, when glucocorticoid therapy was initiated during the second week[2] or after the third week.[3] Thus, the Cochrane analyses indicate that postnatal glucocorticoids are potentially neurotoxic when they are used in the first week after birth to prevent bronchopulmonary dysplasia (BPD). They do not appear to have significant neurotoxicity when used later to manage existing BPD. This observation is supported by the analysis of Doyle et al[4] that revealed that the higher the risk of BPD in the control group, the lower the risk of steroid induced CNS toxicity. (In their report on postnatal steroids, the American Academy of Pediatrics[5] overlooked, or failed to report, the fact that in the studies they quoted there was a significant increase in neurotoxicity only in those studies in which steroids were used in the first week after birth and in the O'Shea study, in which steroids were administered for 6 weeks and in which there was an increased incidence of CP, but not CP or death.)

The questions of optimal dose and duration of glucocorticoid therapy for refractory hypotension have also not been resolved. The usual starting dose of hydrocortisone is approximately 1 mg/kg every 12 hours. It is possible that lower doses are effective. In addition, initial therapy should be as short as possible. The experience with the use of postnatal glucocorticoids for CLD has revealed that the administration of excessive doses for unnecessarily prolonged periods was recommended in a number of studies. Trials evaluating indications, dose, duration, effectiveness, and short- and long-term side effects of the use of glucocorticoids for the management of refractory hypotension in the premature infant are indeed urgently required.

I. Gross, MD

References

1. Halliday HL, Ehrenkranz RA, Doyle LW. Early postnatal (<96 hours) corticosteroids for preventing chronic lung disease in preterm infants. *Cochrane Database Syst Rev.* 2003;1:CD001146.
2. Halliday HL, Ehrenkranz RA, Doyle LW. Moderately early (7-14 days) postnatal corticosteroids for preventing chronic lung disease in preterm infants. *Cochrane Database Syst Rev.* 2003;1:CD001144.
3. Halliday HL, Ehrenkranz RA, Doyle LW. Delayed (> 3 weeks) postnatal corticosteroids for preventing chronic lung disease in preterm infants. *Cochrane Database Syst Rev.* 2003;1:CD001145.
4. Doyle LW, Halliday HL, Ehrenkranz RA, Davis PG, Sinclair JC. Impact of postnatal systemic corticosteroids on mortality and cerebral palsy in preterm infants: effect modification by risk for chronic lung disease. *Pediatrics.* 2005;115:655-661.
5. Blackmon LR, Bell EF, Engle WA, et al, for the Committee on Fetus and Newborn. Postnatal corticosteroids to treat or prevent chronic lung disease in preterm infants. *Pediatrics.* 2002;109:330-338.

Intravenous Morphine and Topical Tetracaine for Treatment of Pain in Preterm Neonates Undergoing Central Line Placement

Taddio A, Lee C, Yip A, et al (Univ of Toronto; Mount Sinai Hosp, Toronto; New York Med College, Valhalla)

JAMA 295:793-800, 2006   13–6

Context.—There is limited evidence of the analgesic effectiveness of opioid analgesia or topical anesthesia during central line placement in neonates, and there are no previous studies of their relative effectiveness.

Objective.—To determine the effectiveness and safety of topical tetracaine, intravenous morphine, or tetracaine plus morphine for alleviating pain in ventilated neonates during central line placement.

Design, Setting, and Participants.—Randomized, double-blind, controlled trial enrolling 132 ventilated neonates (mean gestational age, 30.6 [SD, 4.6] weeks at study entry) and conducted between October 2000 and July 2005 in 2 neonatal intensive care units in Toronto, Ontario.

Interventions.—Prior to central line insertion, neonates were randomly assigned to receive tetracaine (n = 42), morphine (n = 38), or both (n = 31); a separate nonrandomized group of 21 neonates receiving neither tetracaine nor morphine was used as a control group.

Main Outcome Measures.—The primary outcome measure was a pain score for the proportion of time neonates displayed facial grimacing (brow bulge) during different phases of the procedure (skin preparation, needle puncture, and recovery). In randomized neonates, safety assessments included blood pressure, ventilatory support, and local skin reactions.

Results.—Compared with no treatment, pain scores were lower in the morphine and tetracaine-morphine groups during skin preparation (mean difference, −0.22; 95% confidence interval [CI], −0.4 to −0.04; $P = .02$ and −0.29; 95% CI, −0.49 to −0.09; $P = .01$, respectively), and needle

TABLE 3.—Mean Difference in Proportion of Time Brow Bulge Was
Observed During Central Line Placement

	Mean Difference (95% Confidence Interval)	P Value
Skin preparation phase		
Tetracaine vs no analgesia	0.02 (−0.16 to 0.20)	.86
Morphine vs no analgesia	−0.22 (−0.40 to −0.04)	.02
Tetracaine + morphine vs no analgesia	−0.29 (−0.49 to −0.09)	.01
Morphine vs tetracaine	−0.24 (−0.40 to −0.08)	.003
Morphine + tetracaine vs tetracaine	−0.30 (−0.48 to −0.12)	.001
Morphine + tetracaine vs morphine	−0.07 (−0.25 to 0.11)	.45
Needle puncture phase		
Tetracaine vs no analgesia	−0.20 (−0.42 to 0.02)	.09
Morphine vs no analgesia	−0.35 (−0.57 to −0.13)	.003
Tetracaine + morphine vs no analgesia	−0.47 (−0.71 to −0.24)	<.001
Morphine vs tetracaine	−0.15 (−0.35 to 0.05)	.12
Morphine + tetracaine vs tetracaine	−0.27 (−0.49 to −0.05)	.01
Morphine + tetracaine vs morphine	−0.11 (−0.33 to 0.11)	.28

(Courtesy of Taddio A, Lee C, Yip A, et al. Intravenous morphine and topical tetracaine for treatment of pain in preterm neonates undergoing central line placement. *JAMA*. 295:793-800. Copyright 2006, American Medical Association.)

puncture (mean difference, −0.35; 95% CI, −0.57 to −0.13; P = .003 and −0.47; 95% CI, −0.71 to −0.24; P<.001, respectively), but pain scores did not differ statistically for tetracaine alone vs no treatment. Pain scores were lower for morphine and tetracaine-morphine vs tetracaine during the skin preparation phase and for tetracaine-morphine vs tetracaine during needle puncture. Compared with neonates without morphine, morphine-treated neonates required larger increases in ventilation rate in the first 12 hours (mean difference, 3.9/min; 95% CI, 1.3-6.5/min; P = .003). Local skin reactions occurred in 30% of neonates given tetracaine vs 0% for morphine (risk difference, 0.30; 95% CI, 0.19-0.41; P<.001) (Table 3).

Conclusion.—In this study of ventilated neonates undergoing central line placement, morphine and tetracaine plus morphine provided superior analgesia to tetracaine; however, morphine caused respiratory depression and tetracaine caused erythema.

▶ When neonatal intensive care was first applied in the 1960s, the equipment was primitive and so, too, was the approach to pain management. Indeed, awareness of the need to manage pain was below the radar screen. We have come a long way, but are still searching for the optimal management for the many painful procedures to which neonates are subjected. We have become aware, too, that nonpharmacological methods are effective in reducing the signs of pain. The combination of oral sucrose and pacifiers reduce pain scores during procedures, and other simple measures, including facilitated tucking and skin-to-skin contact, might also be effective. For example, Ludington-Hoe et al,[1] working in our own nursery, reported that Kangaroo Care positioning before and during heel stick is a simple and inexpensive analgesic intervention to ameliorate pain in stable premature infants. Boyle et al[2] established that nonnutritive sucking reduced distress responses in infants undergoing screening for retinopathy of prematurity. Stevens et al[3] were able to show that consistent management of painful procedures with sucrose plus pacifier was effective and safe for preterm neonates during their stay in the neonatal intensive care unit. Leslie and Marlow[4] plea for better organization of care to reduce exposure to painful procedures because there is some evidence of long-term improvement in pain sensitivity following the introduction of pain reduction programs. However, Taddio et al draw attention to the risk-benefit ratio. Tetracaine was associated with a great deal of skin irritation and morphine, the most potent and effective analgesic, not surprisingly suppressed the respiratory effort. It will take more diligent observations and further trials to determine the optimal pain management strategies. Until then we will need to combine non-pharmacologic with pharmacologic methods and closely observe the infants for side effects.

A. A. Fanaroff, MD

References

1. Ludington-Hoe SM, Hosseini R, Torowicz DL. Skin to skin contact (Kangaroo Care) analgesia for preterm infant heel stick. *AACN Clin Issues*. 2005;16:373-387.
2. Boyle EM, Freer Y, Khan-Orakzai Z, et al. Sucrose and non-nutritive sucking for the relief of pain in screening for retinopathy of prematurity: a randomised controlled trial. *Arch Dis Child Fetal Neonatal Ed*. 2006;91:F166-F168.
3. Stevens B, Yamada J, Beyene J, et al. Consistent management of repeated procedural pain with sucrose in preterm neonates: is it effective and safe for repeated use over time? *Clin J Pain*. 2005;21:543-548.
4. Leslie A, Marlow N. Non pharmacological pain relief. *Semin Fetal Neonatal Med*. 2006;11:246-250.

Intra- and interindividual variability of glucuronidation of paracetamol during repeated administration of propacetamol in neonates
Allegaert K, de Hoon J, Verbesselt R, et al (Univ Hosp, Leuven, Belgium; Sophia's Children Hosp, Rotterdam, The Netherlands)
Acta Paediatr 94:1273-1279, 2005   13–7

Background.—Major changes in drug clearance and metabolism are observed during infancy, in part based on ontogenic regulation of various metabolic pathways. Since paracetamol provides a good substrate to study UGT (1A6) activity, urinary metabolites of propacetamol were determined in neonates in whom propacetamol was repeatedly administered.

Methods.—Paracetamol glucuronide (APAP-G), paracetamol sulphate (APAP-S) and free paracetamol were determined in urine samples of neonates during repeated administration of propacetamol. Spearman rank and linear multiple regression (MedCal®, Mariakerke, Belgium) were used to study the effect of postnatal age, of postconceptional age and of repeated administration on the relative contribution of APAP-G to overall urine paracetamol (APAP-G + APAP-S + free paracetamol) elimination (G/T ratio).

Results.—147 samples were collected in 23 neonates. Molar median G/T ratio was 14% (range 1–53). Besides increasing G/T ratio with increasing postnatal ($p < 0.0001$) and postconceptional age ($p < 0.01$), repeated administration ($p < 0.01$) also correlated with an increasing G/T ratio, and repeated administration remained significant ($p < 0.01$) after correction of postnatal and postconceptional age in a multiple regression model.

Conclusion.—Major variability in the ontogeny of UGT activity to overall elimination of paracetamol was documented in neonates. Besides postnatal and postconceptional age, a significant effect of repeated administration on UGT activity was documented.

▶ The ontogenic timeline for many physiologic processes involved in human drug metabolism have been well described.[1,2] The availability of highly sensitive and specific methodologies has permitted the description of the initial expression of many drug metabolizing systems and transporters during fetal life and their maturational patterns through birth, infancy, and childhood. Nowhere in the age spectrum of pediatrics are these maturational changes so rapid, diverse, and continuous within a very short period of time than in neonatal practice. Knowledge of these ontogenic patterns serves as the foundation for the design of optimal drug dose regimens for neonatal ICU patients and all pediatric patients.

To date, research and practice has focused on the ontogenic patterns of the cytochrome P450 mono-oxygenase system, a super family of enzymes responsible for the metabolism of a number of endogenous and exogenous substances, including drugs.[1-3] Numerous investigators have described the developmental patterns of enzyme expression in the fetus from the time of initial function to final full activity, relative to patient age. The cytochrome P (CYP) isoforms responsible for the metabolism of drugs commonly used in the neonatal ICU include CYP1A2 (eg, caffeine and theophylline), CYP2C9 (eg, ibuprofen), CYP2C19 (eg, proton pump inhibitors, phenobarb, and indomethacin), CYP2D6 (selective serotonin reuptake inhibitors), and CYP3A4,5,7 (eg, erythromycin, benzodiazepines, dexamethasone, and fentanyl). Although this information has been pivotal to the design of effective dosage regimens for these drugs in neonatal ICU patients, substantial variability in the systemic drug exposure among patients remains when usual weight-based doses are administered.[1-3]

This article by Allegaert and colleagues adds to their research team's series of publications assessing the ontogeny of human phase II drug metabolism. In contrast to CYP-mediated drug metabolism (phase I), phase II reactions are often referred to as biosynthetic because these processes involve the conjugation of endogenous compounds/drugs with molecules (eg, glucuronide, sulfate, glutathione) to enhance product solubility and subsequent elimination via the bile and/or urine.[1,3] Like the CYPs, phase II enzymes metabolize a wide variety of inherently endogenous substances as well as a diverse range of hydrophobic substances introduced into the body by intent or environmental exposure. However, far less is known about the ontogeny of phase II reactions compared with the wealth of data describing phase I activity.[1-3] Nevertheless, pediatric practitioners are very well aware of the importance of these metabolic processes because a phase II enzyme (UGT1A1) is responsible for catalyzing bilirubin conjugation with glucuronic acid for efficient, nontoxic elimination.[4] Commonly used drugs in the neonatal ICU that undergo partial or complete phase II metabolism include acetaminophen, codeine, ibuprofen, morphine, and propofol.

The UGTs catalyze the conjugation of hydrophobic compounds into hydrophilic compounds that are usually inactive or of reduced activity compared with the parent compound. At least 15 different human UGTs have been identified, and based on sequence homologies, they have been divided into 2 distinct families: UGT1 and UGT2. These enzymes are found inside and outside of the liver, and individual enzymes demonstrate broad and overlapping substrate specificities.[1,3,4] The functional capacity of nearly all UGT enzymes is very low at birth, influenced by gestational and postnatal ages and, as shown by Allegaert and colleagues, by substrate exposure (ie, single-dose vs repeated drug administration). Moreover, like certain CYPs that exhibit polymorphic expression (eg, 1A2, 2C19, and 2D6), poor metabolizers have been identified in select UGTs. Thus, it is not surprising that substantial intrapatient and interpatient variability is observed in drug metabolism characteristics for drugs metabolized via a phase II pathway. An increasing number of studies like that of Allegaert and colleagues are appearing and will increasingly appear in the literature assessing the influence of age on phase II enzymatic activity. These and other investigators will continue to study the disposition of therapeutically administered drugs as probes to assess specific UGT and CYP enzyme activity. Acetaminophen, in the present study, was simply the probe to assess UGT1A6 activity, and their finding of substantial variability is consistent with reports evaluating other UGTs in the neonatal period as well as what has been reported in adults.[5] Recognizing that many drugs may undergo metabolic conversion by 1 or more CYPs before undergoing phase II metabolism (eg, acetaminophen, codeine, ibuprofen, and others) via 1 or more UGTs and that many of these enzymes exhibit polymorphic expression, the degree of variability observed is not surprising. Our challenge is to acquire the knowledge that accounts for the multiple interrelationships/dependencies between the many different drug-metabolizing enzymes and transporters and the influence of age and/or disease on these processes. Only with such information can we achieve the goal of designing highly precise, individualized drug dose regimens for individual patients.

M. D. Reed, PharmD, FCCP, FCP

References

1. Johnson TJ. The development of drug metabolizing enzymes and their influence on the susceptibility to adverse drug reactions in children. *Toxicology.* 2003;192:37-48.
2. Blake MJ, Castro L, Leeder JS, Kearns GL. Ontogeny of drug metabolizing enzymes in the neonate. *Semin Fetal Neonatal Med.* 2005;10:123-138.
3. Alcorn J, McNamara PJ. Ontogeny of hepatic and renal systemic clearance pathways in infants: part I. *Clin Pharmacokinet.* 2002;41:959-998.

4. Kaplan M, Hammerman C, Maisels MJ. Bilirubin genetics for the nongeneticist: hereditary defects of neonatal bilirubin conjugation. *Pediatrics.* 2003;111: 886-893.

5. Krishnaswamy S, Hao Q, Al-Rohaimi A, et al. UDP glucuronosyltransferase (UGT) 1A6 pharmacogenetics: II. Functional impact of the three most common nonsynonymous UGT1A6 polymorphisms (S7A, T181A) and R184S). *J Pharmacol Exp Ther.* 2005;313:1340-1346.

14 Miscellaneous

Sudden infant death syndrome and sleeping position in pre-term and low birth weight infants: an opportunity for targeted intervention
Blair PS, for the CESDI SUDI Research Group (Univ of Bristol, England; Royal Victoria Infirmary, Newcastle upon Tyne, England; Nuffield Inst for Health, Leeds, England)
Arch Dis Child 91:101-106, 2006   14–1

Aims.—To determine the combined effects of sudden infant death syndrome (SIDS) risk factors in the sleeping environment for infants who were "small at birth" (pre-term (<37 weeks), low birth weight (<2500 g), or both).

Methods.—A three year population based, case-control study in five former health regions in England (population 17.7 million) with 325 cases and 1300 controls. Parental interviews were carried out after each death and reference sleep of age matched controls.

Results.—Of the SIDS infants, 26% were "small at birth" compared to 8% of the controls. The most common sleeping position was supine, for both controls (69%) and those SIDS infants (48%) born at term or ≥2500 g, but for "small at birth" SIDS infants the commonest sleeping position was side (48%). The combined effect of the risk associated with being "small at birth" and factors in the infant sleeping environment remained multiplicative despite controlling for possible confounding in the multivariate model. This effect was more than multiplicative for those infants placed to sleep on their side or who shared the bed with parents who habitually smoked, while for those "small at birth" SIDS who slept in a room separate from the parents, the large combined effect showed evidence of a significant interaction. No excess risk was identified from bed sharing with non-smoking parents for infants born at term or birth weight ≥2500 g.

Conclusion.—The combined effects of SIDS risk factors in the sleeping environment and being pre-term or low birth weight generate high risks for these infants. Their longer postnatal stay allows an opportunity to target parents and staff with risk reduction messages.

► The authors of this study present their analysis of data collected from the Confidential Enquiry into Stillbirths and Deaths in Infancy Study specifically designed to examine sudden unexpected deaths in infancy (known as the CESDI SUDI study). Sudden infant death syndrome (SIDS) makes up a large subset of sudden unexpected death in infancy. This article is the most recent in a series of articles that have been published using these data to examine a number of variables related to SIDS such as sleeping position, smoking, bed sharing, and sleeping environment.[1-4]

Data from the CESDI SUDI study have been very useful to researchers and have contributed to knowledge about the epidemiology of and risk factors associated with SIDS in part because it is a large, carefully designed and implemented case-control study. For each case identified, there were 4 matched controls. The study covered 5 health regions in England with 473,000 live births during the study period and 363 identified eligible cases. Ninety percent of the families of the infants as well as all families of controls were interviewed by trained researchers who conducted the extensive interview by using standardized forms shortly after the death of the infant. The demographics of the participants closely matched the demographics of the study region. The authors acknowledge that one limitation to the study was the lack of ethnic and racial diversity in the study sample, limiting the degree to which the findings might be generalized to a more diverse population.[3]

In this study, the authors have focused on infant care practices known to be associated with SIDS such as bed sharing, maternal smoking, and infant sleeping position, specifically in infants who are "small at birth." By small at birth they refer to infants born preterm (<37 weeks) and/or low birth weight (<2500 g). The authors found that being born preterm or weighing less than 2500 g put infants at risk for SIDS. In addition, like term infants who were not small, those considered small at birth were at increased risk of SIDS when placed in the nonsupine position. Being small at birth and in the nonsupine position appeared to have a multiplicative affect. Other particularly important risk factors for small-at-birth infants included sleeping with a parent who smoked and sleeping alone in another room. The authors argue that some of these risk factors are modifiable, especially infant sleeping position, and that it is important to educate families of small-at-birth infants to always place their infants in the supine position for sleep. Although some hospital staff members have been shown to be resistant to placing infants in the supine position for sleep,[5] this role modeling in the hospital can change the infant care practices of parents thus decreasing the risk of SIDS in this particularly vulnerable group of infants.[6]

E. R. Colson, MD

References

1. Fleming PJ, Blair PS, Bacon C, et al. Environment of infants during sleep and risk of sudden infant death syndrome: results of the 1993-95 case-control study for confidential inquiry into still births and deaths of infancy. Confidential Enquiry into Stillbirths and Deaths Regional Coordinators and Researchers. *BMJ.* 1996;313:191-195.
2. Blair PS, Fleming PJ, Bensley D, et al. Smoking and the sudden infant death syndrome: results from 1993-95 case control study for confidential inquiry into stillbirths and deaths in infancy. Confidential Enquiry into Stillbirths and Deaths Regional Coordinators and Researchers. *BMJ.* 1996;313;195-198.
3. Leach CE, Blair PS, Fleming PJ, et al. Epidemiology of SIDS and explained sudden infant deaths. CESDI SUDI Research Group. *Pediatrics.* 1999;104:e43.

4. Blair PS, Fleming PJ, Smith IJ, et al. Babies sleeping with parents: case-control study of factors influencing the risk of the sudden infant death syndrome. CESDI SUDI Research Group. *BMJ.* 1999;319:1457-1461.
5. Hein HA, Pettit SF. Back to sleep: good advice for parents but not for hospitals? *Pediatrics.* 2001;107:537-539.
6. Colson ER, Joslin SC. Changing nursery practice gets inner-city infants in the supine position for sleep. *Arch Pediatr Adolesc Med.* 2002;156:717-720.

Longitudinal changes in bone health as assessed by the speed of sound in very low birth weight preterm infants

Tomlinson C, McDevitt H, Ahmed SF, et al (Princess Royal Maternity Hosp, Glasgow; Queen Mother's Hosp, Glasgow; Southern Gen Hosp, Glasgow; et al)

J Pediatr 148:450-455, 2006   14–2

Objective.—To assess longitudinal changes in speed of sound (SOS) in very low birth weight (VLBW) infants and investigate the relationship with markers of osteopathy of prematurity (OP) and clinical illness.

Study Design.—Twenty-five infants were recruited. Eighteen infants, median gestation 27 weeks (range 24–32), median birth weight 957 g (range 625–1500 g), had serial scans. SOS was measured at both tibiae weekly until 35 to 37 weeks corrected gestational age (CGA).

Results.—Initial median SOS standard deviation score (SDS) (Z) score was -0.07 (range -1.3–1.3). SOS correlated with gestation (r, 0.8, $P <.005$), and birth weight (r, 0.67, $P <.005$.) SOS fell from a median of 2923 m/s (2672–3107) at birth to 2802 m/s (2502–2991) at 35 to 37 weeks CGA ($P <.05$). This fall was greater in the 24- to 27-week gestation cohort with a median reduction of 2.2 SDS (1.6, 4.0) compared with 1.3 SDS (0.8–2.2) in those >28 weeks ($P <.05$). There was a negative correlation between SOS, at the end of the study, peak serum alkaline phosphatase (ALP) (r, 0.6, $P <.05$), CRIB (Clinical Risk Index for Babies)/CRIB II scores (both r, 0.6, $P <.05$), and duration of total parenteral nutrition (TPN) (r, 0.58, $P <.05$).

Conclusions.—Although tibial SOS was within the expected range at birth, there was a subsequent failure to gain SOS, and this was most marked in infants of a lower gestation.

▶ Here is another potential application of portable US in the neonatal unit. A larger study may be able to show equivalent or perhaps increased efficacy compared with current biochemical markers. As this was a small study, there was no mention of the use of SOS to predict fractures. Although the final SOS measurements correlated with risk factors and somewhat with biochemical markers, the initial SOS measurements and changes in measurements over the weeks of hospitalization were not able to predict final SOS. By the time one figures out that the final SOS was abnormal, it may perhaps be too late to intervene.

Again, we see that the sickest babies at birth are also the ones at higher risk for later morbidities. As SOS correlated strongly with gestational age, the superiority of in utero bone mineralization is also demonstrated, telling us that when possible, the avoidance of premature delivery is a continued goal. Also, according to the reference ranges used in this study, essentially all infants ended up with an abnormal SOS by discharge. Perhaps in the future an adjusted curve according to gestational age can be constructed, progressing beyond 40 weeks postconceptional age in order to see when "catch up" may occur for most preterm infants. At this time, SOS will remain a research tool until correlation with relevant outcomes can be established and its use as a diagnostic tool can subsequently be found to improve those outcomes.

H. C. Lee, MD

Costs of Newborn Care in California: A Population-Based Study
Schmitt SK, Sneed L, Phibbs CS (Veterans Affairs Palo Alto Health Care System, Calif; Stanford Univ, Calif)
Pediatrics 117:154-160, 2006   14–3

Objective.—We sought to describe the current costs of newborn care by using population-based data, which includes linked vital statistics and hospital records for both mothers and infants. These data allow costs to be reported by episode of care (birth), instead of by hospitalization.

Methods.—Data for this study were obtained from the linked 2000 California birth cohort data. These data ($n = 518,704$), provided by the California Office of Statewide Health Planning and Development (OSHPD), contain infant vital statistics data (birth and death certificate data) linked to infant and maternal hospital discharge summaries. In addition to the infant and maternal hospital discharge summaries associated with delivery, these data include discharge summaries for all infant hospital-to-hospital transfers and maternal prenatal hospitalizations. The linkage algorithm that is used by OSHPD in creating the linked cohort data file is highly accurate. More than 99% of the maternal and infant discharge abstracts were linked successfully with the birth certificates. These data were also linked successfully with the infant discharge abstracts from the receiving hospital for 99% of the infants who were transferred to another hospital. The hospital discharge records were the source of the hospital charges and length-of-stay information summarized in this study. Hospital costs were estimated by adjusting charges by hospital-specific ratios of costs to charges obtained from the OSHPD Hospital Financial Reporting data. Costs, lengths of stay, and mortality were summarized by birth weight groups, gestational age, cost categories, and types of admissions.

Results.—Low birth weight (LBW) and very low birth weight (VLBW) infants had significantly longer hospital stays and accounted for a significantly higher proportion of total hospital costs. The average hospital stay for LBW infants ranged from 6.2 to 68.1 days, whereas the average hospital stay for infants who weighed >2500 g at birth was 2.3 days. Overall, VLBW infants accounted for 0.9% of cases but 35.7% of costs, whereas LBW infants accounted for 5.9% of cases but 56.6% of total hospital costs. Although total maternal and infant costs were similar (~\$1.6 billion), the distribution of maternal costs was much less skewed. For infants, 5% of infants accounted for 76% of total infant hospital costs. Conversely, the most expensive 3% of deliveries accounted for only 17% of total maternal costs.

Conclusions.—The very smallest infants make up a hugely disproportionate share of costs; more than half of all neonatal costs are incurred by LBW or premature infants. Maternal costs are similar in magnitude to newborn costs, but they are much less skewed than for infants. Preventing premature deliveries could yield very large cost savings, in addition to saving lives.

▶ To investigate the costs of neonatal care requires an analytic approach that considers both mother and infant in terms of their total care. For the mother, total care must include prenatal hospitalization as well as natal hospitalization. For the infant, especially in an era of regionalization, the perspective must be one that links all hospital-to-hospital transfers. Finally, from the perinatal point of view, it is important to assess the relative contributions of maternal and infant costs across categories of risk such as birth weight and gestational age. Using an extensively linked California dataset, the authors have addressed these technical difficulties in what will surely become a landmark investigation. While some of the findings provide a quantitative estimate for what has been well-established by clinical experience (eg, VLBW infants account for only 0.9% of cases but 35.7% of costs and the 2.1% of predominantly term infants with a major congenital anomaly account for another 25.5% of costs), the study provides many important new findings, especially when comparing maternal and infant costs across birth weight categories. The authors found that maternal costs tend to be more equally distributed across birth weight than do infant costs, although the total maternal and infant costs are approximately equal. They also point out the importance of prenatal admissions when estimating the costs of birth and report that 1 maternal admission does not result in delivery for every 11 deliveries. While some might question the ultimate validity of estimating costs from hospital charges, the relative differences in magnitude across birth weight and gestational age seem quite reasonable and provide a great deal of insight on costs of hospitalization. This insight, while precise and profound, addresses only 1 aspect of the cost of newborn care: the cost associated with hospitalization. Costs to the family, to the infant's life course, and to society are areas of great concern that remain largely undefined.

J. B. Gould, MD, MPH

---

6 weeks with the von Rosen splint is sufficient for treatment of neonatal hip instability
Lauge-Pedersen H, Gustafsson J, Hägglund G (Lund Univ, Sweden)
Acta Orthop Scand 77:257-261, 2006   14–4

Background.—There is no concensus on the optimal treatment time for unstable hips in the newborn. We analyzed the efficiency of a treatment pro-

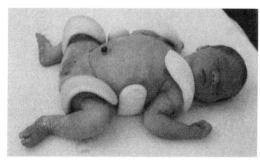

FIGURE 1.—The von Rosen splint. (Courtesy of Lauge-Pedersen H, Gustafsson J, Hägglund. 6 weeks with the von rosen splint is sufficient for treatment of neonatal hip instability. *Acta Orthop Scand.* 2006;77:257-261. Available at http://www.informaworld.com)

gram that has been used for 10 years at our hospital, in which all unstable hips (subluxatable, Barlow-positive and Ortolani-positive) are treated with the von Rosen splint for 6 weeks.

Patients and Methods.—Between 1988 and 1997, 32,171 children were born alive at the hospital. During this period 247 children had a clinically unstable hip diagnosed. 223 of the 247 children underwent a radiographic follow-up after 5–15 years.

Results.—1 patient with bilateral instability and treated with a splint for 6 weeks showed a dislocated left hip at the radiographic examination at 8 months, which is part of the screening program, and needed operative treatment. 1 patient did not follow the treatment program and showed a dislocated hip at the age of 3. Another 4 patients required more treatment than the 6 weeks with the splint.

We found no dysplastic hips at the radiographic follow-up. There was no late dysplasia and there were no late dislocations in children born in Lund between 1988 and 1997 who were diagnosed at other Swedish centers that treat developmental dysplasia of the hip (DDH).

Interpretation.—We conclude that the present screening and 6-week treatment in a von Rosen splint prevent almost all cases of late dysplasia and late dislocation of the hip (Fig 1).

▶ Early detection and treatment of developmental dysplasia of the hip (DDH) is important because it reduces the likelihood of the adverse consequences associated with a late diagnosis. To aid in the early diagnosis and management of DDH, the American Academy of Pediatrics published clinical practice guidelines in 2000.[1] Since about 60% of all unstable hips found on newborn examinations resolve within the first 2 to 4 weeks of life, common practice includes early observation, with or without an ultrasound examination, and then follow-up by an orthopedist if hip joint laxity persists. Initial treatment of DDH is usually a brace, such as the Pavlik harness, that holds the hip in flexion and abduction.

In this article, Lauge-Pedersen et al describe their experience using a standardized management plan that included treatment with the von Rosen splint (Fig 1) for the treatment of neonatal hip instability, defined as subluxatable (unstable, but not dislocatable) and Barlow-positive and/or Ortolani-positive hips. During a 10-year period they identified and treated 247 infants with unstable hips from a population of 32,171 live births; 244 of those infants had stable hips after being treated with the von Rosen splint for 6 weeks. Ninety percent (223) of the treated children had a radiographic follow-up 5 to 15 years later; 217 of them had no evidence of DDH at that time. Thus, the investigators have confirmed the benefit of early identification and management of instability of the neonatal hip with the von Rosen splint on reducing the occurrence of DDH.

R. A. Ehrenkranz, MD

Reference

1. American Academy of Pediatrics. Committee on Quality Improvement, Subcommittee on Developmental Dysplasia of the Hip. Clinical practice guideline: early detection of developmental dysplasia of the hip. *Pediatrics.* 2000;105:896-905.

15 Postnatal Growth and Development/Follow-up

Long term effects of antenatal betamethasone on lung function: 30 year follow up of a randomised controlled trial
Dalziel SR, Rea HH, Walker NK, et al (Univ of Auckland, New Zealand)
Thorax 61:678-683, 2006   15–1

Background.—Antenatal betamethasone is routinely used for the prevention of neonatal respiratory distress syndrome in preterm infants. However, little is known of the long term effects of exposure to antenatal betamethasone on lung function in adulthood.

Methods.—Five hundred and thirty four 30 year olds whose mothers had participated in the first and largest randomised controlled trial of antenatal betamethasone were followed. Lung function was assessed by portable spirometric testing. The prevalence of asthma symptoms was assessed using the European Community Respiratory Health Survey questionnaire.

Results.—Fifty (20%) betamethasone exposed and 53 (19%) placebo exposed participants met the criteria for current asthma (relative risk 0.98 (95% CI 0.74 to 1.30), p = 0.89). 181 betamethasone exposed and 202 placebo exposed participants had acceptable spirometric data. There were no differences in lung function between betamethasone and placebo exposed groups (mean (SD) forced vital capacity in the betamethasone and placebo groups 105.9 (12.0) *v* 106.6 (12.6)% predicted, difference = −0.7 (95% CI −3.2 to 1.8), p = 0.59; mean (SD) forced expiratory volume in 1 second in the betamethasone and placebo groups 98.9 (13.4) *v* 98.5 (13.6)% predicted, difference = 0.3 (95% CI −2.4 to 3.1, p = 0.80)).

Conclusions.—Antenatal exposure to a single course of betamethasone does not alter lung function or the prevalence of wheeze and asthma at age 30.

▶ The random control trials (RCT)[1] of antenatal corticosteroid treatment for prevention of respiratory distress syndrome (RDS) performed after the landmark trial of Liggins and Howie[2] did not change the conclusion that antenatal treatment significantly reduced the risk of developing RDS; the RCTs only narrowed the confidence limits around the risk difference.[3] And, as evident from this report by Dalziel et al, many of the Auckland Steroid Trial participants are still being helpful more than 30 years after the publication by Liggins and Howie. Their participation in this 30-year follow-up study has demonstrated that a single course of antenatal corticosteroids does not alter pulmonary function or the prevalence of asthma in adulthood; good news! Thus, this classic study continues to lead the way by showing us the importance of long-term follow-up of perinatal interventions and encouraging us to follow suit.

R. A. Ehrenkranz, MD

References

1. Crowley PA. Antenatal corticosteroid therapy: a meta-analysis of the randomized trials, 1972-1994. *Am J Obstet Gynecol.* 1995;173:322-335.
2. Liggins GC, Howie RN. A controlled trial of antepartum glucocorticoid treatment for prevention of the respiratory distress syndrome in premature infants. *Pediatrics.* 1972;50:515-525.
3. Sinclair JC. Meta-analysis of randomized controlled trials of antenatal corticosteroid for the prevention of respiratory distress syndrome: discussion. *Am J Obstet Gynecol.* 1995;173:335-344.

Long-term neurodevelopmental outcome and brain volume after treatment for hydrops fetalis by in utero intravascular transfusion
Harper DC, Swingle HM, Weiner CP, et al (Univ of Iowa, Iowa City; Univ of Maryland, Baltimore; Southern Illinois Univ, Springfield)
Am J Obstet Gynecol 195:192-200, 2006   15–2

Objective.—We tested the hypothesis that long-term neurodevelopmental outcomes of successfully treated fetuses with immune hydrops are similar to their unaffected siblings according to a protocol that addresses the underlying pathophysiologic condition.

Study design.—Sixteen of 18 consecutive hydropic fetuses (89%) who were treated in a dedicated fetal medicine unit between July 1985 and October 1995 survived. The transfusion protocol used a 2-step correction over a 2 to 4 day interval, combined with umbilical venous pressure measurements to avoid over transfusion and bicarbonate administration to assure a posttransfusion UV pH of >7.30. Survivors were evaluated at a mean age of 10 years. Statistical analyses included *t*-test, Wilcoxon rank-sum test, Fisher's exact test, and Pearson coefficients.

Results.—Overall, death or major neurologic morbidity occurred in 4 of 18 of the fetuses (22%) who were treated (2/16 of survivors [12.5%]). Among the survivors, the children with immune hydrops had physical, neurologic, and cognitive outcomes statistically similar to their siblings, except for a measure of visual attention. Two of the children (12%) had major neurologic sequelae. Brain volumes were statistically smaller than unrelated control subjects by 8.8%, but these control subjects were not matched for height at testing or gestational age at birth. Both groups had brain volumes within the normal range.

Conclusion.—Intravascular transfusion of fetuses with profoundly anemic immune hydrops results in high survival rates and favorable long-term neuropsychological outcomes.

▶ Whereas a search of the term hydrops fetalis yielded over 2000 references, the combination of hydrops and neurodevelopmental outcome resulted in only this publication by Harper et al. I guess that by definition this becomes a landmark publication. It is reassuring that the 10-year follow-up on these severely compromised fetuses yields such good outcomes and is a ringing endorsement for the advanced technology that made these in utero transfusions possible. Ten-year-olds are not at college and the fact that the brain volumes are smaller is of some concern, but these survival rates for hydrops fetalis are spectacular and I am encouraged because these children are performing at the same level as their peers.

A. A. Fanaroff, MD

Object working memory deficits predicted by early brain injury and development in the preterm infant

Woodward LJ, Edgin JO, Thompson D, et al (Univ of Canterbury, New Zealand; Univ of Melbourne)
Brain 128:2578-2587, 2005   15–3

Children born preterm and of very low birth weight are at increased risk of learning difficulties and educational under-achievement. However, little is known about the specific neuropsychological problems facing these children or their neurological basis. Using prospective longitudinal data from a regional cohort of 92 preterm and 103 full-term children, this study examined relations between term MRI measures of cerebral injury and structural brain development and children's subsequent performance on an object working memory task at the age of 2 years. Results revealed clear between-group differences, with preterm children having greater difficulty encoding new information in working memory than term control children. Within the preterm group, task performance at the age of 2 years was related to both qualitative MRI measures of white matter (WM) injury and quantitative measures of total and regional brain volumes assessed at term equivalent. Bilateral reductions in total tissue volumes (% region) of the following cerebral regions were specifically related to subsequent working memory performance: dorsolateral prefrontal cortex, sensorimotor, parietooccipital and premotor. Associations between total cerebral tissue volumes at term (adjusted and unadjusted for intracranial volume) persisted even after the effects of WM injury were taken into account. This suggests that early disturbance in cerebral development may have an independent adverse impact on later working memory function in the preterm infant. These findings add to our understanding of the neuropathological pathways associated with later executive dysfunction in the very preterm infant.

▶ We have all been impressed and concerned by the major findings on MRI when the preterm infants reach 40 weeks corrected age. Dyet et al[1] noted that diffuse white matter abnormalities and post-hemorrhagic ventricular dilation are common at term and seem to correlate with reduced developmental quotients. Early lesions, except for cerebellar hemorrhage and major destructive lesions did not show clear relationships with outcomes.

This elegant report by Woodward et al translates and relates abnormal structure (decreased volume) in specific areas, with function. We agree that the findings add to "our understanding of the neuropathological pathways associated with later executive dysfunction in the very preterm infant." But how do we preserve brain volume; how do we explain the infants who have these lesions without alterations in executive function, and are there any ways to restore these functions if they are identified in a timely manner?

The answers will emerge with continued follow-up of this important cohort. My colleague, Maureen Hack, who has followed preterm very low birth weight infants through to adulthood reminds me constantly that we are not able to predict the ultimate outcome, so I will remain optimistic for these children.[2-4]

A. A. Fanaroff, MD

References

1. Dyet LE, Kennea N, Counsell SJ, et al. Natural history of brain lesions in extremely preterm infants studied with serial magnetic resonance imaging from birth and neurodevelopmental assessment. *Pediatrics.* 2006;118:536-548.
2. Hack M, Costello DW. Decrease in frequency of cerebral palsy in preterm infants. *Lancet.* 2007;369:7-8.
3. Wilson-Costello D, Friedman H, Minich N, et al. Improved neurodevelopmental outcomes for extremely low birth weight infants in 2000-2002. *Pediatrics.* 2007;119:37-45.
4. Hack M, Klein N. Young adult attainments of preterm infants. *JAMA.* 2006; 295:695-696.

Cerebral Palsy Among Children Born After In Vitro Fertilization: The Role of Preterm Delivery—A Population-Based, Cohort Study
Hvidtjørn D, Grove J, Schendel DE, et al (Univ of Aarhus, Denmark; Ctrs for Disease Control and Prevention, Atlanta, Ga; Aarhus Univ Hosp, Denmark)
Pediatrics 118:475-482, 2006   15–4

Objective.—Our aim was to assess the incidence of cerebral palsy among children conceived with in vitro fertilization and children conceived without in vitro fertilization.

Methods.—A population-based, cohort study, including all live-born singletons and twins born in Denmark between January 1, 1995, and December 31, 2000, was performed. Children conceived with in vitro fertilization (9255 children) were identified through the In Vitro Fertilization Register; children conceived without in vitro fertilization (394,713) were identified through the Danish Medical Birth Register. Cerebral palsy diagnoses were obtained from the National Register of Hospital Discharges. The main outcome measure was the incidence of cerebral palsy in the in vitro fertilization and non-in vitro fertilization groups.

Results.—Children born after in vitro fertilization had an increased risk of cerebral palsy; these results were largely unchanged after adjustment for maternal age, gender, parity, small-for-gestational age status, and educational level. The independent effect of in vitro fertilization vanished after additional adjustment for multiplicity or preterm delivery. When both multiplicity and preterm delivery were included in the multivariate models, preterm delivery remained associated strongly with the risk of cerebral palsy.

Conclusions.—The large proportions of preterm deliveries with in vitro fertilization, primarily for twins but also for singletons, pose an increased risk of cerebral palsy.

▶ In vitro fertilization (IVF) treatment has been associated with an increased incidence of cerebral palsy (CP), but whether the increase is due to associations with IVF—including multiple gestations, small-for-gestational-age status, or prematurity—or IVF itself is unclear. This insightful study helps tease out the association, suggesting that the culprit is not IVF per se but prematurity, which is seen at an increased rate among IVF twin *and* singleton pregnancies.

The study is impressive in its scope and encompasses the strengths and shortcomings of large, population-based cohort studies. The Danish Medical Birth Register contains data on all births in Denmark. Since 1994, fertility clinics in Denmark have been required to report each treatment cycle to a national IVF Register. A National Register of Hospital Discharges contains data on hospital inpatient discharge codes and outpatient diagnoses. The authors obtained and linked extensive data from these databases for this analysis. The effect of assisted-reproduction on CP may have been underestimated in this study. IVF rates increased during the study period, which resulted in shorter follow-up among children born after IVF. In addition, the study group included only IVF; pregnancies resulting from hormonal treatments with intrauterine insemination or intercourse were included in the nonexposed group. We do not know how these treatments, with an attendant increase in multiple births, would affect the outcome of this study.

Regardless, the finding that prematurity among IVF pregnancies consistently and independently conferred an increased risk for CP among singletons (and more so among twins) lends weight to the argument for single-embryo transfer and the need for continued research into preterm birth prevention.

D. J. Lyell, MD

Factors Associated With Neurodevelopmental Outcome at 2 Years After Very Preterm Birth: The Population-Based Nord-Pas-de-Calais EPIPAGE Cohort

Fily A, for the EPIPAGE Nord-Pas-de-Calais Study Group (Hôpital Jeanne de Flandre, Lille, France; et al)

Pediatrics 117:357-366, 2006

15–5

Objective.—We sought to (1) evaluate at 2 years the postsurfactant era developmental outcome of children who were born before 33 weeks of gestational age (GA) in the Nord-Pas-de-Calais area in France in 1997 and (2) identify risk factors of poor developmental quotient (DQ). Children were part of the EPIPAGE study, which included all of these births in 9 French regions.

Methods.—A prospective observational study was conducted of all births before 33 weeks in 1997. Risk factors of poor DQ were obtained from a multiple linear regression, and results were expressed as DQ differences with 95% confidence intervals.

Results.—A total of 546 births were included in the study. A total of 461 (84.4%) had a clinical evaluation at 2 years of age, and 380 (69.6%) had an assessment with the use of the Brunet-Lezine scale of infant development. Their mean GA was 29.9 weeks (29.7–30.1 weeks), and mean birth weight was 1378 g (1338–1418 g). A total of 9% had a recognizable pattern of cerebral palsy, 0.2% were blind, and 0.8% required hearing aids. The mean DQ was 94 ± 11 and decreased from 97 at 32 weeks to 86 at 24 to 25 weeks. After multivariate analysis, children who were born at 24 to 25 weeks had a mean DQ reduction of 11 points (−20 to −1) compared with those who were born at 32 weeks, but minor differences were found from 26 to 32 weeks. Boys had a DQ 4 points lower than girls (−7 to −1).

Conclusion.—In this study, the outcome of extremely preterm infants was poor. After 25 weeks, outcome was related mainly to the sociocultural level of the family and to the presence of severe cerebral ultrasound abnormalities. Consequently, in the postsurfactant era, we have to propose follow-up programs to children who are born extremely preterm and to concentrate our efforts on children with less-than-optimal social and family setting.

▶ Fily et al remind us that ongoing outcome studies of children born prematurely are important as NICU care continues to evolve with medical advances. Using a prospective observational design, the authors measured neurodevelopmental outcome in infants born at less than 33 weeks' gestational age in the postsurfactant era and determined risk factors for poor outcome using multivariate analyses. The impact of gestational age on outcome was analyzed, and study results suggest that extreme prematurity (24 or 25 weeks' gestation) continues to be associated with significantly increased risk for developmental delay. Study limitations include a regional cohort with high unemployment and poor education among parents, which differs from other regions in France; significant differences in gender, parental employment, and maternal smoking between children who completed developmental testing (69.6% of enrolled subjects) and children who did not have follow-up testing; and a small number of children representing extreme prematurity in the 24- to 25-week range (19 of 546), given that the authors made conclusions with respect to this group. Despite these limitations, conclusions were consistent with previous studies. This study, which measures outcome in the postsurfactant era, suggests that although neonatal viability has improved with medical advancements, long-term disability continues to be an unresolved issue. This is especially true as the prevalence of infants born extremely premature rises. Thus, despite medical advancements, there is still plenty of work to be done to improve neonatal outcomes and an ongoing need for follow-up studies.

This study also identified maternal, family, child, and social factors that increase the risk for poor outcome. Parental unemployment and severe cerebral ultrasound abnormalities were highly significant. Importantly, the authors observed that the impact of parental unemployment, and thus socioeconomic status, on developmental outcome is comparable to the impact of extreme prematurity. The next step is to translate this information into intervention studies to determine whether concentrated resources and early intervention can alter a path believed to be destined as high risk. If we know which children are at highest risk, let's do more for them.

T. L. Sutcliffe, MD, MSc, FRCPC

The Impact of Modest Prematurity on Visual Function at Age 6 Years: Findings From a Population-Based Study
Robaei D, Kifley A, Gole GA, et al (Univ of Sydney; Univ of Queensland, Brisbane, Australia)
Arch Ophthalmol 124:871-877, 2006   15–6

Objective.—To determine the effects of modest low birth weight and prematurity on visual function of children predominantly aged 6 years.

Methods.—Children with a birth weight of 1500 to 2499 g were considered exposed to a modest low birth weight (n = 82) and were compared with children with a birth weight of 2500 g or more (n = 1386). Exposure to modest prematurity, 32 to 36 weeks' gestation (n = 115), was similarly analyzed and compared with birth at term, 37 or more weeks' gestation (n = 1446). Logarithm of the minimum angle of resolution visual acuity was measured in both eyes. Cycloplegic autorefraction (cyclopentolate), cover testing, and dilated fundus examinations were performed.

Results.—A modest low birth weight increased the risk of amblyopia (relative risk [RR], 5.1; 95% confidence interval [CI], 2.2-12.0), strabismus (RR, 3.7; 95% CI, 1.5-9.1), and anisometropia (RR, 3.7; 95% CI, 1.2-11.1), together with an increased risk of uncorrected visual acuity in the lowest quartile (RR, 1.7; 95% CI, 1.3-2.2). Modest prematurity increased the risk of amblyopia (RR, 4.5; 95% CI, 1.9-10.6), strabismus (RR, 2.6; 95% CI, 1.1-6.0), and uncorrected visual acuity in the lowest quartile (RR, 1.5; 95% CI, 1.1-2.0).

Conclusion.—Modest degrees of low birth weight and prematurity may be associated with increased ophthalmic morbidity at age 6 years.

▶ Several studies have reported an increased incidence of visual problems—including myopia, strabismus, amblyopia, and anisometropia—in the very low birth weight (<1500 g) and preterm infant with a gestational age less than 32 weeks. The American Academy of Pediatrics recommends ophthalmologic examination and follow-up for these infants. However, much less is known about visual outcomes in infants with modestly low birth weight (1500-2500 g) or those born between 32 and 36 weeks' gestation. This is an important outcome measure as these infants comprise a much higher percentage of babies in the low birth weight (<2500 g) and/or preterm (<37 weeks' gestation) category than those who are extremely premature.

In this study conducted in Australia, the investigators sought to determine the incidence of ocular morbidity in this group of infants. A population-based survey of the results of eye examinations in 6-year-old children with birth weights between 1500 and 2500 g or gestational age between 32 and 36 weeks was conducted. Data collected included measurements to assess ocular morbidities, including myopia, strabismus, amblyopia, hyperopia, astigmatism, anisometropia, and stereoscopic vision. The "exposed" group consisted of 82 children with birth weights between 1500 and 2499 g and 1386 children with birth weights greater than 2500 g, whereas the "control" group consisted of 115 children with gestational age between 32 and 36 weeks and 1446 children born at more than 36 weeks' gestation. Among the selected visual outcomes that were measured, exposed infants were found to have a 3- to 5-fold increased risk of amblyopia as well as an increased risk of anisometropia and strabismus. Although visual acuity tended to be in the lowest quartile in both modest preterm and low birth weight children, it was not statistically different compared with the more than 37-week gestational age or more than 2500-g infant. Similarly, there was no significantly increased risk of myopia or hyperopia. Exposed infants also showed a nonsignificant trend toward increased astigmatism. Infants who were both low birth weight and premature had the highest prevalence of ocular morbidity, followed by low birth weight infants (term or preterm). The modestly preterm infant with a birth weight greater than 2500 g was less likely to be affected. These data indicate both prematurity and low birth weight are risk factors for ocular morbidity.

Prior studies have shown that infants in this category tend to have a higher incidence of learning disorders and behavioral abnormalities, possibly secondary to subtle cortical defects of perinatal hypoxic-ischemic injury. The pathogenesis of amblyopia in the context of prematurity/low birth weight has not been determined but may have a similar etiology to that of the above conditions. Another possibility is there may be other causative factors, such as diet or maternal smoking, that were not evaluated in this study. The findings of this study highlight the importance of long-term ophthalmologic surveillance examinations in the borderline preterm or low birth weight infant.

A. Madan, MD

Impact of Prenatal and/or Postnatal Growth Problems in Low Birth Weight Preterm Infants on School-Age Outcomes: An 8-Year Longitudinal Evaluation

Casey PH; Whiteside-Mansell L, Barrett K, et al (Univ of Arkansas for Med Sciences, Little Rock; Univ of Arkansas, Little Rock)
Pediatrics 118:1078-1086, 2006   15–7

Objective.—The objective of this study was to assess the 8-year growth, cognitive, behavioral status, health status, and academic achievement in low birth weight preterm infants who had failure to thrive only, were small for gestational age only, had failure to thrive plus were small for gestational age, or had normal growth.

Methods.—A total of 985 infants received standardized evaluations to age 8; 180 infants met the criteria for failure to thrive between 4 and 36 months' gestational corrected age. The following outcome variables were collected at age 8: growth, cognitive, behavioral status, health status, and academic achievement. Multivariate analyses were performed among the 4 growth groups on all 8-year outcome variables.

Results.—Children who both were small for gestational age and had failure to thrive were the smallest in all growth variables at age 8, and they also demonstrated the lowest cognitive and academic achievement scores. The children with failure to thrive only were significantly smaller than the children with normal growth in all growth variables and had significantly lower IQ scores. Those who were small for gestational age only did not differ from those with normal growth in any cognitive or academic achievement measures. There were no differences among the 4 groups in behavioral status or general health status.

Conclusion.—Low birth weight preterm infants who develop postnatal growth problems, particularly when associated with prenatal growth problems, demonstrate lower physical size, cognitive scores, and academic achievement at age 8. There does not seem to be an independent affect of small for gestational age status on 8-year cognitive status and academic achievement when postnatal growth is adequate.

▶ Children born prematurely often experience periods of poor weight gain, either before birth or during childhood. This large, multisite, well-executed, longitudinal study of 985 children enrolled in the Infant Health and Development Project describes growth, health status, cognitive test scores, academic achievement, and behavioral characteristics of the low birth weight, premature infants as a function of growth patterns. Small for gestational age (SGA) was defined as weight less than the 10th percentile on the Lubchencho curves. Failure to thrive (FTT) was defined as lower than average weight gain velocity, indicated by weight less than the 5th percentile for corrected age at least 2 time points and weight gain velocity less than the mean on appropriate curves. The authors subdivided the sample into 4 groups: SGA/FTT, FTT, SGA, and normal. Children in the SGA/FTT group had the lowest weight, height, and head circumference at age 8 years. They also had lower intelligence scores, receptive vocabulary, visual-motor function, and academic achievement scores at age 8 years. In general, the FTT group had poorer outcomes than did the SGA group, although they were both worse than the normal group. Before nutritional interventions are changed, particularly after birth for children born prematurely, it is important to recognize that these data represent correlations, which do not imply causality. It is possible that weight gain either prenatally or after birth is a marker for multiple adverse factors, such as malnutrition, poor health, genetic disorders, and interactional feeding problems, all of which could contribute to the findings of this study. In addition, maternal height and weight were lower in the FTT and SGA/FTT groups in comparison with the SGA and normal groups, which suggests that familial factors may also contribute to weight, height, and, possibly, the cognitive and academic outcomes. An intervention study that randomizes assignment to usual or enhanced nutrition may elucidate whether weight gain itself contributes to outcomes.

H. M. Feldman, MD, PhD

A non-handicapped cohort of low-birthweight children: Growth and general health status at 11 years of age
Elgen I, Johansson KA, Markestad T, et al (Univ of Bergen, Norway)
Acta Paediatr 94:1203-1207, 2005   15–8

Aims.—To describe and compare physical growth, current health status, functional limitations and neurodevelopmental impairments (defined as low IQ, school problems or psychiatric disorder) at 11 y of age in a population of non-handicapped low-birthweight (LBW) children with that of normal-birthweight (NBW) children.

Methods.—A population-based sample of 130 LBW children (weighing less than 2000 g at birth) without major handicaps, and a random sample of 131 NBW children born at term. Somatic and mental health and cognitive abilities were assessed through questionnaires to parents, a physical examination, standardized tests of cognitive function (WISC-R) and a semi-structured interview (Children Assessment Schedule).

Results.—General somatic health status was similar for the LBW and NBW children. The LBW children were shorter (mean difference −2.5 cm; 95% CI −0.9 to −4.2) and had a smaller head circumference (mean difference −0.8 cm; 95% CI −0.4 to −1.1) but similar weights and body mass indices. Differences and similarities in anthropometric measures were the same at 5 and 11 y of age. The LBW children had higher systolic (mean difference 3.2 mmHg; 95% CI −0.6 to −0.3) but similar diastolic blood pressure. A higher proportion of LBW children had decreased visual acuity and hearing impairment. Forty per cent of LBW children had neurodevelopmental impairments, compared to 20% of NBW children (OR 2.6; 95% CI 1.5 to 4.5).

Conclusion.—At 11 y of age, survivors of moderately low birthweight without major handicaps may have generally good health, but are at risk of neurodevelopmental impairments.

▶ Population-based studies describing the long-term outcomes of LBW infants are preferred because they provide the best estimates of the incidence of selected problems. Therefore, this paper by Elgen et al, in which growth and general health outcomes at 11 years of age were reported in a population-based sample of all surviving infants weighing less than 2000 g at birth born between April 1, 1986 and August 8, 1988, caught my eye. There were 217 liveborn infants during the study period; 21 infants with major handicaps were excluded from evaluation (12 cerebral palsy, 8 chromosomal aberrations, and 1 deaf). A control population of NBW children was randomly identified, and comparisons of the LBW and NBW cohorts have been the subject of a number of reports[1-5] by these investigators. At 5 years of age, 174 (80%) of 217 of the eligible LBW children were examined; at 11 years of age 130 (75%) of 174 eligible LBW children and 130 (76%) of 170 eligible NBW children were examined. Among the LBW children examined at 11 years of age, 50 were VLBW and 80 weighed between 1500 and 2000 g at birth.

The authors reported that while both the moderately LBW and NBW groups had generally good health at 11 years of age, the LBW children were at greater risk of neurodevelopmental impairments. Because there are limited follow-up studies involving moderately LBW infants, especially at 11 years of age, these observations are important. Nonetheless, their generalizability may be limited because only 60% of the original LBW cohort were examined at 11 years of age.

R. A. Ehrenkranz, MD

References

1. Elgen I, Sommerfelt K. Low birthweight children: coping in school? *Acta Paediatr.* 2002;91:939-945.
2. Elgen I, Sommerfelt K, Markestad T. Population based, controlled study of behavioural problems and psychiatric disorders in low birthweight children at 11 years of age. *Arch Dis Child Fetal Neonatal Ed.* 2002;87:F128-F132.
3. Sommerfelt K, Ellertsen B, Markestad T. Parental factors in cognitive outcome of non-handicapped low birthweight infants. *Arch Dis Child Fetal Neonatal Ed.* 1995;73:F135-F142.
4. Sommerfelt K, Troland K, Ellertsen B, Markestad T. Behavioural problems in low-birthweight preschoolers. *Dev Med Child Neurol.* 1996;38:927-940.
5. Sommerfelt K, Troland K, Ellertsen B. Neuropsychological performance in low birth weight preschoolers: a population-based, controlled study. *Eur J Pediatr.* 1998;157:53-58.

Long-Term Neurodevelopmental Outcome and Exercise Capacity After Corrective Surgery for Tetralogy of Fallot or Ventricular Septal Defect in Infancy

Hövels-Gürich HH, Konrad K, Skorzenski D, et al (Aachen Univ of Technology, Germany; Inst for Medical Research and Information Processing, Aachen, Germany)

Ann Thorac Surg 81:958-967, 2006   15–9

Background.—The purpose of this prospective study was to assess whether neurodevelopmental status and exercise capacity of children 5 to 10 years after corrective surgery for tetralogy of Fallot or ventricular septal defect in infancy was different compared with normal children and influenced by the preoperative condition of hypoxemia or cardiac insufficiency.

Methods.—Forty unselected children, 20 with tetralogy of Fallot and hypoxemia and 20 with ventricular septal defect and cardiac insufficiency, operated on with combined deep hypothermic circulatory arrest and low flow cardiopulmonary bypass at a mean age of 0.7 ± 0.3 years (mean $\pm$ SD), underwent, at mean age 7.4 ± 1.6 years, standardized evaluation of neurologic status, gross motor function, intelligence, academic achievement, language, and exercise capacity. Results were compared between the groups and related to preoperative, perioperative, and postoperative status and management.

Results.—Rate of mild neurologic dysfunction was increased compared with normal children, but not different between the groups. Exercise capacity and socioeconomic status were not different compared with normal children and between the groups. Compared with the normal population, motor function, formal intelligence, academic achievement, and expressive and receptive language were significantly reduced ($p < 0.01$ to $p < 0.001$) in the whole group and in the subgroups, except for normal intelligence in ventricular septal defect patients. Motor dysfunction was significantly higher in the Fallot group compared with the ventricular septal defect group ($p < 0.01$) and correlated with neurologic dysfunction, lower intelligence, and reduced expressive language ($p < 0.05$ each). Reduced New York Heart Association functional class was correlated with lower exercise capacity and longer duration of cardiopulmonary bypass ($p < 0.05$ each). Reduced socioeconomic status significantly influenced dysfunction in formal intelligence ($p < 0.01$) and academic achievement ($p < 0.05$). Preoperative risk factors such as prenatal hypoxia, perinatal asphyxia, and preterm birth, factors of perioperative management such as cardiac arrest, lowest nasopharyngeal temperature, and age at surgery, and postoperative risk factors as postoperative cardiocirculatory insufficiency and duration of mechanical ventilation were not different between the groups and had no influence on outcome. Degree of hypoxemia in Fallot patients and degree of cardiac insufficiency in ventricular septal defect patients did not influence the outcome within the subgroups.

Conclusions.—Children with preoperative hypoxemia in infancy are at higher risk for motor dysfunction than children with cardiac insufficiency.

Corrective surgery in infancy for tetralogy of Fallot or ventricular septal defect with combined circulatory arrest and low flow bypass is associated with reduced neurodevelopmental outcome, but not with reduced exercise capacity in childhood. In our experience, the general risk of long-term neurodevelopmental impairment is related to unfavorable effects of the global perioperative management. Socioeconomic status influences cognitive capabilities.

▶ This study is part of a new era in pediatric surgical literature as long-term neurodevelopmental function replaces survival as the primary outcome variable. The authors provide important information regarding motor, language, and cognitive function; academic performance; neurologic exam; and exercise capacity in school-aged children, who underwent repair of tetralogy of Fallot (TOF) or ventricular septal defects (VSD) during infancy with cardiopulmonary bypass and deep hypothermic circulatory arrest. Additionally, they examined whether outcome is influenced by preoperative hypoxemia or cardiac insufficiency. Study results show that TOF and VSD groups are similar to normal controls with respect to exercise capacity; however, they differ from controls in motor function, language skills, and academic achievement. Patients with TOF also differ with respect to cognitive function and have greater motor impairment compared with the VSD group. Due to the increased impairment in the TOF group, the authors conclude that children with preoperative hypoxemia are at increased risk for motor dysfunction compared with children with preoperative cardiac insufficiency; however, one should be cautious with these conclusions of causality as additional factors may be associated with both TOF and increased risk for impairment. Additional studies are needed to determine specific causes for developmental delay in children with repaired congenital heart defects. Other contributing factors may include atypical brain development and preoperative, perioperative, and postoperative management, which may be unique for different cardiac anomalies. Children with obvious genetic syndromes were excluded from the study; however, aberrant brain development may occur in the absence of recognizable syndromes. Overall, the authors provide important data to the field because long-term follow-up, rather than short-term follow-up, has been shown to be necessary to appreciate developmental outcome after repair of congenital heart defects.[1]

T. L. Sutcliffe, MD, MSc, FRCPC

Reference

1. McGrath E, Wypij D, Rappaport LA, Newburger JW, Bellinger DC. Prediction of IQ and achievement at age 8 years from neurodevelopmental status at age 1 year in children with D-transposition of the great arteries. *Pediatrics*. 2004;114:e572-e576.

Blood Pressure Among Very Low Birth Weight (<1.5 kg) Young Adults

Hack M, Schluchter M, Cartar L, et al (Rainbow Babies and Childrens Hosp, Cleveland, Ohio; Univ Hosps, Cleveland, Ohio; Case Western Reserve Univ, Cleveland, Ohio)
Pediatr Res 58:677-684, 2005   15–10

Our objective was to compare the blood pressure of 20-y-old very low birth weight (VLBW; <1.5 kg) individuals with that of normal birth weight (NBW) control individuals. The population included 195 VLBW (92 female and 103 male) and 208 NBW (107 female and 101 male) individuals who were born between 1977 and 1979. Independent effects of birth weight status (VLBW *versus* NBW) and within the VLBW cohort of intrauterine growth (birth weight z score) were examined *via* multiple regression analyses. VLBW individuals had a higher mean systolic blood pressure (SBP) than NBW control individuals (114 ± 11 *versus* 112 ± 13 mm Hg). SBP for VLBW female infants was 110 ± 9 *versus* NBW 107 ± 12 and for VLBW male individuals was 118 ± 11 *versus* NBW 117 ± 11 mm Hg. After adjustment for gender, race, and maternal education, the difference in SBP between VLBW and NBW individuals was 1.9 mm Hg but was 3.5 mm after also adjustment for later size (20-y weight and height z scores), which reflects catch-up growth. For female individuals, the difference in SBP between VLBW and NBW individuals was significant both unadjusted and adjusted for later size, whereas for male individuals, the difference was significant only after adjustment for later size. Intrauterine growth did not have a significant effect on SBP within the VLBW group, even after adjustment for later size. VLBW individuals, specifically female individuals, have a higher SBP than NBW control individuals. This is not explained by intrauterine growth failure (Table 2).

► It is interesting that there was no correlation between small for gestational age status as a marker for intrauterine growth and later blood pressure in this study as well as previous studies. In considering the "fetal origins hypothesis," one would think that there would be an impact on adult blood pressure for fetuses that had been in a suboptimal environment in utero manifesting as growth restriction. As such, although birth weight may have an impact on later blood pressure, this effect does not appear to stem from the forces that influence intrauterine growth. This impact of birth weight, which is more significant in females, is small but worth noting, and further investigation will be needed to determine the etiology of this risk. However, considering the other factors that may influence risk for adult cardiovascular disease, such as diet and activity, general practitioners in developed countries can probably counsel both low and NBW patients in a similar fashion.

As challenging as it may be to follow a cohort over such a long span, this sort of study certainly bears repeating over time, as perinatal care has changed over the past 20 years and continues to do so. Changes continue to occur in regard to the types of patients who are being born and surviving as well as in changes in treatments, such as antenatal and postnatal steroid use and nutri-

TABLE 2.—Comparison of Very Low Birth Weight and Normal Birth Weight Young Adult and Maternal Blood Pressure and Growth

	Males			Females		
	Very Low Birth Weight (n = 103)	Normal Birth Weight (n = 101)	P Value	Very Low Birth Weight (n = 92)	Normal Birth Weight (n = 107)	P Value
Young Adult						
Age (years)	20.2 ± 0.5	20.1 ± 0.4	.01	20.1 ± 0.4	20.1 ± 0.4	.62
Blood Pressure (mm Hg)						
Systolic	117.5 ± 10.6	116.9 ± 11.0	.66	110.4 ± 9.1	107.2 ± 12.1	.03
Diastolic	73.7 ± 8.6	73.1 ± 8.6	.65	72.5 ± 8.5	72.1 ± 8.9	.78
Chronic Illness	18 (18%)	16 (16%)	.45	22 (24%)	14 (13%)	.04
Asthma	8 (8%)	6 (6%)	.41	7 (8%)	2 (2%)	.05
Growth Measures						
Weight (kg)	69.2 ± 13.9	79.9 ± 16.7	.000	64.9 ± 16.8	67.6 ± 18.3	.28
Weight z-score*	−0.35 ± 1.25	0.53 ± 1.06	.000	0.26 ± 1.17	0.45 ± 1.16	.25
Height (cm)	173.7 ± 7.9	177.0 ± 6.8	.001	161.7 ± 7.3	163.0 ± 7.0	.20
Height z-score*	−0.44 ± 1.10	0.03 ± 0.95	.001	−0.26 ± 1.13	−0.06 ± 1.08	.20
BMI (kg/m^2)	22.9 ± 4.2	25.5 ± 4.9	.000	24.7 ± 5.2	25.4 ± 6.2	.37
BMI z-score*	−0.33 ± 1.24	0.42 ± 1.09	.000	0.42 ± 0.93	0.45 ± 1.24	.88
Maternal Data†	(n = 79)	(n = 85)		(n = 79)	(n = 94)	
Age	44.5 ± 5.1	46.6 ± 5.3	.01	44.5 ± 5.2	45.1 ± 4.7	.39
Blood Pressure						
Systolic	123.1 ± 13.6	124.1 ± 18.4	.71	124.0 ± 13.8	120.1 ± 13.5	.07
Diastolic	81.2 ± 9.1	80.8 ± 13.5	.81	81.0 ± 10.2	79.5 ± 9.4	.30
Height						
Height (cm)	161.6 ± 6.4	163.4 ± 5.9	.06	162.2 ± 7.1	163.1 ± 6.9	.48
Height z-score*	−0.26 ± 0.98	0.01 ± 0.91	.06	−0.17 ± 1.09	−0.04 ± 1.07	.43

*Using CDC weight norms (Kuczmarski RJ, Ogden CL, Grummer-Strawn LM, et al. CDC growth charts: United States. *Adv Data*. 2000;314:1-27.)
†For mothers with blood pressure measurements at 20 years.
(Courtesy of Hack M, Schluchter M, Carrar L, et al. Blood pressure among very low birth weight (<1.5 kg) young adults. *Pediatr Res*. 2005;58:677-684. Reprinted with permission from Lippincott William & Wilkins at http://lww.com.)

tional regimens. Perhaps, as the cohort of infants that survive include those who were previously at the margins of viability, intrauterine and immediate postnatal influences will become more important.

H. C. Lee, MD

Reduced Lung Function at Birth and the Risk of Asthma at 10 Years of Age
Håland G, for ORAACLE (Ullevål Univ, Oslo, Norway; et al)
N Engl J Med 355:1682-1689, 2006   15–11

Background.—Reduced lung function in early infancy has been associated with later obstructive airway diseases. We assessed whether reduced lung function shortly after birth predicts asthma 10 years later.

Methods.—We conducted a prospective birth cohort study of healthy infants in which we measured lung function shortly after birth with the use of tidal breathing flow-volume loops (the fraction of expiratory time to peak tidal expiratory flow to total expiratory time $[t_{PTEF}/t_E]$) in 802 infants and passive respiratory mechanics, including respiratory-system compliance, in 664 infants. At 10 years of age, 616 children (77%) were reassessed by measuring lung function, exercise-induced bronchoconstriction, and bronchial hyperresponsiveness (by means of a methacholine challenge) and by conducting a structured interview to determine whether there was a history of asthma or current asthma.

Results.—As compared with children whose t_{PTEF}/t_E shortly after birth was above the median, children whose t_{PTEF}/t_E was at or below the median were more likely at 10 years of age to have a history of asthma (24.3% vs. 16.2%, P=0.01), to have current asthma (14.6% vs. 7.5%, P=0.005), and to have severe bronchial hyperresponsiveness, defined as a methacholine dose of less than 1.0 μmol causing a 20% fall in the forced expiratory volume in 1 second (FEV_1) (9.1% vs. 4.9%, P=0.05). As compared with children whose respiratory-system compliance was above the median, children with respiratory compliance at or below the median more often had a history of asthma (27.4% vs. 14.8%; P=0.001) and current asthma (15.0% vs. 7.7%, P=0.009), although this measure was not associated with later measurements of lung function. At 10 years of age, t_{PTEF}/t_E at birth correlated weakly with the maximal midexpiratory flow rate (r=0.10, P=0.01) but not with FEV_1 or forced vital capacity.

Conclusions.—Reduced lung function at birth is associated with an increased risk of asthma by 10 years of age.

▶ The authors conducted a prospective birth cohort study on 802 healthy term infants born in Oslo, Norway, in 1992. These awake, nonsedated infants all had lung function assessed by a noninvasive method shortly after birth (mean age 2.7 ± 0.9 days). Measures included tidal breathing flow volume loops and passive respiratory mechanics to measure respiratory system compliance. A 10-year follow-up study of 614 children who could be contacted was then conducted and spirometry, methacholine challenge testing, allergy skin testing, and an exercise challenge test were performed. Asthma diagnosis was made by medical history using the ISAAC core questionnaire. Children who had t_{PTEF}/t_E (fraction of expiratory time to peak tidal expiratory flow) measured shortly after birth that was below the group median, were more likely to have a history of (24.3% vs 16.2%) or current asthma (14.6% vs 7.5%) compared to those with t_{PTEF}/t_E above the median. These children also had increased methacholine sensitivity, but the measures in the newborn period did not correlate with spirometric measures at age 10 years. The authors conclude that low lung function measured in the immediate newborn period is correlated with the later development of asthma and airway hyperresponsiveness. This is an intriguing finding that is consistent with similar studies performed on somewhat older infants (3-6 months). It is clear that low lung function in infancy, before the development of any respiratory infection, is associated with persistent and recurrent wheezing in childhood. The study by Håland suggests a complex measure, t_{PTEF}/t_E, that is dependent not only on airway caliber, but also respiratory control and mechanics of the chest wall, when reduced below a population median, may indicate later development of reversible forms of airway obstruction in childhood. However, t_{PTEF}/t_E did not correlate with standard spirometric measures of obstruction, such as FEV_1, FVC or results of exercise challenge tests. The latter are measures that predict morbidity and mortality due to airway obstruction later in life. In addition, other host intrinsic factors and a multiplicity of environmental exposures and infections during infancy and childhood can, no doubt, influence outcome in both those with normal and low pulmonary function at birth. Lastly, the absence of a proven intervention that can be applied early in life to alter the natural history of recurrent wheezing or asthma further limits the utility of this or any other technique for early diagnosis. Still, the ability to readily measure lung function in early infancy helps provide a better understanding of the factors that contribute to the development of obstructive lung diseases.

C. M. Kercsmar, MD

Lung Function and Exercise Capacity in Young Adults Born Prematurely
Vrijlandt EJLE, Gerritsen J, Boezen HM, et al (Beatrix Children's Hosp Groningen, The Netherlands; Univ Med Ctr Groningen, The Netherlands; Univ of Groningen, The Netherlands)
Am J Respir Crit Care Med 173:890-896, 2006   15–12

Rationale.—Limited information is available about the long-term outcome of lung function and exercise capacity in young adults born prematurely.

Objective.—To determine long-term effects of prematurity on lung function (volumes, diffusing capacity) and exercise capacity in ex-preterms compared with healthy peers.

Methods.—In a prospective cohort study, children born with a gestational age of less than 32 wk and/or a birth weight under 1,500 g were followed up for 19 yr. Participants (n = 42; mean gestational age, 30 wk, and mean birth weight, 1,246 g) and healthy term control subjects (n = 48) were recruited for lung function and exercise tests.

Measurements.—Spirometry, bodybox (TLC_{box}), diffusing capacity (DL_{CO}), bicycle ergometer test.

Main Results.—Preterm birth was associated with lower FEV_1 (preterms, 95% predicted, vs. controls, 110% predicted; p < 0.001), $DL_{CO}sb$ (88% predicted vs. 96% predicted, p = 0.003), and exercise capacity (load, 185 vs. 216 W; p < 0.001; anaerobic threshold: mean, 1,546 vs. 1,839 ml/min; p < 0.001) compared with control subjects at follow-up. No differences between the groups were found in TLC_{box}, peak oxygen consumption ($\dot{V}O_2$), and breathing reserve. No significant differences in lung function and exercise parameters were found between preterms with and without bronchopulmonary dysplasia.

Conclusions.—Long-term effects of prematurity were airway obstruction and a lower CO diffusing capacity compared with control subjects, although mean lung function parameters were within the normal range. Ex-preterms had a lower exercise level, which could not be explained by impaired lung function or smoking habits, but might be due to impaired physical fitness.

▶ In this article, the authors address an issue that is of great significance to neonatologists and pediatricians engaged in the care of preterm infants. The authors seek to determine the effect of prematurity on both lung function and exercise capacity. The study identified all infants born in 1983 weighing less than 1500 g and performed pulmonary function tests and exercise testing when the subjects had reached 19 years of age.

The primary conclusions of the study are that young adults born prematurely have greater airflow obstruction, diminished diffusion capacity of carbon monoxide, and decreased exercise capacity compared with the control population in the study. Despite the seemingly straightforward conclusions, the findings should be interpreted with at least some degree of caution.

The study population was recruited from only 99 of the 959 eligible participants. Among the 99 invited to participate, only 42 opted to enter the study, representing data from only 4% of the eligible study population. The authors do not address whether and how the participants might represent a random sample. Moreover, the control group was identified and recruited by the study group, which makes it difficult to ensure that systematic bias was not introduced into the study. Further concerns regarding the presence of relevant differences between the control and study groups include the higher number of smokers and maternal smoking in the preterm group versus the control group. Perhaps the most significant confounding variable in the study is the absence of a diagnosis of asthma in the preterm group, despite clear pulmonary function testing data indicating significant airflow limitation in the preterm group compared with the control group. Current data suggest that airflow limitation likely derives from chronic inflammation that should be treated with long-term inhaled corticosteroids. Whether the present findings would be similar in the presence of long-term and appropriate anti-inflammatory therapy would shine still further light on a relatively murky issue.

The article provides clear evidence that preterm, low birth weight infants are at greater risk of obstructive lung disease than their full-term peers. Whether the exercise tolerance is affected is unclear, as the inability to tolerate exercise may derive from deconditioning, obstructive lung disease, or both. Overall, the study provides important information, although its strength is diminished by attempts to address issues for which the study is not appropriately powered.

D. N. Cornfield, MD

Low Birth Weight, a Risk Factor for Cardiovascular Diseases in Later Life, Is Already Associated With Elevated Fetal Glycosylated Hemoglobin at Birth
Pfab T, Slowinski T, Godes M, et al (Ctr for Cardiovascular Research/Inst of Pharmacology, Berlin)
Circulation 114:1687-1692, 2006   15–13

Background.—It remains unclear whether the association between low birth weight and insulin resistance in adulthood has its origin in utero or whether it develops later in life depending on predisposition and exogenous factors.

Method and Results.—Total glycosylated hemoglobin (TGH) was quantified at delivery in 1295 mother/child pairs serving as a surrogate of maternal and fetal glycemia. Multivariable regression analysis considering gestational age at delivery, the child's sex, maternal body mass index, and smoking during pregnancy revealed that an increase in TGH by 1% in the child was significantly associated with a mean birth weight reduction of 135 g (P<0.0001), whereas the same increase in the mother was associated with a mean birth weight increase of 88 g (P<0.0001). The ratio of fetal/maternal TGH suggests that lighter newborns have a higher percentage of TGH than would be expected from maternal TGH.

Conclusions.—The study demonstrates for the first time in a large population that there is an inverse association between TGH of a newborn and its birth weight. This might be due to increased insulin resistance in newborns with lower birth weight. Our data suggest that the pathophysiological mechanisms linking prenatal growth and postnatal sensitivity to insulin are present as early as before birth.

▶ That low birth weight is a risk factor for cardiovascular diseases in later life is now pretty well established. The hypothesis is that reprogramming of the fetus for a circumstance of deprivation sets a stage for later metabolic consequences that become apparent as fuels are introduced in relative excess after birth. There may be truth to this hypothesis, but this work demonstrates something even more profound: a measurable metabolic consequence already exists for the low birth weight infant as reflected by the inverse association between TGH of the newborn and birth weight, which suggests that lighter newborns have a higher percentage of glycosylated hemoglobin, already reflecting insulin resistance. In some sense, this is nothing new to the neonatologist, who already knows that low birth weight infants with hyper- glycemia may have insulin resistance. The situation is conceptually complex, however, because elevated TGH levels in the mother are usually correlated directly with the birth weight of the infant in normal pregnancies and in dia- betic pregnancies; that is, the fetal blood glucose concentration is usually regarded as a passive reflection of the maternal glucose level, and the con- sequence is predictable for the fetus in terms of growth. It is only in the circumstance of the intrauterine growth–restricted infant that the inability to respond to the glucose load may reflect a fundamental alteration in insulin resistance that leads to a difference in the way fuels are used. What is new about this study is that the data suggest that the fetal response to similar maternal glucose levels may not be uniform and reflects a fundamental change in the intrauterine growth–restricted fetal circumstance with respect to the ability to handle a glucose load. The study does not address this issue directly, but the evidence is highly suggestive that this is the case. The study brings more credence to the Barker hypothesis and suggests that circum- stances in utero can permanently influence long-term fuel utilization. I sus- pect that a genetic predisposition to this vulnerability also exists. As the au- thors point out, an alternative way of understanding the data is that genetically determined insulin resistance results in low insulin–mediated fetal growth and elevated blood glucose levels in utero. Nonetheless, the metabolic con- sequences are profound: much is determined in the womb before we en- counter the challenges of the environment around us.

D. K. Stevenson, MD

Transition of Extremely Low-Birth-Weight Infants From Adolescence to Young Adulthood: Comparison With Normal Birth-Weight Controls
Saigal S, Stoskopf B, Streiner D, et al (McMaster Univ, Hamilton, Ont, Canada; Univ of Toronto; Michigan State Univ, East Lansing)
JAMA 295:667-675, 2006   15–14

Context.—Traditionally, educational attainment, getting a job, living in- dependently, getting married, and parenthood have been considered as markers of successful transition to adulthood.

Objective.—To describe and compare the achievement and the age at at- tainment of the above markers between extremely low-birth-weight (ELBW) and normal birth-weight (NBW) young adults.

Design, Setting, and Participants.—A prospective, longitudinal, popu- lation-based study in central-west Ontario, Canada, of 166 ELBW partici- pants who weighed 501 to 1000 g at birth (1977-1982) and 145 sociodemo- graphically comparable NBW participants assessed at young adulthood (22-25 years). Interviewers masked to participant status administered vali- dated questionnaires via face-to-face interviews between January 1, 2002, and April 30, 2004.

Main Outcome Measures.—Markers of successful transition to adulthood, including educational attainment, student and/or worker role, independent living, getting married, and parenthood.

Results.—At young adulthood, 149 (90%) of 166 ELBW participants and 133 (92%) of 145 NBW participants completed the assessments at mean (SD) age of 23.3 (1.2) years and 23.6 (1.1) years, respectively. We included participants with neurosensory impairments (ELBW vs NBW: 40 [27%] vs 3 [2%]) and 7 proxy respondents. The proportion who graduated from high school was similar (82% vs 87%, *P* = .21). Overall, no statistically significant differences were observed in the education achieved to date. A substantial proportion of both groups were still pursuing postsecondary education (47 [32%] vs 44 [33%]). No significant differences were observed in employment/school status; 71 (48%) ELBW vs 76 (57%) NBW young adults were permanently employed (*P* = .09). In a subanalysis, a higher proportion of ELBW young adults were neither employed nor in school (39 [26%] vs 20 [15%], *P* = .02 by Holm's correction); these differences did not persist when participants with disabilities were excluded. No significant differences were found in the proportion living independently (63 [42%] vs 70 [53%], *P* = .19), married/cohabitating (34 [23%] vs 33 [25%], *P* = .69), or who were parents (16 [11%] vs 19 [14%], *P* = .36). The age at attainment of the above markers was similar for both cohorts.

Conclusion.—Our study results indicate that a significant majority of former ELBW infants have overcome their earlier difficulties to become functional young adults.

▶ Proverb: All good things come to those who wait.

As a parent, my long-term goal for my own children has been to have them graduate from school, become employed, and move on with their independent lives. The impressive longitudinal study to young adulthood by Saigal et al, allows us to see these long-term outcomes in a cohort of ELBW survivors. It also reinforces 2 important concepts: (1) neurodevelopmental and educational outcomes become more reliable with increasing age; and (2) ELBW infants without evidence of significant neonatal brain injury can recover from the stresses of preterm birth and prolonged NICU care when exposed to an advantaged environment and comprehensive intervention and education support services.

In Saigal et al's cohort, the proportion of ELBW young adults who graduated from high school was similar to the NBW controls (82 and 87%), and no significant differences were observed in employment, marital status, or independent living, despite the fact that 27% of the ELBW young adults had disabilities. In reviewing prior reports of this cohort, a third of the ELBW children were performing in the moderate low to low range on the Vineland at kindergarten age[1]; this percent decreased to 15% at age 8.[2] In adolescence, their mean IQ was 89 ± 19, and 58% were either receiving education assistance or had repeated a grade.[3] The finding that outcomes of adaptation to adult life experience for ELBW young adults were similar to term controls at 22 to 25 years, therefore, was unexpected good news. A second finding of interest was that the ELBW young adults had achieved levels of education, employment status, and job classification status similar to their parents. This may be related, in part, to the fact that this Canadian population was relatively advantaged.

Within a United States cohort of VLBW children evaluated at age 3, 4½, 6, and 8 years, significant improvement in cognitive and language test scores was observed between 3 and 8 years.[4] Improvements in test scores were associated with higher maternal education, 2-parent household, and early intervention services if the mother had less than a 12th grade education. Hack et al[5] also reported that rates of impairment defined as MDI or KABC less than 70 dropped from 39% at 20 months CA to 16% at 8 years for ELBW infants.

Outcome studies of premature infants in young adulthood are rare. These studies are difficult to accomplish because of long-term tracking and the associated costs. Hack et al[6] reported outcomes of VLBW infants in Cleveland at 20 years of age compared with term controls. Her VLBW adults, who were of lower socioeconomic status, were less likely to have graduated from high school or to be enrolled in a secondary school, and they had lower IQs, and more sensory impairments compared with term controls. Hack et al[7] also examined the mental health status of this cohort at 20 years of age. Although both VLBW men and women reported fewer delinquent behaviors than NBW control subjects, there were increased rates of psychopathology among VLBW survivors compared with control subjects. It is readily apparent that outcomes of importance that reflect successful adaptation to the adult world are quite different from the traditional neurodevelopmental outcome studies at younger ages.

I believe the important conclusion of the current study is that the majority of ELBW survivors in this cohort had an innate potential for resiliency and recovery. It will take another 10 to 20 years to know whether the micro preemies born since the 1990s have this same potential for successful adaptation to the adult world. What is apparent is that there is a need to continue to explore the mechanisms that contribute to recovery of this population with increasing age.

B. Vohr, MD

References

1. Saigal S, Szatmari P, Rosenbaum P, Campbell D, King S. Intellectual and functional status at school entry of children who weighed 1000 grams or less at birth: a regional perspective of births in the 1980s. *J Pediatr.* 1990;116:409-416.
2. Saigal S, Szatmari P, Rosenbaum P, Campbell D, King S. Cognitive abilities and school performance of extremely low birth weight children and matched term control children at age 8 years: a regional study. *J Pediatr.* 1991;118:751-760.
3. Saigal S, Hoult LA, Streiner DL, Stoskopf BL, Rosenbaum PL. School difficulties at adolescence in a regional cohort of children who were extremely low birth weight. *Pediatrics.* 2000;105:325-331.
4. Ment LR, Vohr B, Allan W, et al. Change in cognitive function over time in very low-birth-weight infants. *JAMA.* 2003;289:705-711.
5. Hack M, Taylor HG, Drotar D, et al. Poor predictive validity of the Bayley Scales of Infant Development for cognitive function of extremely low birth weight children at school age. *Pediatrics.* 2005;116:333-341.
6. Hack M, Flannery DJ, Schluchter M, Cartar L, Borawski E, Klein N. Outcomes in young adulthood for very-low-birth-weight infants. *N Engl J Med.* 2002;346: 149-157.

7. Hack M, Youngstrom EA, Cartar L, et al. Behavioral outcomes and evidence of psychopathology among very low birth weight infants at age 20 years. *Pediatrics.* 2004;114:932-940.

Personality in Young Adults Who Are Born Preterm

Allin M, Rooney M, Cuddy M, et al (King's College, London; Mercy Univ Hosp, Grenville Place, Cork, Ireland; Royal Free and Univ College Med School, London)
Pediatrics 117:309-316, 2006   15–15

Introduction.—Very preterm birth (VPT; <33 weeks' gestation) is associated with later neuromotor and cognitive impairment, reduced school performance, and psychiatric morbidity. Several follow-up studies have demonstrated increased anxiety and social rejection and reduced self-esteem in preterm children and adolescents, but few studies have examined the effects of preterm birth on adult personality.

Methods.—We assessed 108 VPT individuals and 67 term-born controls at ages 18 to 19 years with the Eysenck Personality Questionnaire-Revised, short form (EPQ-RS). This questionnaire rates 3 dimensions of personality: extraversion (sociability, liveliness, sensation seeking); neuroticism (anxiety, low mood, low self-esteem); and psychoticism (coldness, aggression, predisposition to antisocial behavior). A fourth scale, "lie," which measures dissimulation, is also derived.

Results.—VPT individuals had significantly lower extraversion scores, higher neuroticism scores, and higher lie scores than term-born controls, after controlling for age at assessment and socioeconomic status. *P* scores were not significantly different between the 2 groups. There was a gender difference in that the increased neuroticism and decreased extraversion scores were accounted for mainly by VPT females. Associations between EPQ-RS scores and neonatal status, adolescent behavioral ratings, and body size at 18 to 19 years were assessed by using Kendall partial correlations, correcting for age at assessment and socioeconomic status. Gestational age, indices of neonatal hypoxia, and neonatal ultrasound ratings were not correlated with EPQ-RS scores. Birth weight was weakly associated with increased lie scores. Rutter Parents' Scale score, a measure of adolescent psychopathology, was associated with an increased neuroticism score. Poor social adjustment in adolescence was associated with an increased lie score. Height and weight at 18 to 19 years were not associated with EPQ-RS, but reduced occipitofrontal circumference was associated with both decreased extraversion and increased lie scores.

Conclusions.—Young adults who are born VPT have different personality styles from their term-born peers. This may be associated with an increased risk of psychiatric difficulties.

▶ The authors find differences in the personalities of young adults who are born preterm, complementing the previously reported observations of Hack et al.[1] Interestingly, less risk-taking and antisocial behaviors, which distinguish the VLB group from the control group, can be attributed primarily to the girls. Good sense, it seems, tracks with gender, and this influence of gender on behavior (as a surrogate for personality) is not lost in individuals with a history of prematurity. The causes of personality differences are, of course, complex and interacting, and there are many genetic and environmental influences to consider. Amazingly, reduced extraversion and increased neuroticism for female young adults who were born preterm still emerge as measurable long-term consequences of preterm birth. Such associations, even without understanding the causation, are important to appreciate to provide appropriate advice to young adults who were born preterm and who face the challenges of an adult world that requires assertiveness and self-confidence.

D. K. Stevenson, MD

Reference

1. Hack M, Flannery D, Schluchter M, Cartar L, Borawski E, Klein N. Outcomes in young adulthood for very-low-birth-weight infants. *N Engl J Med.* 2002;346: 149-157.

A Functional Magnetic Resonance Imaging Study of the Long-term Influences of Early Indomethacin Exposure on Language Processing in the Brains of Prematurely Born Children

Ment LM, Peterson BS, Meltzer JA, et al (Yale Univ, New Haven, Conn; Columbia College of Physicians and Surgeons, New York; Brown Med School, Providence, RI; et al)
Pediatrics 118:961-970, 2006

15–16

Background.—Previous studies have demonstrated that indomethacin lowers the incidence and decreases the severity of intraventricular hemorrhage, as well as improves the cognitive outcome, in prematurely born male infants.

Objective.—The purpose of this work was to use functional magnetic resonance imaging to test the hypothesis that neonatal indomethacin treatment would differentially affect brain activation across genders in school-aged, prematurely born children during performance of a language task.

Methods.—Forty-seven prematurely born children (600–1250-g birth weight) and 24 matched term control subjects were evaluated using a functional magnetic resonance imaging passive language task and neurodevelopmental assessments that included the Wechsler Intelligence Scale for Children-III and the Peabody Picture Vocabulary Test-Revised. Neural activity was assessed during both phonologic and semantic processing in the functional magnetic resonance imaging protocol.

Results.—Neurodevelopmental assessments demonstrated significant differences in full-scale, verbal, and performance intelligence quotient, as well as Peabody Picture Vocabulary Test scores, between the preterm and term control subjects. Rates of perinatal complications did not differ significantly across preterm treatment groups, but male preterm subjects randomly assigned to saline tended to have lower Peabody Picture Vocabulary Test-Revised scores than did all of the other preterm groups. During phonological processing, a significant treatment-by-gender effect was demonstrated in 3 brain regions: the left inferior parietal lobule, the left inferior frontal gyrus (Broca's area), and the right dorsolateral prefrontal cortex.

Conclusions.—These data demonstrate a differential effect of indomethacin administration early in postnatal life on the subsequent development of neural systems that subserve language functioning in these male and female preterm infants.

▶ The use of functional imaging to determine the long-term effects of neonatal interventions on the developing CNS represents great progress. It is intriguing to be able to combine structural and functional changes as the complexities of the CNS are unraveled. Potential limitations of the Ment study include the sample size (as large as any functional MRI report) and selection bias within the study group, which they assiduously avoided.

Ment's series confirms the gender differences in the response to indomethacin that Ohlsson et al[1] documented from the Trial of Indomethacin Prophylaxis in Preterms (TIPP) study and their own findings where gender influenced the rate of intraventricular hemorrhage (IVH) and cognitive school performance. Ohlsson reported both a strong negative effect of indomethacin in female preterm infants, as well as a weaker positive one in male subjects. Ment notes, "The current study extends this work by identifying language processes that indomethacin may uniquely affect and by demonstrating brain regions that may serve as targets for the effects of indomethacin in the brains of prematurely born boys. The biological mechanisms of indomethacin and its effect on corticogenesis remain to be explored." There is evidence that suggests the presence of inborn gender differences in the response to injury of the developing CNS and is attributable to intrinsic properties of individual cells.[2] We will await the results of further exploration of this topic.

A. A. Fanaroff, MD

References

1. Ohlsson A, Roberts RS, Schmidt B, et al. Male/female differences in indomethacin effects in preterm infants. *J Pediatr.* 2005;147:860-862.
2. Du L, Bayir H, Lai Y, et al. Innate gender based proclivity in response to cytotoxicity and programmed cell death pathway. *J Biol Chem.* 2004;279:38563-38570.

Catch-down growth during infancy of children born small (SGA) or appropriate (AGA) for gestational age with short-statured parents

Völkl TMK, Haas B, Beier C, et al (Friedrich-Alexander-Univ of Erlangen-Nuremberg, Germany)

J Pediatr 148:747-752, 2006   15–17

Objective.—We analyzed postnatal growth in children with familial short stature (FSS) with regard to small (SGA) or appropriate (AGA) for gestational age status at birth.

Study Design.—We studied 96 otherwise healthy short-statured children (58 males; SGA: n = 41, AGA: n = 55). At least one of the parents was short-statured. Cross-sectional data for length/height and weight for the first 4 years of age were collected retrospectively.

Results.—AGA children had a mean length of 0.09 ± 1.02 standard deviation score (SDS) at birth, −1.57 ± 1.16 SDS after 1 year of age, and −2.36 ± 0.72 SDS after 4 years. SGA children had a mean length of −2.04 ± 1.06 SDS at birth, −2.70 ± 1.12 SDS at 1 year of age, and −3.05 ± 0.86 SDS at 4 years. The loss of length SDS within the first 2 years of life was greater in AGA than in SGA children. SGA children were significantly shorter than AGA children at all of the study points ($p < .001$) (Fig 1).

Conclusions.—Children with an FSS background born AGA show catch-down growth to their lower familial range during the first 2 years of life. SGA children did not catch up to their AGA peers at any time.

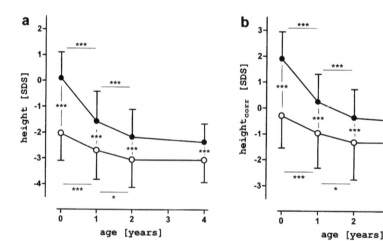

FIGURE 1.—Longitudinal growth pattern of AGA (filled circles) and SGA (open circles) children during the first 4 years of life. Chartes show height SDS (a) and height SDS corrected for target height (b). The level of significance is indicated by three ($p < .001$), two ($p < .01$), or one asterisk ($p < .05$). (Courtesy of Völkl TMK, Haas B, Beier C, et al. Catch-down growth during infancy of children born small (SGA) or appropriate (AGA) for gestational age with short-statured parents. *J Pediatr.* 148:747-752. Copyright 2006 by Elsevier.)

▶ This report by Völkl and colleagues confirms the widely held pediatric belief that a child's adult height is greatly influenced by parental height but focuses on growth between birth and 4 years of age in children of parents with idiopathic short stature. The investigators studied 96 children between 5 and 10 years of age who were evaluated for short stature in a Pediatric Endocrine Clinic; 41 of the children had been SGA at birth. All the children were healthy, had at least 1 parent with short stature (height less than −2.0 SDS), and had "familial short stature defined as height SDS less than −2.0 but within the normal range of parental height according to calculated target height." As shown in Figure 1, there was a significant decline in height SDS during the first 2 years of life in both SGA and AGA children, but that decline was greater in AGA infants. Furthermore, although similar growth patterns were evident by 4 years of age, the SGA infants remained smaller then their AGA peers.

Since Latal-Hajnal et al[1] have recently demonstrated that postnatal growth rather than the appropriateness of weight for gestational age at birth is associated with neurodevelopmental outcomes in VLBW infants, these observations by Völkl and colleagues suggest that awareness of parental stature may be important in understanding postnatal growth patterns and the likelihood of adverse neurodevelopmental outcomes in VLBW infants. Specifically, the finding by Latal-Hajnal et al that VLBW AGA infants who were less than 10th percentile at 2 years of age were more likely to have neurodevelopmental impairments than VLBW SGA infants who remained less than 10th percentile might be modulated in the presence of parental short stature.

R. A. Ehrenkranz, MD

Reference

1. Latal-Hajnal B, von Siebenthal K, Kovari H, Bucher HU, Largo RH. Postnatal growth in VLBW infants: significant association with neurodevelopmental outcome. *J Pediatr.* 2003;143:163-170.

16 Ethics

Restriction of Ongoing Intensive Care in Neonates: A Prospective Study
Hentschel R, Lindner K, Krueger M, et al (Univ of Freiburg, Germany; Univ of Basel, Switzerland)
Pediatrics 118:563-569, 2006   16–1

Objective.—The purpose of this work was to record the current practice of restricting ongoing intensive care in severely ill newborns.

Methods.—This was a prospective observational study over a 30-month period of consecutive newborns for whom restriction of ongoing intensive care was taken into consideration, discussed, or decided on. A standardized form recorded patients' medical condition, the type of restriction decided on, parents' wishes, and their information level. The research was conducted in a neonatal unit of a level III university children's hospital, with no interventions.

Results.—Forty patients were enrolled, 25 were preterm, 21 had either a genetic defect or an inborn malformation. Restriction of ongoing intensive care was decided on for 32 patients with a great variety of specified recommendations. Thirty-six patients died during the observation period. In general, parents were well informed; however, their wishes concerning restriction of ongoing intensive care were unknown in ~25% of cases.

Conclusions.—The decision-making process for restriction of ongoing intensive care is well established, but the role of parents needs to be defined.

▶ This article describes the practice of restriction of ongoing intensive care (RIC) with regard to such therapies as cardiopulmonary resuscitation and mechanical ventilation in the newborn ICU in the University Children's Hospital in Freiberg, Germany. Many such descriptions exist in the medical literature, but these authors rightly point out that most have relied on questionnaires and self-report data. This study presumably provides a higher level of objectivity, through the use of an "embedded researcher" who observed and recorded clinical management as well as discussions without taking part in either.

The patient data presented do not provide sufficient basis for a reader's judgment as to the appropriateness of RIC decisions, but some insights into the decision-making process are provided. Of particular interest is the use of "ethics rounds" for certain patients, which generally included physicians and a nurse, but not necessarily anyone with expertise in the field of ethics. This could reflect a lack of availability or an unfortunate belief that such individuals could not substantially contribute to the discussion. The most common justification cited for RIC was "futility," which is a justification now largely avoided by many ethicists and others because of a lack of consensus over its meaning and concerns over its misuse. In particular, concern exists that futility may sometimes be invoked by physicians to preclude a more difficult (but valuable) discussion of the predicted benefits and burdens of treatment with parents and with one another.

Because the embedded researcher did not speak with parents, no reliable data exist regarding their understanding, which is a weakness of the study that the authors acknowledge. In several cases, it was unknown whether parents agreed with the decision for RIC. This could be inappropriate, but one can envision situations in which it might be reasonable. For example, if (1) the medical team planned RIC based on their assessment of the best interest of the child; and (2) parents were informed, understood, and voiced no objections, then, perhaps in certain cases, it is not necessary to require the parents to say more.

In their discussion, the authors rightly observe that "it is debatable how far parents should have the privilege to prioritize their own interests against the hypothetical interests of the child." Debate needs to occur and needs to include practicing neonatologists alongside ethicists and others. Although the primacy of the patient's best interest is often invoked in our policies and teaching, it has long been suggested that the interests of others, such as family, are also a valid consideration. Ethical judgments regarding RIC in certain cases may depend on the relative weight we assign to these sometimes competing interests.

Retrospective studies based on questionnaires provide information on what we think we do in difficult situations. This article provides a better insight into what we do. Ethics, however, is the study of what we ought to do. While it is helpful to get a clearer look at current practice, the real ethical work lies in critical consideration of the relevant principles, competing interests, and potential moral justifications for RIC. The authors apparently plan to publish ethical analyses of some cases from this study. Such analyses are rarely as succinct as quantitative studies, but we neonatologists should take the time to read and discuss them.

M. R. Mercurio, MD, MA

SUGGESTED READING

Hardwig J. What about the family? In: Hardwig J, Hentoff N, Callahan D, eds. *Is There a Duty to Die?* New York, NY: Routledge; 2000:29-43.

Helft PR, Siegler M, Lantos J. The rise and fall of the futility movement. *N Engl J Med.* 2000;343:293-296.

▶ In the literature, but not, I imagine, in real neonatal ICU life, a gap exists in the discussion of ethical decision making regarding withdrawal of life-sustaining measures: from the initial focus on delivery room resuscitation decisions, we move to end-of-life decision making when things have become clearly evident of either impending death/nonsurvivability or survival with a poor predicted outcome. This study, to a degree, looks at that interim period from the medical team's perspective.

What is new and interesting here is the methodology of an "embedded researcher" (from the authors' Institute of Medical Ethics) who observed the process after one or more members of the medical team articulated an ethical issue. A medical ethics round was convened, during which RIC was taken into consideration, discussed, or decided, and the team incorporated the wishes and attitudes of the parents (as perceived by the medical staff in informal talks with them, apart from 8 infants in whom parental wishes were not known). The methodology, the authors believe, enabled the gathering of standardized information in a naturalistic and ethically neutral way. A decision was conveyed to parents, and as the authors state, "the position of parents concurred more or less with the recommendations of the ethics round; in no case was there a strict opposition to the group's decision." The methodology also enabled examination of those cases in which RIC was discussed for not only those who died but also those who survived; however, this is not developed further.

The authors describe the statistical data evaluation of 40 severely ill infants; a deeper ethical analysis of each case is not their purpose here. The findings are consistent with other studies in many respects: reasons for raising a discussion of RIC were categorized into either futility in a physiologic sense or the more neurologic quality-of-life outcome, and most were in the former category; the most frequent decision was for a "no CPR" order. The findings also highlighted a number of other interesting points: infants with complex multisystem disorders were often the focus, whereas the limits of viability were less often the focus than assumed; also, discussions appeared to take place earlier in the infant's course, as "inevitability of death" was not quoted as a prompt for the RIC discussion.

The study was not designed to directly solicit parents' views: dare I suggest an analogy to "embedded" war correspondents who detail the actions of the units in which they are embedded but who cannot roam freely among the people (the parents). The authors acknowledge the lack of information on the parents' situation and are very concerned about how to promote parental participation in the decision-making process. However, I think a lot of other embedded data can be found herein: how the team functioned, how easy was it to gain consensus, was the ethicist or the senior neonatologist the dominant decider, what role did nurses play in discussion, how did the team feel after a decision was reached? I am sure rich data within this study could be explored further.

J. Hellmann, MB, BCh, FCP(SA), FRCPC

Matters of Spirituality at the End of Life in the Pediatric Intensive Care Unit

Robinson MR, Thiel MM, Backus MM, et al (Children's Hosp, Boston; Beverly Hosp, Mass; Harvard Med School, Boston)
Pediatrics 118:719-729, 2006   16–2

Objective.—Our objective with this study was to identify the nature and the role of spirituality from the parents' perspective at the end of life in the PICU and to discern clinical implications.

Methods.—A qualitative study based on parental responses to open-ended questions on anonymous, self-administered questionnaires was conducted at 3 PICUs in Boston, Massachusetts. Fifty-six parents whose children had died in PICUs after the withdrawal of life-sustaining therapies participated.

Results.—Overall, spiritual/religious themes were included in the responses of 73% (41 of 56) of parents to questions about what had been most helpful to them and what advice they would offer to others at the end of life. Four explicitly spiritual/religious themes emerged: prayer, faith, access to and care from clergy, and belief in the transcendent quality of the parent-child relationship that endures beyond death. Parents also identified several implicitly spiritual/religious themes, including insight and wisdom; reliance on values; and virtues such as hope, trust, and love.

Conclusions.—Many parents drew on and relied on their spirituality to guide them in end-of-life decision-making, to make meaning of the loss, and to sustain them emotionally. Despite the dominance of technology and medical discourse in the ICU, many parents experienced their child's end of life as a spiritual journey. Staff members, hospital chaplains, and community clergy are encouraged to be explicit in their hospitality to parents' spirituality and religious faith, to foster a culture of acceptance and integration of spiritual perspectives, and to work collaboratively to deliver spiritual care.

▶ Bioethics is often accused of using reason and facts without formal reference to religious traditions (even if bioethics and bioethicists are informed by them). While secular moral principles and modes of reasoning may be tenable in bioethical discussion, we cannot ignore matters of religion or the more inclusive term of *spirituality* in clinical deliberations with parents in end-of-life discussions in ICUs.

The findings in this qualitative study were gathered from a questionnaire completed by parents 12 to 45 months after their child's death. Interestingly, it showed the emergence of 4 explicitly spiritual/religious themes: prayer, faith, access to and care from clergy, and belief in the transcendent quality of the parent–child relationship that endures beyond death. However, other significant themes that the authors believe have a religious/spiritual dynamic also emerged. These included finding meaning, hope, trust, and love. Finding meaning is a very subjective view, constructed by parents over time and typically after difficult soul-searching. Similarly, hope is considered important, even though it may change from hope for a cure to hope for comfort and dignity at life's end. Trust is a spiritual dynamic, be it trust in God or secular resources, and may include the health care team itself. Love was interpreted by many parents from simple acts of kindness and gestures of compassion.

The implications from this study are that health care teams need to consider whether they have or need to create an environment that is hospitable to and supportive of prayer, that they identify parents' model of faith and customize spiritual care, that clinical staff recognize parents' spiritual needs and provide access to hospital chaplains as well as community clergy and, on a deeper level, in end-of-life discussions appreciate that parents' religious/spiritual perspectives may stem from their trying to protect a life that they believe has been entrusted divinely to their care. Glib statements regarding the "meaning" of a child's life or death should be avoided by clinicians and chaplains alike. Regarding hope, care providers may benefit families by helping members identify and articulate what they are hoping for at any given time in the child's illness; expressions of kindness and compassion enable families to feel supported and not only help parents to access sources of hope, trust, and meaning but also have long-term benefits on parental bereavement.

In a related vein, see the recent study by Grossoehme et al,[1] who conducted a survey of Midwestern pediatricians to explore the disparity between believing in the relevance of spirituality and religion in clinical practice and its actual application.

J. Hellmann, MB, BCh, FCP(SA), FRCPC

Reference

1. Grossoehme DH, Ragsdale JR, McHenry CL, Thurston C, DeWitt T, VandeCreek L. Pediatrician characteristics associated with attention to spirituality and religion in clinical practice. *Pediatrics.* 2007;119:e117-e123.

Parents' experiences of sharing neonatal information and decisions: Consent, cost and risk
Alderson P, Hawthorne J, Killen M (Univ of London; Univ of Cambridge, England)
Soc Sci Med 62:1319-1329, 2006   16–3

This paper is about the care of babies with confirmed or potential neurological problems in neonatal intensive care units. Drawing on recent ethnographic research, the paper considers parents' experiences of sharing information and decisions with neonatal staff, and approaches that support or restrict parents' involvement. There are growing medicolegal pressures on practitioners to inform parents and involve them in their babies' care. Data are drawn from observations in four neonatal units in southern England, and interviews with the parents of 80 babies and with 40 senior staff. The paper compares standards set by recent guidance, with parents' views about their share in decision-making, their first meetings with their babies, 'minor' decision-making, the different neonatal units, being a helpless observer and missed opportunities. Parents' standards for informed decisions are summarised, with their reported views about two-way decision-making, and their practical need to know. Whereas doctors emphasise distancing aspects of the consent process, parents tend to value 'drawing together' aspects.

▶ Consent, as a vital protection against negligence and abuse and a means of maintaining high standards of care, became increasingly important in the aftermath of 2 major inquiries in the United Kingdom, such that concerns were raised that virtually every neonatal test or procedure should be preceded by a formal parental consent process. The issue of which procedures require formal consent is, of course, endemic to all neonatal ICUs, such that I think lessons are to be learned here, not only about consent per se but also about communication in general.

The information gathered from a "Foretelling Futures" ethnographic study[1] determining neurologic outcomes in neonatal patients was used, not to question the importance of informed and voluntary consent but to show how vital consent procedures are and to give a more nuanced appreciation of parents' views from their experiences of sharing information, decisions, and approaches that restrict or support parental involvement in their infants' care.

Interviews with the parents of 80 babies (the major focus of this article) revealed that, while the "big" decisions, such as to intubate or operate on a baby, involve informed consent, these are relatively rare. Parents wanted some control over events when this was realistic but did not want to be asked to consent to every procedure. They often felt overwhelmed when asked to consent for routine and minor procedures and felt they were given the illusion that they could or should say stop when there was no real choice and no time to learn more about each procedure. Attempting to transfer responsibility to parents in such situations could be both invalid and unkind. It was also clear that the more the staff offered time and information to listen to parents, the easier it was for parents to discuss questions and dilemmas on fairly equal terms. How uncertain prognoses are framed, how some caregivers treat the provision of information as an emergency in and of itself, how awareness by staff of the stressful context in which parents find themselves, and how agreements are honored, despite changing staff schedules, are some of the numerous factors that affect parental involvement in more formal decisions and consent.

Both the complexity of parents' responses and the nature of this analytical (and not statistical) study preclude simple categorization of parents into 2 groups who either want to be informed or not informed: parents' experience of their infant's neurologic outcome allows only one of a number of potential outcomes, parents' views change over time, and parents whose babies die can recall events very differently. Nevertheless, the authors describe an overall difference between the "distancing" approach used by physicians and the parental emphasis on the "drawing together" aspects in the content, ethos, and form of consent, which should be a 2-way informed agreement between fairly equal partners with established mutual trust and respect. The authors' fear is that current guidance appears to be driven by economic concerns to prevent costly litigation rather than to raise standards of communication and relationships between doctors and parents. The message, I believe, from these observations is that requiring consent for all interventions, however minor, devalues consent and that, if information sharing and relationship building opportunities are utilized, informed consent for every test or procedure is not advisable. It should be limited to those situations in which the conditions for legally valid consent are met: only then should responsibility for risk be transferred from practitioner to parent.

J. Hellmann, MB, BCh, FCP(SA), FRCPC

Reference

1. Alderson P, Ehrich K, Hawthorne J, Killen M, Warren I, for the Social Science Research Unit. Foretelling futures: dilemmas in neonatal neurology. Institute of Education, University of London Web site. Available at: http://ioewebserver.ioe.ac.uk/ioe/cms/get.asp?cid=11991&11991_0=12017. Accessed: May 1, 2007.

Subject Index

Electroencephalography (EEG)
  compromised activity in very preterm
    infants, early low cardiac output
    and, 113
End-of-life decisions
  nature and role of spirituality in, 330
Endotoxin shock
  intratracheal recombinant surfactant
    protein D for prevention in
    newborn preterm lamb, 154
Endotracheal intubation
  low-dose dexamethasone for facilitation
    of extubation among chronically
    ventilator-dependent neonates, 128
  mivacurium with fentanyl for
    facilitation in the neonatal intensive
    care unit, 130
  nonemergent, premedication with
    atropine and fentanyl vs. atropine,
    fentanyl, and mivacurium, 282
  prediction of successful extubation in
    very low birth weight infants, 129
Epidural analgesia
  with and without fentanyl in labor,
    effect on breastfeeding, 81
Epidural hematoma
  intracranial, in newborn infants, 165
Epinephrine
  endotracheal vs. intravenous, for
    neonatal cardiopulmonary
    resuscitation in the delivery room,
    74
Escherichia coli
  early-onset invasive infections in
    neonates, intrapartum antibiotic
    therapy as risk factor for, 88
Extremely low birth weight (ELBW)
    infants
  acute intestinal perforation in, timing
    and type of surgical management,
    213
  arterial stiffness in, 107
  blood pressure at age 20 years, 312
  candidiasis in, risk factors, mortality
    rates, and neurodevelopmental
    outcomes at 18 to 22 months, 96
  costs of care in California, 294
  cranial ultrasound for detection of
    impaired growth of the corpus
    callosum in, 175
  early low cardiac output and
    compromised EEG activity in, 113
  effects of hypercapnia on cerebral
    autoregulation during mechanical
    ventilation in, 141
  genetic polymorphisms of hemostasis
    genes and primary outcome of, 63

immediate vs. delayed cord clamping in,
    intraventricular hemorrhage and
    late-onset sepsis incidence and, 76
  longitudinal changes in bone health as
    assessed by the speed of sound in,
    293
  milrinone for low systemic blood flow
    in, 112
  nosocomial staphylococcal sepsis in,
    INH-A21 for prevention of, 94
  patent ductus arteriosus in
    combined treatment with nitric oxide
      synthase inhibitor and
      indomethacin, 117
    prevalence of spontaneous closure,
      115
  personality in young adults born as,
    321
  postnatal steroid administration in,
    prospective evaluation, 283
  prediction of successful extubation, 129
  refractory hypotension in, "stress dose"
    of hydrocortisone for rescue
    treatment, 110
  survival advantage with cesarean
    delivery, 69
  survival and major neonatal
    complications in infants born after
    22-23 vs. 24 weeks gestation, 55
  sustainable use of nasal continuous
    positive airway pressure in, 127
  tracheotomy in, indications and
    outcomes, 151
  transfusion in, restrictive vs. liberal
    hemoglobin threshold for, 250

F

Familial short stature
  postnatal growth in children small or
    appropriate for gestational age at
    birth, 324
Fetal alcohol syndrome
  alteration in $GABA_A\alpha_5$ expression as
    mechanism of alcohol-induced
    learning dysfunction in, 191
Fetus
  anemia, Doppler ultrasonography vs.
    amniocentesis for prediction of, 17
  biometry measurement, cumulative sum
    analysis in assessment of trainee
    competence in, 28
  cerebral injury after fetoscopic laser
    surgery treatment of twin-to-twin
    transfusion syndrome, 14
  congenital heart defects
    absences of pulmonary valve, prenatal
      diagnosis and outcome, 121

Author Index